304
Current Topics in Microbiology and Immunology

Editors

R.W. Compans, Atlanta/Georgia
M.D. Cooper, Birmingham/Alabama
T. Honjo, Kyoto · H. Koprowski, Philadelphia/Pennsylvania
F. Melchers, Basel · M.B.A. Oldstone, La Jolla/California
S. Olsnes, Oslo · P.K. Vogt, La Jolla/California
H. Wagner, Munich

S. A. Plotkin (Ed.)

Mass Vaccination: Global Aspects – Progress and Obstacles

With 40 Figures and 27 Tables

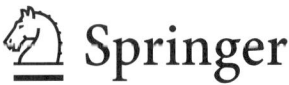

Stanley A. Plotkin, MD
Sanofi Pasteur
4650 Wismer Road
Doylestown, PA 18901
USA

e-mail: stanley.plotkin@sanofipasteur.com

Legend to the cover figure by Oliver Rosenbauer, WHO, Geneva: Women and their children queue up to register at an immunization post in Togo. The children receive four life-saving interventions at once – polio and measles vaccination, deworming tablets and insecticide-treated nets to prevent malaria.
Photo credit: Marko Kokic, Canadian Red Cross

Library of Congress Catalog Number 72-152360

ISSN 0070-217X
ISBN-10 3-540-29382-5 Springer Berlin Heidelberg New York
ISBN-13 978-3-540-29382-8 Springer Berlin Heidelberg New York

This work is subject to copyright. All rights reserved, whether the whole or part of the material is concerned, specifically the rights of translation, reprinting, reuse of illustrations, recitation, broadcasting, reproduction on microfilm or in any other way, and storage in data banks. Duplication of this publication or parts thereof is permitted only under the provisions of the German Copyright Law of September, 9, 1965, in its current version, and permission for use must always be obtained from Springer-Verlag. Violations are liable for prosecution under the German Copyright Law.

Springer is a part of Springer Science+Business Media
springeronline.com
© Springer-Verlag Berlin Heidelberg 2006
Printed in Germany

The use of general descriptive names, registered names, trademarks, etc. in this publication does not imply, even in the absence of a specific statement, that such names are exempt from the relevant protective laws and regulations and therefore free for general use.
Product liability: The publisher cannot guarantee the accuracy of any information about dosage and application contained in this book. In every individual case the user must check such information by consulting the relevant literature.

Editor: Simon Rallison, Heidelberg
Desk editor: Anne Clauss, Heidelberg
Production editor: Nadja Kroke, Leipzig
Cover design: design & production GmbH, Heidelberg
Typesetting: LE-TEX Jelonek, Schmidt & Vöckler GbR, Leipzig
Printed on acid-free paper   SPIN 11560043   27/3150/YL – 5 4 3 2 1 0

Preface

Mass immunization is the *blitzkrieg* of vaccination practice. It serves to rapidly protect populations, both because of the high coverage achieved and because of the herd immunity thereby induced. However, as in war, mass immunization campaigns must be conducted intelligently, with careful strategy and strong attention to logistics of supply and deployment. If conducted badly, mass immunization may fail or even be counter-productive.

In this volume, some of the most successful practitioners of mass immunization tell us about its art and science. David Heymann and Bruce Aylward of WHO begin the book with a theoretical and practical overview of mass immunization. Michael Lane, who participated in the successful effort to eradicate smallpox relates how this was done using mass vaccination and other strategies. Application of mass immunization by the US military is covered by John Grabenstein and Remington Nevin, who have a large experience in these matters. Karen Noakes and David Salisbury recount the striking successes of mass immunization in the United Kingdom. The global control of the clostridia that produce diphtheria toxin is described by Charles Vitek. Hepatitis A is decreasing dramatically under the impact of large-scale vaccination, as Francis André illustrates. The French experience with Hepatitis B vaccination has been mixed, and François Denis and Daniel Levy-Bruhl explain the circumstances. Influenza vaccination is an annual example of large-scale campaigns, the complexity of which is recounted by Benjamin Schwartz and Pascale Wortley. Ciro de Quadros describes the eminently successful effort by the Pan American Health Organization to eliminate measles from the Americas through mass immunization. Mexican scientists are attempting to develop the aerosol route for mass measles vaccination, as illustrated for us by José Luis Valdespino-Gomez and his coworkers. The huge effort to eradicate polio, with its many complications, is reviewed by Roland Sutter and Chris Maher. Susan Reef describes the advancing effort to eliminate rubella and its congenital disease by rapid immunization of children and adults. Typhoid is a disease that often breaks out under adverse conditions, and mass immunization is important in control, as elucidated by Myron Levine. Finally, Gregory Glenn and Richard Kenney recount the efforts to develop transcutaneous delivery of vaccine to assist in mass immunization.

This volume emphasizes that vaccination is always both a matter of individual and community protection, and that massive public health efforts are often needed to control infectious diseases in the most effective manner.

Doylestown, Pennsylvania, April 2006 *Stanley A. Plotkin*

List of Contents

Mass Vaccination: When and Why 1
    D. L. Heymann and R. B. Aylward

Mass Vaccination and Surveillance/Containment
in the Eradication of Smallpox 17
    J. M. Lane

Mass Immunization Programs: Principles and Standards 31
    J. D. Grabenstein and R. L. Nevin

Immunization Campaigns in the UK 53
    K. Noakes and D. Salisbury

Diphtheria 71
    C. R. Vitek

Universal Mass Vaccination Against Hepatitis A 95
    F. E. André

Mass Vaccination Against Hepatitis B: The French Example 115
    F. Denis and D. Levy-Bruhl

Mass Vaccination for Annual and Pandemic Influenza 131
    B. Schwartz and P. Wortley

Is Global Measles Eradication Feasible? 153
    C. A. de Quadros

Measles Aerosol Vaccination 165
    J. L. Valdespino-Gómez, M. de Lourdes Garcia-Garcia,
    J. Fernandez-de-Castro, A. M. Henao-Restrepo, J. Bennett,
    and J. Sepulveda-Amor

Mass Vaccination Campaigns for Polio Eradication:
An Essential Strategy for Success 195
    R. W. Sutter and C. Maher

Rubella Mass Campaigns 221
    S. Reef

Mass Vaccination to Control Epidemic and Endemic Typhoid Fever 231
    M. M. Levine

Mass Vaccination: Solutions in the Skin 247
    G. M. Glenn and R. T. Kenney

Subject Index 269

List of Contributors

(Addresses stated at the beginning of respective chapters)

André, F. E. 95
Aylward, R. B. 1

Bennett, J. 165

de Lourdes Garcia-Garcia, M. 165
de Quadros, C. A. 153
Denis, F. 115

Fernandez-de-Castro, J. 165

Glenn, G. M. 247
Grabenstein, J. D. 31

Henao-Restrepo, A. M. 165
Heymann, D. L. 1

Kenney, R. T. 247

Lane, J. M. 17

Levine, M. M. 231
Levy-Bruhl, D. 115

Maher, C. 195

Nevin, R. L. 31
Noakes, K. 53

Reef, S. 221

Salisbury, D. 53
Schwartz, B. 131
Sepulveda-Amor, J. 165
Sutter, R. W. 195

Valdespino-Gómez, J. L. 165
Vitek, C. R. 71

Wortley, P. 131

Mass Vaccination: When and Why

D. L. Heymann (✉) · R. B. Aylward

World Health Organization, 1211 Geneva 27, Switzerland
heymannd@who.int

1	The Concept of Mass Vaccination	2
2	Mass vaccination in the Twentieth Century—Smallpox Eradication	3
3	Routine Immunization and Mass Vaccination Today—A Necessary Alliance	4
4	Preventing Emerging Outbreaks	5
4.1	Meningitis	6
4.2	Influenza	7
4.3	Yellow Fever	8
4.4	Displaced Persons	8
4.5	Threat of Deliberately Caused Outbreaks	9
5	Mass Vaccination to Accelerate Disease Control	10
5.1	New Vaccine Introduction	11
5.2	Eradication	12
5.3	Mortality Reduction	13
5.3.1	Measles	13
5.3.2	Maternal and Neonatal Tetanus	13
6	Mass Vaccination in the Twenty-First Century	13
	References	14

Abstract With increased demand for smallpox vaccination during the nineteenth century, vaccination days—early mass vaccination campaigns—were conducted over time-limited periods to rapidly and efficiently protect maximum numbers of susceptible persons. Two centuries later, the challenge to rapidly and efficiently protect populations by mass vaccination continues, despite the strengthening of routine immunization services in many countries through the Expanded Programme on Immunization strategies and GAVI support. Perhaps the most widely accepted reason for mass vaccination is to rapidly increase population (herd) immunity in the setting of an existing or potential outbreak, thereby limiting the morbidity and mortality that might result, especially when there has been no routine vaccination, or because populations have been displaced and routine immunization services disrupted. A second important use of mass vaccination is to accelerate disease control to rapidly increase coverage with a new vaccine at the time of its introduction into routine immunization programmes, and to attain the herd immunity levels required to meet international targets for eradication and mortality reduction. In the twenty-first century, mass vaccination and routine immunization remain a necessary alliance for attaining both national and international goals in the control of vaccine preventable disease.

1
The Concept of Mass Vaccination

Ever since the practice of variolation was used to prevent serious smallpox infection in China and India sometime about A.D. 1000 [1], vaccination of populations at risk of infectious diseases has remained a challenge. In 1796, Edward Jenner took smallpox vaccination a step further by inoculating humans with material from lesions of cowpox from milkmaids, rather than from smallpox lesions, thus pre-empting the requirement of direct vaccination from a person with smallpox. By the beginning of the nineteenth century still further advances were made, when the practice of vaccination used material from cowpox lesions dried on threads as a vaccine that could then be sent throughout the United Kingdom and to other parts of the world [2]. Vaccination thus became portable—it no longer required direct person-to-person inoculation, and vaccines could be easily transported to vaccinate persons at risk.

Vaccination against smallpox soon became compulsory in Europe with Bavaria, Denmark and Sweden adopting vaccination laws between 1807 and 1816. The Vaccination Acts in Great Britain later in the nineteenth century made vaccine universal, free and mandatory in that country, and vaccination officers enforced them. Those who refused vaccination for any reason were fined. Mandatory smallpox vaccination was soon accepted by many other countries, either through school entry laws or legislation pertaining to young children and families [3].

With increased demand for vaccination, general vaccination days were held in Europe and many other parts of the world where person-to-person vaccination, and vaccination using impregnated threads, was replaced by vaccination directly from cowpox lesions on cows. These vaccination days were early mass vaccination campaigns—vaccination over time-limited periods to provide protection rapidly and efficiently to maximum numbers of susceptible persons. By 1820, Sweden had been able to decrease smallpox by over a hundredfold by mass vaccination [4], and it soon became evident that vaccination not only offered individual protection—it could also be used to prevent infection among those not vaccinated because of an overall decrease in the number of infected persons, reducing the net rate of transmission of the smallpox virus. This principal of herd immunity has become an important benefit of mass campaigns—susceptible persons can either gain protection directly by being vaccinated, or indirectly by having their risk of infection reduced as transmission of the infectious agent decreases among those vaccinated.

Since Jenner's time, mass vaccination campaigns have become a common, and frequently controversial, element of communicable disease control programmes in developing as well as industrialized countries worldwide. This chapter briefly reviews the recent evolution of mass vaccination and the sometimes-uneasy alliance that has emerged between mass vaccination and routine immunization services. Based on this experience, the subsequent sections propose a broad framework for policy makers in evaluating the potential role of mass vaccination in their efforts to control vaccine-preventable diseases.

2
Mass vaccination in the Twentieth Century—Smallpox Eradication

By the twentieth century it was understood that achieving herd immunity could in itself be an important goal of mass vaccination programmes as it could stop person-to-person transmission of an infectious agent. It was further understood that if the infectious agent had no reservoir other than humans, zero transmission among humans worldwide could be equated with eradication of the disease it caused.

In 1967, the member states of the World Health Organization (WHO) resolved to intensify smallpox eradication efforts throughout the world [5], and countries that had not yet interrupted smallpox transmission agreed to supplement routine immunization programmes with mass vaccination campaigns. Smallpox vaccination was not without its complications however. Complications associated with primary smallpox vaccination ranged from vaccinial eruption at sites of the body that are or have previously been eczematous, to generalized vaccinia infection and post-vaccinal encephalitis leading to permanent neurological disability or death. With a case fatality rate for post-vaccinial encephalitis of approximately 30%, the risk of fatal complication from smallpox vaccine was approximately one per million doses of vaccine administered, complications being most severe in children under the age of 2 years [6].

Despite the risks from primary smallpox vaccination the benefits of eradication were clear: 31 countries still had endemic smallpox in 1967 at the time of the resolution to intensify eradication efforts, an estimated two to three million persons in those countries would die from smallpox that year, and uncounted others would be left with severe facial scarring, corneal scarring and blindness [7]. There was no doubt that smallpox eradication would save lives and that the death and disability prevented would be considerable, as would the financial savings associated with foregone medical treatment costs and the cessation of smallpox vaccination [8, 9].

In 1977, after 10 years of intensified country activities to eradicate smallpox, the last naturally occurring chain of human-to-human smallpox transmission had occurred. Three years later, in 1980, an independent global commission certified that smallpox had been eradicated from the world. The smallpox eradication programme became the first public health programme to achieve worldwide equity in the benefits of a vaccine. That equity was achieved in large part through mass vaccination.

3
Routine Immunization and Mass Vaccination Today— A Necessary Alliance

The fundamental reason that mass vaccination was required to eradicate smallpox was that routine vaccination services in many developing countries lacked the infrastructure needed to vaccinate a sufficient number of their population to attain the herd immunity required to interrupt transmission of the smallpox virus. During the 1970s, as the smallpox eradication programme continued, there was increasing dialogue in WHO expert advisory groups about ensuring equitable distribution of other vaccines in developing countries, such as the DPT vaccine and the newly developed measles and rubella vaccines. These discussions focused on the intensity of the effort required for mass vaccination, the cost of sustaining mass vaccination efforts, and the potential for better sustainability if immunizations were routinely made available along with other maternal and child health services. The outcome of these discussions was the development of the WHO Expanded Programme on Immunizations (EPI) in 1974, the goal of which is to establish and/or strengthen routine immunization programmes in developing countries [10–12].

The overall strategy of the EPI was to increase and sustain the percentage of children who were protected against selected diseases for which vaccines existed. It established common strategies for planning, implementation and evaluation of the effectiveness of national immunization programmes, and introduced these strategies in developing countries through standardized training programmes. In 1977 the World Health Assembly resolved to provide four vaccines (multi-antigen, diphtheria, pertussis and tetanus vaccine; trivalent oral polio vaccine; measles; and BCG) to children throughout the world. By 1990, 16 years after EPI was first established, it was estimated that nearly

80% of children in the world had been vaccinated, some countries having achieved this goal through supplementary mass vaccination campaigns that had received substantial support from bilateral, multilateral, nongovernmental and international organizations [13, 14].

Sustainability of this extraordinary achievement began to wane in many developing countries soon after 1990, due to non-sustained external support, and internal factors such as civil disturbance and war. By 2003 it was estimated that vaccination coverage globally was 75%, ranging from 80% or more in industrialized countries to less than 56% in much of sub-Saharan Africa. Seventeen of the poorest countries in the world were reaching fewer than 50% of children. Obstacles to vaccinating children through routine immunization programmes included poor quality planning, inadequate funding of peripheral staff and operational costs (resulting in low quality and unreliable services), and inadequate monitoring and supervision of immunization activities [15].

In an effort to help countries overcome these obstacles and strengthen immunization services in 75 of the poorest countries with low coverage, the Global Alliance for Vaccines and Immunization (GAVI) was established in 2000 [16]. GAVI provides incremental funding for immunization services, with continuity in funding linked to improvements in the percentage of children immunized. It also provides finances for the introduction of new vaccines into routine immunization programmes in most of these countries. Despite strengthening routine immunization services in many countries through EPI strategies and GAVI support, the need for mass vaccination remains, both for preventing emerging outbreaks, and for accelerating disease control programmes.

In all mass vaccination activities, except for those involving oral polio vaccine, auto-disable syringes are the method of choice for vaccinating. Puncture-resistant containers for collecting disabled needles and syringes must also be available. Multiple-use jet injectors are only used when public health authorities determine that the benefit outweighs the slight, but real risk of transmission of blood-borne infections [17].

4
Preventing Emerging Outbreaks

Perhaps the most widely accepted reason for using mass vaccination is to rapidly increase population (herd) immunity in the setting of an existing or potential infectious disease outbreak, thereby limiting the morbidity and mortality that might result. The rationale for using a mass vaccination approach is particularly strong when the incidence of an epidemic prone disease

Table 1 Mass vaccination to prevent emerging outbreaks

Mass vaccination category	Objective of mass vaccination	Examples	Comment
Response to an emerging epidemic	Rapidly limit the morbidity and mortality due to the documented presence of a vaccine-preventable disease	Meningitis campaigns in sub-Saharan Africa, annual influenza campaigns in industrialized countries, yellow fever campaigns in sub-Saharan Africa and Latin America	Particularly important when the antigen is not delivered through routine immunization programmes
Displaced persons	Rapidly establish population immunity when risk occurs	Measles immunization in refugee camps	Compensate for lack of routine services
Threat of deliberately caused outbreaks	Rapidly establish population immunity when risk is perceived	Smallpox vaccination in response to a real or perceived threat.	May serve as event deterrent

is beginning to rise and when there has been no routine vaccination because the vaccines are unsuitable for routine use, or because populations have been displaced and routine immunization services disrupted (Table 1).

4.1
Meningitis

Meningococcal meningitis is one of a number of diseases for which mass vaccination is a standard, proven element of epidemic control. Although meningococcal meningitis occurs throughout the world the largest epidemics occur in the semi-arid areas of 12 sub-Saharan African countries, designated the African meningitis belt [18]. Most countries within the meningitis belt experience increased transmission each year during the dry period, with large epidemics occurring every 8–12 years during the past 50 years, particularly in regions with extensive communication and mixing of populations.

Meningitis epidemics in sub-Saharan Africa are generally caused by serogroup A organisms, although W135 serogroups have been recently shown to also play a role. Meningococcal vaccines are based on capsular polysaccharide antigens. They are not routinely used in early childhood because of their general lack of efficacy in infants and young children, those at greatest risk of infection and disease [19].

When increased transmission of meningitis occurs in sub-Saharan Africa, epidemiological surveillance is important to determine when the threshold of transmission that generally leads to epidemics has been reached. Once reached, mass vaccination is begun and targeted at a broad age range, sometimes the whole population. Rapidly organized and conducted mass vaccination campaigns effectively protect susceptible individuals and can often interrupt epidemic transmission within 2 or 3 weeks. Mass vaccinations are usually provided by mobile vaccination teams or fixed vaccination stations at health centres or other community facilities [20]. If newly developed meningococcal conjugate vaccines are shown to be protective in infants and young children, meningococcal vaccination could eventually be included in national immunization programmes in areas at high risk of meningococcal disease [21].

4.2
Influenza

Influenza vaccines are not included in routine immunization programmes because of the need to alter the vaccine's composition each year, making it necessary to rapidly vaccinate populations at risk before the epidemic season for influenza begins. Each year seasonal influenza occurs during the winter months in both the northern and southern hemisphere. It is estimated that up to 500 000 persons die each year from seasonal influenza, mainly those over the age of 60 years (WHO). The influenza virus is highly unstable and regularly mutates through a process called antigenic drift. Because antigenic drift decreases the efficacy of the influenza vaccine, the recommended antigenic composition of vaccines is altered each year based on prevalent virus strains. The composition is altered once in February, for the influenza season that will begin 11 months later, and again in August for the influenza season in the southern hemisphere.

As soon as altered influenza vaccines become available each year, they are provided to the population at risk (usually the elderly, and in some countries to health workers as well) prior to the epidemic season and by mass vaccination at fixed health facilities, mainly in industrialized countries [22, 23]. Recently the provincial government of Ontario in Canada recommended vaccination of populations of all ages with influenza vaccine prior to the influenza season. This experience will provide a comparative evaluation of the approach being used in most other countries. Although it is known that seasonal influenza occurs in developing countries, further study is needed to understand the target population and vaccination strategy required to optimize the impact of mass vaccination.

At times, an antigenic shift occurs when a new pandemic influenza virus enters human populations, usually from an avian source. The new virus strain must then be used to develop a new vaccine because little, if any cross immunity is anticipated from existing influenza vaccines. New vaccines for pandemic influenza are targeted at the entire population, and are provided in mass campaigns.

4.3
Yellow Fever

Yellow fever occurs sporadically in 33 countries in Africa and 11 countries in South America. A severe epidemic of human-to-human transmission is most likely to occur when conditions allow the density of mosquito vector populations to substantially increase, as often happens during the rainy season. Epidemiological surveillance is a key strategy for limiting yellow fever epidemics by rapidly identifying human infections when they occur. Mosquito control is also an effective supplemental prevention strategy. However, the most effective means of preventing yellow fever epidemics is through vaccination at 9 months of age using the vaccine as part of routine immunization programmes [24], and yellow fever vaccine is integrated into routine immunization programs in some, but not all countries at risk.

If routine immunization at 9 months of age does not reach the level needed for herd immunity in the general population, epidemic transmission is a risk and mass vaccination is required to fill the gap in immunity. The target population for mass vaccination, once yellow fever has been identified in human populations, is the entire population living or working in the area from which the infection has been identified. In the event of limited financial resources or vaccine supply, the primary target population is usually children aged from 9 months to 14 years after which adults at risk are also vaccinated. Vaccinations are generally provided through house-to-house campaigns, during which there is active questioning to determine whether additional human infections are occurring. As with any epidemic, planning and implementation of mass vaccination must begin as soon as possible after an outbreak is confirmed, and emergency supplies of 17D yellow fever vaccine ordered immediately.

4.4
Displaced Persons

Sudden and massive influxes of people with varied backgrounds and immunization status can occur during civil disturbance, war and natural disasters.

In such situations routine immunization activities are often not available and, where displaced populations live in close proximity, and where sanitation and water supplies may be compromised, they create a particularly rife environment for epidemics of vaccine preventable diseases. Major vaccines used in mass campaigns among displaced persons are measles, meningococcal meningitis, and yellow fever vaccines. Mass vaccination for measles is usually conducted immediately after displaced persons congregate, particularly if vaccine coverage rates are estimated to be less than 80%. The target population is often extended, to a lower age limit of 6 months and an upper limit of 14 years, with revaccination of infants when they reach 12 months of age. Mass vaccination for meningitis and yellow fever is conducted if risk factors for epidemics are present, while studies of the applicability of the new cholera and typhoid vaccines in displaced populations are currently underway in several geographic areas to evaluate their usefulness in mass campaigns among displaced persons [25].

4.5
Threat of Deliberately Caused Outbreaks

There is a variety of circumstances under which public health authorities gauge the risk of a deliberately-caused epidemic or biologic threat to be sufficent to warrant preventive action. Mass vaccination campaigns are then sometimes conducted as a deterrent, and/or to prevent a deliberately caused outbreak should one be planned or occur. Some countries perceive a particular threat from disease such as smallpox and/or anthrax, and have begun to stockpile vaccines against these perceived threats that would be used for mass vaccination of entire populations should such a threat materialize [26].

Strategies for the use of these vaccines vary, but most countries state as the first priority mass vaccination of primary responders such as health workers, followed by mass vaccination of the general population if the deliberately-used infectious agent has the potential to spread from person to person. The strategies for mass vaccination may, however, be much more complex than for other indications due to the deterrent nature and thus the need to be as safe as possible. For example, because infection with HIV has been associated with generalized vaccinia and death after smallpox vaccination, strategies of preventive mass vaccination using smallpox vaccine need to incorporate the ability to avoid vaccination of HIV infected persons, and to provide them protection by other means such as passive immunization with vaccinia immune globulin [27].

5
Mass Vaccination to Accelerate Disease Control

A second important use of mass vaccination strategies is to accelerate disease control to rapidly increase coverage with a new vaccine at the time of its introduction into routine immunization programmes, or to attain the herd immunity levels required to meet international targets for eradication and mortality reduction. Since the late 1980s, international accelerated disease control targets have been established for eradication, for mortality reduction, and for heightened control of infectious diseases. Reaching these targets requires rapidly increasing population immunity, usually with the goal of interrupting human-to-human transmission of the causative infectious agent. Mass vaccination campaigns are a particularly important element of these efforts as the vaccination coverage levels required to achieve herd immunity, especially in densely populated areas, often exceed the coverage rates from routine immunization programmes (Table 2).

Table 2 Mass vaccination to accelerate disease control

Mass vaccination category	Objective of mass vaccination	Examples	Comment
New vaccine introduction	Rapidly optimize the impact of a new antigen and/or minimize potential side effects associated with its introduction	Rubella campaigns (e.g. targeting children and women < 45 years)	One-time supplement at time of initiation of routine childhood immunization with a new vaccine
Disease eradication	Achieve population immunity needed during time-limited period to interrupt transmission	National Immunization Days (NIDs) for polio eradication	Essential if coverage required for herd immunity exceeds that of routine immunization coverage or goals
Mortality reduction	Accelerate achievement of specific national or international disease control goals	Measles morbidity and mortality reduction campaigns, neonatal tetanus elimination campaigns	Sometimes continued as a transition or temporary strategy while routine immunization is strengthened

5.1
New Vaccine Introduction

During the past 60 years more than 20 new vaccines have become available. Mass vaccination can be a key element of new vaccine introduction, the goal being to quickly reduce the proportion of susceptible persons at risk at the time the new vaccine is introduced into the routine immunization programme. The impact of the mass campaign is to equalize population immunity levels, thus preventing a potential exacerbation of the disease that is targeted because of a sudden change in its transmission patterns or other epidemiological characteristic that might occur by vaccinating only a portion of the susceptible population through routine immunization programmes.

At the time of new vaccine introduction, persons considered susceptible and at risk of infection are vaccinated in mass vaccination campaigns to 'mop up' or protect all those who were susceptible. Mass vaccination is then ended, and the vaccines remain incorporated in routine immunization programmes to vaccinate susceptible persons as they enter the cohort of susceptibility (usually at birth).

A clear example of this strategy first occurred in the 1950s when the Salk inactivated polio vaccine was first licensed. Initially it was offered in mass campaigns to all populations considered at risk of polio, then incorporated into routine childhood immunization programmes to ensure that children entering the birth cohort were fully protected.

Although routine childhood immunization against rubella is now a standard component of vaccination programmes in industrialized countries, the vaccine has until recently seen limited uptake in developing countries. Decision-making on whether or not to introduce rubella vaccine was complicated by concern that routine childhood immunization against the disease could shift the average age of infection to older girls, inadvertently increasing, at least transiently, the risk of disease in pregnant women and thus the incidence of congenital rubella syndrome. Consequently, the introduction of routine childhood immunization against rubella is accompanied by a one-time mass campaign, targeting all girls less than 15 years of age, and in some countries all women of childbearing age [28].

It is likewise recommended standard practice to accompany the introduction of yellow fever vaccine into routine childhood immunization programmes with a one-time mass vaccination campaign. In these campaigns children aged less than 15 years are targeted to prevent yellow fever epidemics that could continue because of the immunization gap that would occur until immunized childhood cohorts reach adulthood [29].

5.2
Eradication

Polio vaccination has been included in routine immunization programmes since the licensing of the Salk and Sabin vaccines. In 1988, when the target to eradicate polio was set, an increasing number of countries had already interrupted human-to-human transmission of wild poliovirus by using oral poliovirus vaccine (OPV) in routine immunization programmes. In many countries in Latin America, where routine immunization programmes had not ever achieved high level control it was demonstrated that by supplementing routine immunization with mass vaccination these tropical and semi-tropical developing countries could rapidly interrupt transmission.

The mass vaccination strategy currently used in polio eradication targets all children under the age of 5 years, during National Immunization Days or Weeks in which OPV is administered to children through fixed sites with house-to-house mop-up campaigns that sometimes target a broader age group if required to interrupt the final chains of transmission. In some densely populated areas, interrupting poliovirus transmission has required well over 90% coverage in up to seven mass vaccination campaigns each year. Areas with low standards of sanitation and high population densities have required the most campaigns.

Prior to conducting mass vaccination, district level micro-planning is used to identify areas where children under the age of 5 years may be living and to prepare maps that are used by social mobilizers and vaccinators as they pass from community to community and house to house. The oral route of OPV administration allows the widespread use of health workers, school teachers and community volunteers trained in short courses to administer polio vaccine during the campaigns. Worldwide interruption of human-to-human transmission of wild poliovirus is presently targeted for 2005. At the time this chapter was written mass vaccination was being further intensified in the six countries that remained polio-endemic, in six countries that had re-established polio transmission due to imported virus, and in other countries to control outbreaks following polio importation [30].

Despite the impact of the global polio eradication initiative to date, the use of mass vaccination strategies with the endpoint of eradication remains an uneasy alliance with routine immunization programmes, largely due to the massive marginal and opportunity costs associated with eliminating the final chains of human-to-human transmission. This debate has led to the establishment of careful and comprehensive criteria for considering future eradication programmes, particularly the need for explicit and appropriate cost–benefit analysis in advance, as well as the capacity to sustain sufficient societal and political support throughout [31, 32].

5.3
Mortality Reduction

5.3.1
Measles

Although measles vaccine is universally included in routine immunization programmes in developing countries, targeting children between the ages of 9 and 12 months, there is frequent failure of children to seroconvert to measles vaccine because of the presence of maternal antibody to measles. Once maternal antibody disappears the window of opportunity to effectively vaccinate children before natural infection is short and operationally difficult to exploit. Mass vaccination campaigns are a frequently used strategy to overcome this problem [33].

Based on the age profile of measles susceptibility, a one-time nationwide catch-up campaign is conducted in Latin American countries to reduce population susceptibility and interrupt transmission. Usually all children aged less than 15 years are targeted, regardless of prior measles immunization status. Follow-up mass vaccination campaigns, targeting children aged less than 5 years, are then conducted every 3–5 years thereafter, giving those who have not previously seroconverted a second opportunity. Countries that are achieving very high coverage through their routine immunization programmes generally provide the 'second opportunity' prior to school entry.

5.3.2
Maternal and Neonatal Tetanus

To prevent maternal and neonatal tetanus, mass vaccination campaigns with tetanus toxoid are conducted in high-risk areas that are delineated using surveillance data and the prevalence of clean birth and delivery practices. In most countries with an explicit maternal and neonatal tetanus elimination goal, districts are now ranked from highest to lowest risk of the diseases. Multiple rounds of mass vaccination are often required, targeting young girls and women of childbearing age, to rapidly boost immunity against tetanus [34].

6
Mass Vaccination in the Twenty-First Century

In the 200 years since Edward Jenner first opened the door to disease control through mass vaccination, much attention has been given to establishing and strengthening primary health services through which childhood immunizations can be delivered on a routine, ongoing basis. At the same time, mass vaccination campaigns, conducted over short time periods, continue to play an important role in the control of vaccine preventable diseases, in both industrialized and developing country settings. Mass vaccination is particularly important for preventing emerging outbreaks of vaccine-preventable diseases, rapidly boosting population immunity in emergency settings, optimizing the impact of a new vaccine, achieving very high herd immunity levels to achieve international disease control goals (especially eradication), and, in some settings, to efficiently supplement routine immunization of young children. Mass vaccination and routine immunization are a necessary alliance for attaining both national and international goals in the control of vaccine preventable diseases.

References

1. Hopkins DR (1983) Princes and peasants: Smallpox in history. University of Chicago Press, Chicago
2. Fenner F, Henderson DA, Arita I, Jezek Z, Ladnyi ID (1988) Smallpox and its eradication. World Health Organization, Geneva p 263
3. McLeod RM (1967) Law, Medicine and public opinion: the resistance to compulsory health legislation 1870–1907. Public Law 1967:6: 107–128, 189–211
4. Edwards EJ (1902) A concise history of small-pox and vaccination in Europe. London, Lewis
5. World Health Organization, 1966. World Health Assembly 19.16
6. Fenner F, Henderson DA, Arita I, Jezek Z, Ladnyi ID (1988) Smallpox and its eradication. World Health Organization, Geneva, pp 296–309
7. Fenner F, Henderson DA, Arita I, Jezêk X, LadnyiI D (1988) Developments in Vaccination and Control: Smallpox and its Eradication. World Health Organization, Geneva, p 175
8. Fenner F, Henderson DA, Arita I, Jezêk X, LadnyiI D (1988) Developments in Vaccination and Control: Smallpox and its Eradication. World Health Organization, Geneva, p 1363–1365
9. Barrett S, Hoel M (2003) Optimal disease eradication. Frisch Centre, University of Oslo 203 (HERO working paper 23/2003)
10. Sencer JD, Axnick NW (1973) Cost benefit analysis. Immunological Standardization 22:37–46
11. Gonzalez CL (1965) Mass campaigns and general health services. World Health Organization, Geneva. Public Health Papers, no. 29
12. Mills A (2005) Mass campaigns versus general health services: what we have learnt in 40 years about vertical versus horizontal approaches. Bull World Health Org 83(4): 315–316

13. Henderson RH, Keja K, Galazka AM, Chan CA (1990) Reaping the benefits: getting vaccines to those who need them. In: Woodrow GC, Levine MM (eds). New Generation vaccines. Marcel Dekker, New York, pp 69–82
14. Henderson RH, Keja J, Hayden G, et al. (1988) Immunizing children of the world: progress and prospects. Bull World Health Org 66:535–543
15. Keegan R, Bilous J (2004) Current issues in global immunizations. Seminars in Pediatric Infectious Diseases. Elsevier, Amsterdam
16. Muraskin W (2004) The global alliance for vaccines and immunization: is it a new model for effective public-private cooperation in international public health? Am J Public Health 94:11:1922-1925
17. World Health Organization. "First, do no harm". Introducing auto-disable syringes and ensuring injection safety in immunization systems of developing countries. WHO/V&B/02.26
18. Greenwood BM (1987) The epidemiology of acute bacterial meningitis in tropical Africa. In: Williams JD, Brunie J (eds). Bacterial meningitis. Academic Press, London, pp 61–91
19. Reingold AL, Broome CV, Hightower A, et al. (1985) Age specific differences in duration of clinical protection after vaccination with meningococcal polysaccharide A vaccine. Lancet 2:112–118
20. Schwartz B, Moore PS, Broome CV (1989) Global epidemiology of meningococcal disease. Clin Microbiol Rev 2:S118–S124
21. World Health Organization. Control of Epidemic meningococcal disease. WHO practical guidelines: second edition:WHO/EMC/BAC/98.3
22. Stohr K (2004) Influenza. In: Heymann DL (ed). Control of communicable diseases manual 18th edition, an official report of the American Public Health Association
23. Heymann DL (2005) Preparing for a New Global Threat—Part I. YaleGlobal, 26 January 2005. http://yaleglobal.yale.edu/display.article?id=5174
24. World Health Organization, 2000. Yellow Fever. WHO/EPI/GEN/98.11, WHO/CDS/EDC/2000.2
25. Connolly MA, Gayer M, Ryan MJ, Salama P, Spiegel P, Heymann DL (2004) Communicable Diseases in Complex Emergencies–impacts and challenges. Lancet 364:1974-83
26. World Health Organization (2004) Public health response to biological and chemical weapons, second edition
27. Heymann DL (2004) Smallpox containment updated: considerations for the 21st century. Int J Infect Dis 8(S2):S15–S20 (ISSN 1201–9712)
28. World Health Organization. Control of rubella and congenital rubella syndrome in developing countries. WHO/V&B/00.03
29. World Health Organization. Yellow Fever. WHO/EPI/GEN/98.11, WHO/CDS/EDC/2000.2
30. Heymann DL, Aylward RB (2004) Perspective article. Global Health: Eradicating Polio. New Engl J Med 351(13):1275–1277
31. Melgaard B, Creese A, Aylward B, Olivé J-M, Maher C, Okwo-Bele J-M, Lee JW (1998) Disease eradication and health systems development. Bull World Health Org (Suppl 2): 28–31
32. Dowdle WR (1998) The principles of disease elimination and eradication. Bull World Health Org (Suppl 2) :22–25

33. Bielik R, Madema S, Taole A, Kutsulukuta A, Allies E, Eggers RN, Ngcobo N, Nxumalo M, Shearley A, Mabuzane E, Kufa E, Okwo-Bele J-M (2002). First 5 years of measles elimination in southern Africa: 1996–2000. Lancet 359(9137):1564–1568
34. World Health Organization. Field manual for neonatal tetanus elimination. WHO/V&B/99.14

Mass Vaccination and Surveillance/Containment in the Eradication of Smallpox

J. M. Lane (✉)

869 Clifton Road NE, Atlanta, GA 30307-1223, USA
mikelane869@yahoo.com

1	Background	18
2	Initial Plans for Mass Vaccination Against Measles and Smallpox in West Africa	18
3	Contrasting Epidemiology of Measles and Smallpox in West Africa	19
4	Observations Leading to Increased Importance of Surveillance and Outbreak Containment	20
5	Change in Strategy, 1968	21
6	Elements of the Surveillance/Outbreak Containment Strategy	22
7	Results in West Africa	23
8	Results in Asia	24
9	Validation by Mathematical Modeling	25
10	Summary and Conclusions	26
	References	26

Abstract The Smallpox Eradication Program, initiated by the WHO in 1966, was originally based on mass vaccination. The program emphasized surveillance from the beginning, largely to track the success of the program and further our understanding of the epidemiology of the disease. Early observations in West Africa, bolstered by later data from Indonesia and the Asian subcontinent, showed that smallpox did not spread rapidly, and outbreaks could be quickly controlled by isolation of patients and vaccination of their contacts. Contacts were usually easy to find because transmission of smallpox usually required prolonged face-to-face contact. The emphasis therefore shifted to active searches to find cases, coupled with contact tracing, rigorous isolation of patients, and vaccination and surveillance of contacts to contain outbreaks. This shift away from mass vaccination resulted in an acceleration of the program's success.

1
Background

During 1967–1969, the World Health Organization's Smallpox Eradication Program shifted emphasis from mass vaccination to surveillance and containment. The shift evolved from early field experiences by the Center of Disease Control (CDC) staff who improvised new approaches based on their developing understanding of the epidemiology of smallpox, and the relative ease of its control. This chapter summarizes these data and experiences, and comments on the results of the initial efforts in surveillance and containment.

In 1964 the World Health Organization (WHO) Expert Committee on Smallpox mandated 100% vaccination coverage to eradicate smallpox, rather than an 80% level of herd immunity as previously claimed (WHO 1964). These experts assumed that smallpox was highly contagious and would therefore find isolated pockets of susceptible population. The committee emphasized the need to measure levels of immunity by developing methods of rapid and reliable assessment of vaccination coverage. Around the same time, jet injector technology was being developed for rapid point-of-collection immunization (Millar et al. 1969; Roberto et al. 1969; Neff et al. 1969). Coincidentally, trials in the early 1960s, which showed the safety and efficacy of measles vaccine in Africa, led many West African public health advocates to request assistance with measles control. (Meyer et al. 1964) These developments set the stage for the West African measles/smallpox campaign.

2
Initial Plans for Mass Vaccination Against Measles and Smallpox in West Africa

The initial plan for the smallpox eradication/measles control program was to do mass vaccination of the entire population for smallpox, and all children under the age of 5 years for measles. The program used mobile teams going village to village, with collection point vaccination. Measles had a high case fatality rate in sub-Saharan Africa, about 5%. (Morley 1967) There was therefore considerable interest in the successful trial of measles vaccine in Upper Volta (now Burkina Faso). This led USAID to advocate a measles vaccination campaign through West Africa (Meyer et al. 1964). CDC agreed to provide technical assistance to this campaign if smallpox eradication was added to the effort (Fenner et al. 1988). Simultaneous childhood measles and universal smallpox vaccination was started in 1967, using collection-point mass vaccination with jet injector guns as the main strategy. Collection point mass vaccination utilized the jet guns maximally, and helped the logistics of handling measles vaccine, which required careful refrigeration. The jet guns were cumbersome and made house-to-house visitation awkward. Collection point mass immunization and treatment methods had been successfully used throughout much of West Africa to control yellow fever and yaws, so that public health authorities were comfortable with mass vaccination concepts (Hopkins 1985; Tomori 2002).

CDC and WHO were vitally interested in adding disease surveillance to the effort, mostly as a method of assessing the results of the smallpox and measles immunization program. Surveillance and outbreak investigations also allowed direct comparison of the epidemiology of measles and smallpox in similar communities. While superficially similar, the epidemiology of measles and smallpox in West Africa proved to be quite different.

3
Contrasting Epidemiology of Measles and Smallpox in West Africa

Measles in West Africa was highly infectious and had about a 5% case fatality rate (Morley 1967). The median age of attack was less than 2 years. Virtually all children got the disease. Transmission was common in gathering places such as markets, schools, or other gathering places. It was difficult to trace chains of transmission. In large urban areas such as the city of Dakar, measles would exhaust all susceptibles and require continual re-introductions from outside the city to maintain transmission (Rey et al.1968). One case often caused six or more new cases. Once the disease was introduced into a household or compound, the attack rate among exposed susceptibles was usually nearly 100%.

Smallpox was much less infectious. The median age of attack was in the mid-teens or early 20s (Foege et al. 1975). Chains of transmission were easy to trace. Most transmission was to intimate household contacts (Henderson and Yekpe 1969). One case rarely spread the disease to as many as three others. Very small tribal groups, as few as 200 or so, often sustained transmission for six or more generations (Imperato et al. 1973). In individual compounds with extended family groups, the interval between the onset of the first case and the onset of the last case was frequently 6 weeks, and often was 8 weeks (Foege et al. 1975). The two viral exanthems, although superficially similar, behaved very differently in the community.

4
Observations Leading to Increased Importance of Surveillance and Outbreak Containment

Four observations led the CDC to give increased emphasis on surveillance of smallpox and rapid containment of outbreaks. First, in early 1967 Dr William H. Foege, who had agreed to head the smallpox and measles efforts in the Eastern State of Nigeria, detected a substantial epidemic of smallpox in several communities in Ogoja Province. The initial shipments of vaccine had not arrived. He called upon a network of friends and medical missionaries in the area, and suggested that they use their very limited supplies of vaccine to vaccinate close contacts of cases and possibly attenuate the outbreak. To his delight the outbreak was rapidly eliminated (Foege et al. 1975). In retrospect Dr C.W. Dixon had observed similar results in Tripolitania shortly after World War II. He rapidly eliminated a substantial outbreak among the Arab population with very limited supplies of glycerinated lymph vaccine. He vaccinated occupants of tents in which cases were found, telling his workers to vaccinate residents of surrounding tents only if there was sufficient vaccine. Dixon coined the term 'ring vaccination', which has become synonymous with the vaccination strategy of surveillance/containment (Dixon 1948).

Second, shortly after the Ogoja Province outbreak showed that smallpox was relatively easy to eliminate with vaccination of small numbers of close contacts, Dr Foege and his colleagues conducted a textbook mass vaccination campaign in the Eastern Nigerian city of Abakaliki. Independent field assessment with a carefully drawn sample of the city showed that 88% of the population had been effectively vaccinated, with the major cutaneous reactions that WHO used as criteria for 'take'. Shortly thereafter there was an outbreak of 33 cases of smallpox in the city (Thompson and Foege 1968). This observation cast doubt on the ability of mass vaccination alone to eliminate the disease.

Third, while these observations were being made in West Africa, data from several studies of the epidemiology and viral shedding of Asian Variola major became available. These studies showed that the vast majority of spread was to persons with very close prolonged face-to-face contact with obviously sick patients. Most transmission occurred during the first 5 or 6 days of the rash when the patient was prostrate and visibly ill. Secondary household attack rates among susceptibles were as low as 36% in the seasonal downswing of the disease, and the highest recorded was only 88% during the seasonal increase. Rarely did any patient spread smallpox to more than three other patients, perhaps in part because they were too sick to be effectively mobile (Rao et al. 1968; Mack et al. 1972; Sommer and Foster 1974; Heiner et al. 1971;

Thomas et al. 1971). Joint US, UK, and Indian researchers used plates of viral culture medium placed near patients in a smallpox hospital to show that viral shedding was detected only within 6 feet of the patient. Virus was not shed during the first 2 or 3 days of the prodrome when the patients were very ill, but had not yet developed an enanthem in the back of the nose and throat (Downie et al. 1965).

Finally, review of the epidemiology of imported smallpox in Europe from 1950 to 1971 yielded similar data on the relatively slow spread of the disease. There were very few large outbreaks. Indeed 13 of 47 importations resulted in no spread at all. The average number of cases per importation was just 15. Over 50% of cases acquired smallpox in hospital, when undiagnosed very sick patients were not fully isolated (Mack 1972). In commenting on this study the author wrote "It is my judgment that under contemporary conditions smallpox cannot be said to live up to its reputation. Far from being a quick-footed menace, it has appeared as a plodding nuisance with more bark than bite." Mack has subsequently pointed out that smallpox probably would have been eliminated in developed nations, even without vaccine, by prompt isolation of patients (Mack 2003).

5
Change in Strategy, 1968

During the fall of 1968, the CDC program in West Africa, led by Dr Foege, changed its strategy for smallpox eradication. Foege and his colleagues reasoned that the relatively slow spread of smallpox, with the ease of aborting outbreaks by vaccination of contacts, made the disease susceptible to control by actively searching for cases and concentrating on vaccinating their household and village contacts. Foege was also impressed by the marked seasonality of the disease. He believed that if outbreaks could be found during the West African seasonal low in September through January, and chains of transmission broken by patient isolation and/or vaccination of close contacts, a large decrease in the seasonal high from February through June would result from a fairly small effort. In India less than 1% of villages were infected at any one time, suggesting that only modest numbers of vaccinations were necessary if reporting could be improved (National Institute of Communicable Diseases of India 1968). CDC thus laid plans for intensive active surveillance in the fall of 1968 and early winter of 1969 (Foege et al. 1971).

6
Elements of the Surveillance/Outbreak Containment Strategy

The surveillance and outbreak control strategy is conceptually simple, but required several changes in emphasis from the straightforward mass vaccination technique. Improvements in surveillance were central to the effort. Passive reporting through the medical care system was very poor in the newly emerging nations of West Africa. Reporting efficiency in Nigeria was only about 5% of actual cases, and was poor in other areas of West Africa (Henderson et al. 1973). Instead of relying on formal medical reports, CDC teams went to markets and schools, and showed pictures of typical cases of smallpox, inquiring whether anyone had seen similar patients in their village in recent weeks. They quickly learned that tribal and civil authorities knew more about the health conditions in the villages than the medical hierarchy. Surveillance became an active search, rather than passive reliance on traditional disease notification by medical personnel.

A second element is improved isolation of patients. Patient isolation can be very effective in controlling smallpox since patients are not infectious during the first 3 days or so of the prodrome, and transmission is usually only to contacts with prolonged direct face-to-face exposure. Indeed one experienced observer suggests that in developed countries smallpox could be eradicated by isolation alone (Mack 2003). Many tribes in West Africa hid cases because they had learned that isolation in smallpox hospitals was tantamount to a death sentence. Medical and nursing care was poor in most African smallpox hospitals, and patients were not given good food and fluids. Family members could do a better job of nursing patients, and particularly feeding them, given that there was no actual therapy for smallpox. A system of home isolation with careful education of family members and villagers, coupled with vaccination of caregivers, replaced forced hospitalization.

A third element is identification of contacts. This proved easy once contacts realized that being vaccinated might save them from developing smallpox. Many of the CDC operations officers in the program had been sexually transmitted disease investigators in the US, and were experienced in interviewing and contact tracing.

A fourth element is vaccinating the contacts. The biology and immunology of smallpox allows contacts to be spared the disease if they are vaccinated within about 3 days after contact (Massoudi et al. 2003; Kennedy et al. 2004). CDC staff quickly realized that vaccinating contacts with the jet injector guns was cumbersome and time consuming, whereas all workers in the program could carry several vials of vaccine and containers of sterile bifurcated needles. They could vaccinate contacts wherever and whenever they were found. Fully

100% of contacts had to be vaccinated, which meant that teams often made multiple visits to infected villages, including staying at night to vaccinate villagers who had gone to markets or were engaged in remote agricultural activities.

A fifth element of the new strategy is placing contacts under careful and close surveillance, so that they can be isolated as soon as they develop early prodromal symptoms of smallpox (smallpox is not infectious until 3 or 4 days after the beginning of the febrile prodrome). Surveillance could be accomplished by program team members, local health workers, or village officials trained to do the task.

The final element of the surveillance/containment strategy is vaccinating the 'second ring', i.e., the contacts of contacts. In practice this often meant vaccinating an entire village once the initial contacts had been carefully identified and vaccinated. The second ring was vaccinated in case there was a vaccine failure in one of the first ring contacts, or a failure to identify a contact already infected.

7
Results in West Africa

The shift from mass vaccination to surveillance and outbreak containment rapidly accelerated smallpox eradication. Figure 1 shows the secular trend of smallpox in the 19 nations of West and Central Africa, displayed on a semi-log scale as the ratio of observed cases to those expected from the mean of the 7 years from 1960 to 1967. This corrects for the sharp seasonal trend observed in the historical data. When active search began in the fall of 1968, there was an immediate increase in cases detected. This was followed by a rapid decline, with smallpox being finally eradicated more than 18 months in advance of the original target date (Foege et al. 1971; Foege 1996)

In late 1967, during the tensions leading to, and then the actual conduct of, the Biafra Civil War, the Eastern State of Nigeria shifted from mass vaccination to surveillance and containment and interrupted transmission in just 5 months, with only 750 000 of the state's 12 million population vaccinated (Foege et al. 1975). Sierra Leone had the highest incidence of reported smallpox in all of Africa in 1967, and started its mass vaccination program a year later than most of the other West African nations. It eradicated smallpox rapidly, and indeed three of its four largest outbreaks, and seven of its 13 administrative districts, cleared smallpox completely before the planned beginning of mass vaccinations (Hopkins et al. 1971). Mali eradicated smallpox with barely 51% of its population vaccinated (Foege et al. 1975). There were similar success stories in Guinea, Togo, Upper Volta, and Northern Nigeria.

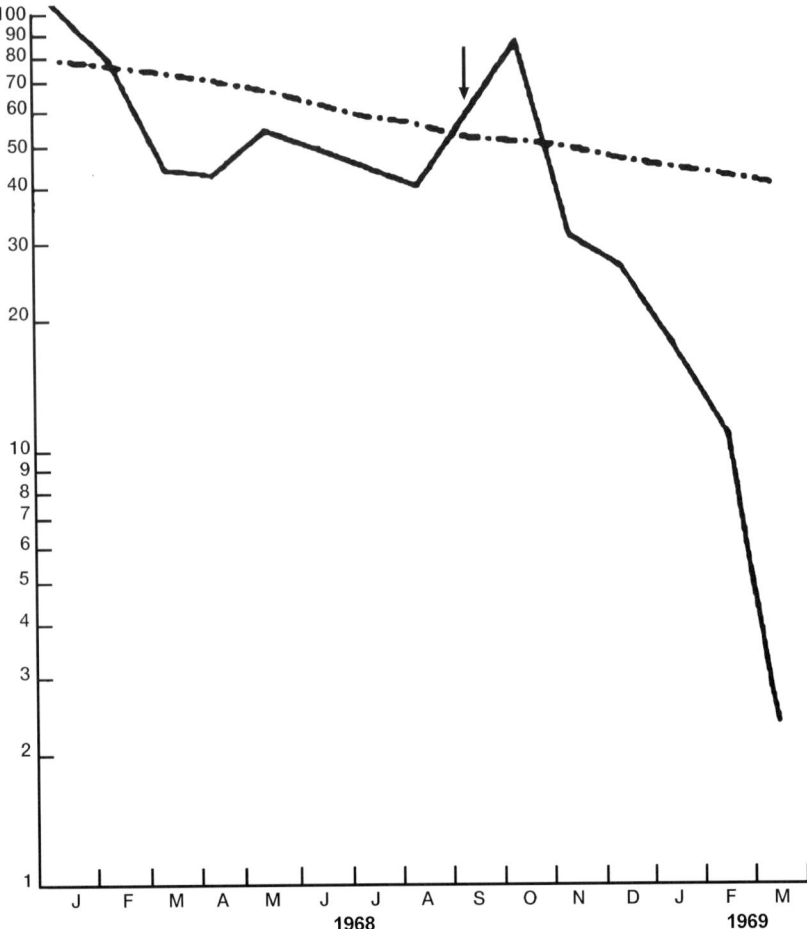

Fig. 1 The percentage of the population not vaccinated in the smallpox eradication program areas of West and Central Africa (*broken line*) compared with the ratio (%) of reported smallpox cases to cases expected from the 1960–67 monthly average (*solid line*). The *arrow* marks the start of surveillance-containment activities

8
Results in Asia

The results of the emphasis on surveillance and outbreak control in West Africa were sufficiently impressive so that WHO urged other nations, particularly in Asia, to adopt the strategy as a mainstay of their eradication programs. The success of these measures is well documented in the definitive history of the WHO Smallpox Eradication Programme (Fenner et al. 1988). In the Indonesian province of West Java, a fortuitous experiment took place in which Bogor regency did surveillance/containment alone, Bandung regency did surveillance/containment combined with mass vaccination efforts aimed at reducing the backlog of unvaccinated population, and Tjirebon regency first did mass vaccination to reduce the backlog, followed by surveillance/containment. The outcome convinced Indonesian authorities of the superiority of surveillance/containment, and they were instrumental in helping WHO convince Indian program leaders to adopt the strategy.

The Asian efforts included improvements and extensions of the basic steps in the surveillance/outbreak containment methods. In India increasing rewards were made for reporting bona fide cases of smallpox, with increasing values (25 to 50 to 100 rupees) as the final cases were found. In Bangladesh family health workers lived for nearly 2 weeks in each infected village to assist with vaccination, and guards were posted at houses where infected patients were isolated. Surveillance built in measures of the time from the onset of each patient's illness to the time of report, the time between initiating control measures and the onset of the last case in the outbreak, and similar methods of documenting the speed of finding cases and contacts. The time taken to control outbreaks became the measure most closely monitored, other than the actual decline of cases itself.

9
Validation by Mathematical Modeling

In 2002 concerns about the use of smallpox as a bioterrorist weapon led to planning for handling outbreaks with unnatural sources. Kaplan and his colleagues constructed a mathematical model of smallpox outbreaks, and claimed that surveillance and outbreak containment methods did not work as well as mass vaccination. His model included several aspects that are not consistent with historical experience; only 50% of contacts were found, patients spread the disease during the asymptomatic period of their infection, and quarantine and isolation of patients and contacts was not fully effective (Kaplan et al. 2002). Several other investigators, using a variety of different mathematical modeling methods but employing realistic biological parameters consistent with historical field experience, have found that surveillance and containment methods works better than mass vaccination in virtually all scenarios (Meltzer et al. 2001: Halloran et al. 2002: Bozette et al. 2003; Eichner 2003; Eubank et al. 2004; LeGrand et al. 2004: Porco et al. 2004; Glasser et al. 2005).

10
Summary and Conclusions

Unique biologic and epidemiologic aspects of smallpox allow it to be rapidly eliminated by surveillance and outbreak containment techniques. Patients have a characteristic visible rash, which is easy for non-medical personnel to recognize. The disease is not infectious in the early stages of the prodrome, while the patients are very sick. This keeps patients from being mobile and spreading the virus. The vast majority of spread is to very close contacts, who are thus easy to identify. Vaccination early in the incubation period is effective in stopping the development of the illness. Emphasis on finding cases, isolating them, and vaccinating their contacts accelerated the eradication of smallpox, and allowed de-emphasis of mass vaccination methods. Surveillance and careful isolation of patients may be important in other diseases spread by large droplet respiratory secretions, such as SARS.

In the author's opinion, a terrorist attack in the US using smallpox should not prompt mass vaccination. Mass vaccination with current first generation vaccinia strains would cause considerable morbidity and mortality (Lane and Goldstein 2003). It would be unnecessary given the efficiency and ease of surveillance and containment in a nation with sophisticated communications systems (Mack 2003; Lane and Goldstein 2003). If widespread simultaneous releases of large volumes of aerosolized smallpox took place in several cities, mass vaccination might become politically inevitable, but during the campaign contacts of known cases would still be ethically and epidemiologically the most important people to receive vaccination. Thus surveillance and containment methods would have to accompany any mass vaccination efforts, and should receive the highest priority. The post 9/11 efforts to create a cadre of vaccinated health care workers in the U.S. was not a mass vaccination effort, but rather an attempt to selectively immunize people known to be at high risk of exposure to smallpox in an attack given the frequency of nosocomial spread.

References

Bozzette SA, Boer R, Bhatnagar V, Brower JL, Keeler EB, Morton SC, Stoto MA (2003) A model for a smallpox-vaccination policy. N Engl J Med 348:416–425

Dixon CW (1948) Smallpox in Tripolitania, 1946; an epidemiological and clinical study of 500 cases, including trials of penicillin treatment. J Hygiene 46:35–77

Downie AW, Meikeljohn M, St Vincent L, Rao AR, Sundara Babu BV, Kempe CH (1965) The recovery of smallpox virus from patients and their environment in a smallpox hospital. Bull World Health Org 33:615–622

Eichner M (2003) Case isolation and contact tracing can prevent the spread of smallpox. Am J Epidemiol 158:118–128

Eichner M, Dietz K (2003) Transmission potential of smallpox: estimates based on detailed data from an outbreak. Am J Epidemiol 158:110–117

Eubank S, Guclu H, Kumar VS. Marathe MV, Srinivasan A, Toroczkai Z, Wang N (2004) Modelling disease outbreaks in realistic urban social networks. Nature 429:180–184

Fenner F, Henderson DA, Arita I, Jezek Z, Ladnyi ID (1988) Smallpox and its Eradication. World Health Orgianization, Geneva

Foege WH (1996) Commentary: Smallpox eradication in West and Central Africa revisited. Bull World Health Org 76:233–235

Foege WH, Millar JD, Lane JM (1971) Selective epidemiologic control in smallpox eradication. Am J Epidemiol 94:311–315

Foege WH, Millar JD, Henderson DA (1975) Smallpox eradication in West and Central Africa. Bull World Health Org 52:209–222

Foster SO (1977) Smallpox eradication: lessons learned in Bangladesh. WHO Chronicle 31(6):245–247

Gani R, Leach S (2001) Transmission potential of smallpox in contemporary populations. Nature 414:748–751

Glasser J, Foster SO, Millar JD, Lane JM (2005) Evaluating public health responses to re-introduced smallpox via dynamic, socially structured, and spatially distributed meta-population models. Am J Epidemiol (in press)

Halloran ME, Longini IM Jr, Nizam A, Yang Y (2002) Containing bioterrorist smallpox. Science 298:1428–1433

Henderson RH, Yekpe M (1969) Smallpox transmission in southern Dahomey. A study of a village outbreak. Am J Epidemiol 90:423–428

Henderson RH, Davis H, Eddins DL, Foege WH (1973) Assessment of vaccination coverage, vaccination scar rates, and smallpox scarring in five areas of West Africa. Bull World Health Org 48:183–194

Heiner GG, Fatima N, McCrumb FR (1971) A study of intrafamilial transmission of smallpox. Am J Epidemiol 94:316–26

Hopkins DR (1985) Control of yaws and other endemic trepanematoses: implementation of vertical and/or integrated programs. Rev Infect Dis 7S:338–342

Hopkins DR, Lane JM, Cummings EC, Thornton JN, Millar JD (1971) Smallpox in Sierra Leona II: the 1968–69 eradication program. Am J. Trop Med and Hyg 20:697–704

Imperato PJ, Sow O, Benitieni F (1973) The persistence of smallpox in remote unvaccinated villages during eradication programme activities. Acta Tropica 30:261–268

Kaplan EH, Craft DL, Wein LM (2002) Emergency repose to a smallpox attack: The case of mass vaccination. Proc Nat Acad Sci USA 99:10935–10940

Kennedy JS, Frey SE. Yan L, Rothman AL, Cruz J, Newman FK, Orphin L, Belshe RB, Ennis FA (2004) Induction of human T cell-mediated immune responses after primary and secondary smallpox vaccination. J Infect Dis 190:1286–1294

Lane JM, Goldstein J (2003) Evaluation of 21st-century risks of smallpox vaccination and policy options. Annals of Int Med 138:488–493

Legrand J, Vibound C, Boelle PY, Valleron AJ, Flahault A (2004) Modeling responses to a smallpox epidemic taking into account uncertainty. Epidemiol Infect 132:19–25

Mack TM (1972) Smallpox in Europe 1950–1971. J Infect Dis 125:161–169

Mack TM (2003) A different view of smallpox and vaccinia. New Engl J Med 348:460–463

Mack TM, Thomas DB, Ali A, Khan MM (1972) Epidemiology of smallpox in West Pakistan I acquired immunity and the distribution of disease. Am J Epidemiol 95:157–168

Massoudi, MS, Barker L, Schwartz B (2003) Effectiveness of postexposure vaccination for the prevention of smallpox: results of a Delphi analysis. J Infect Dis 188:973–976

Meltzer MI, Damon I, LeDuc JW, Millar JD (2001). Modeling potential responses to smallpox as a bioterrorist weapon. Emerg Infect Dis 7:959–969

Meyer HM, Hostetler DD, Bernheim BC, Rogers NG, Lambin P, Chassary A, Labusquiere R, Smadel JE (1964) Response of Volta children to live attenuated measles vaccine. Bull World Health Org 30:769–781

Millar JD, Foege WH (1969) Status of eradication of smallpox (and control of measles) in West and Central Africa. J Infect Dis 120:725–732

Millar JD, Roberto RR, Wulff H, Wenner HA, Henderson DA (1969) Smallpox vaccination by intradermal jet injection. I Introduction, background, and results of pilot studies. Bull World Health Org 41:749–760

Morley DC, Martin WJ, Allen I (1967) Measles in West Africa. West Afr Medl J Nigerian Pract 16:24–31

Mukherjee MK, Sarkar JK, Mitra AS (1974) Pattern of intrafamilial transmission of smallpox in Calcutta, India. Bull World Health Org 51:219–215

National Institute of Communicable Diseases of India (1968) Evaluation of the National Smallpox Eradication Program in Karnal District, Haryana. New Delhi

Neff JM, Millar JD, Roberto RR, Wulff Hl (1969) Smallpox vaccination by intradermal jet injection. III Evaluation in a well vaccinated population Bull World Health Org 41:771–778

Porco TC, Holbrook KA, Fernyak SE, Portnoy DL, Reiter R, Aragon TJ (2004) Logistics of community smallpox control through contact tracing and ring vaccination: a stochastic network model. BMC Publ Health 4:34

Rao AR, Jacob ES, Kamalakshi S, Appaswamy S, Bradbury (1968) Epidemiological studies of smallpox. A study of intrafamilial transmission in a series of 254 infected families. Ind J Med Res 56:1826–1854

Rey M, Cantrelle P, Lafaix C, Mar ID, Sow A, Agboton Y (1968) Lessons of an experimental campaign of vaccination against measles in the urban environment. (in French) Bulletin de la Societe Medicale d Afrique Noire de Langue Francaise. 13:291–231

Roberto RR, Wulff H, Millar JD (1969) Smallpox vaccination by intradermal jet injection. II Cutaneous and serological responses to primary vaccination in children. Bull World Health Org 41:761–769

Sommer A, Foster SO (1974) The 1972 Smallpox outbreak in Khulna municipality, Bangladesh 1. Methodology and epidemiologic findings. Am J Epidemiol 99:291–302

Thomas DB, McCormack WM, Arita I, Khan MM, Islam S, Mack TM (1971) Endemic smallpox in rural East Pakistan. I. Methodology, clinical and epidemiological characteristics of cases and intravillage transmission. Am J Epidemiol 93:361–372

Thompson D, Foege WH (1968) Faith Tabernacle Smallpox Epidemic, Abakaliki, Nigeria. WHO/SE/68.3
Tomori O (2002) Yellow fever in Africa: public health impact and prospects for control in the 21st century. Biomedica 22:178–210
World Health Organization (1964) WHO expert committee on smallpox First Report Technical Report Series No. 283

Mass Immunization Programs: Principles and Standards

J. D. Grabenstein[1] (✉) · R. L. Nevin[2]

[1] Military Vaccine Agency, US Army Medical Command,
5113 Leesburg Pike, Suite 402, Falls Church, VA 22041, USA
john.grabenstein@us.army.mil

[2] Army Medical Surveillance Activity, US Army Center for Health Promotion and Preventive Medicine, Washington, DC, USA

1	Introduction	32
2	Applications for Mass Immunization	33
3	Policy Making and Planning	35
4	Military Cohorts as Examples	37
5	Implementation Issues	38
5.1	Objectives and Standards	40
5.2	Facility, Equipment, and Supplies	40
5.3	Prepare Staff	42
5.4	Invite Potential Vaccinees	43
5.5	Educate Vaccinees	43
5.6	Customize Procedures	44
5.7	Screen for Contraindications	45
5.8	Double-Check Safeguards	45
5.9	Immunize	46
5.10	Observe	46
5.11	Document	47
5.12	Check Quality	47
6	Conclusion	48
	References	49

Abstract Mass immunization involves delivering immunizations to a large number of people at one or more locations in a short interval of time. Good mass immunization programs apply planning and quality standards that maximize return on resources invested and provide the greatest individual benefits when immunizing many people in a short period of time. These programs can be used to counter contagious outbreaks, adopted as a repeated means of sustained healthcare delivery, or applied where many people move through a specific place in a short interval of time. Relevant quality standards address appropriate facilities and supplies, training of professional and paraprofessional staff, education of potential vaccinees and methods to screen them for contraindications to immunization, safeguards against anaphylaxis and syncope, documentation, safety surveillance, and a quality-improvement program. Successful mass immunization programs require early planning that builds on existing competencies. As the number of available vaccines increases, prioritizing which vaccines to administer during mass campaigns requires consideration of effectiveness, safety, and a cost–benefit equation from both the individual and community perspectives. Mass immunization campaigns aim to maximize the health of a population, but such campaigns need to be customized based on individual contraindications to immunization. Mass immunization programs need to be conducted ethically, with considerations of benefit versus risk and the need for detailed education of healthcare workers and vaccinees.

The views expressed are those of the authors and do not represent the official position of the US Department of Defense or Department of Army.

1
Introduction

Active immunization is the deliberate effort to prevent infection by evoking disease-specific immune responses. Active immunization uses an agent similar to a pathogen, but less risky. The practice of administering whole or subunit microbes as vaccines dates back over 1,000 years, to early efforts to prevent smallpox [1, 2]. In human history, the preeminent forms of infectious disease control have been sanitation and immunization [3–6]

Mass immunization is a term used in diverse ways in the medical literature. The most frequent use of the term, and the definition adopted here, is delivering immunizations to a large number of people at one or more locations in a short interval of time. A common understanding is that mass immunization campaigns involve more people passing through the immunization process than is the usual baseline rate. Similar, but less commonly used terms are pulse immunization, repeated pulse immunization, surge immunization, or cluster immunization [7]. Mass immunization is the technique employed during National Immunization Days conducted in many developing countries as part of the World Health Organization's (WHO) Expanded Program on Immunization (EPI) [2, 8].

This chapter will focus on principles and quality standards that give the greatest return on investment and the greatest individual benefits when immunizing many people in a short period of time. It can be a challenge to apply these standards in austere field situations, but program managers have a responsibility to do their best with the resources available to them. As with most other applications of preventive medicine, immunization reflects a population-based intervention to reduce disease that may have rare adverse consequences for an individual. For that reason, we will discuss contraindication screening and adverse event management.

Mass immunization has been used to refer to the administration of multiple immunizations at the same clinical encounter. In this chapter, we refer to that common practice as simultaneous or concurrent immunization.

We consider the term mass immunization to be misapplied if used to describe immunization recommended for essentially all members of a large cohort, with the cohort typically defined by age, gender, or occupation. We consider that to be a policy of universal immunization for that cohort.

2
Applications for Mass Immunization

The situations in which mass immunization techniques can be applied are summarized in Table 1. The first mass immunization programs occurred when multiple people received variola inoculation or, later, Jenner's smallpox vaccine to prevent smallpox during community outbreaks [1, 2]. Mass immunization in response to outbreaks has been successfully used in the twentieth century to control outbreaks of smallpox [1, 2], measles [2, 9], meningococcal meningitis [10, 11], poliomyelitis [8, 12], diphtheria [13], hepatitis B [14], yellow fever [2, 15], and other infections. Public-health planners debate the

Table 1 Applications of mass immunization

- In response to outbreaks, such as smallpox, measles, meningococcal meningitis, poliomyelitis, or other contagious infections
- As a repeated or iterative means of healthcare delivery, such as where people do not have ready access to routine immunization services
- At gateways, where many people arrive at a specific place in a short interval of time, such as students at a school, military personnel at a training camp, workers at a new job, religious pilgrims, or refugees
- When a new vaccine becomes available or when a new immunization policy is implemented

Definition: Mass immunization – immunizing a large number of people at one or more locations in a short interval of time merits and cost-effectiveness of using mass immunization as a tool to control typhoid fever or cholera outbreaks [16, 17].

Because of the emergent nature of contagious outbreaks, mass immunization programs in such settings must be fielded rapidly and may lack intricate planning. In contrast, other mass immunization campaigns are adopted as a repeated means of sustained healthcare delivery, such as in developing regions where people do not have ready access to routine immunization services. In such settings, a mass immunization campaign can benefit from a deliberate planning process.

Other applications of mass immunization procedures occur where a large number of people arrive at or move through a specific place in a short interval of time or on a recurring basis. Examples include new cohorts of students arriving at a school, military trainees arriving at a training camp, workers starting a new job, religious pilgrims [10, 18, 19], refugees, and the public coming to places offering influenza immunization.

Mass immunization may also be employed soon after a new vaccine becomes available or when a new immunization policy is first implemented. For example, when a vaccine is first distributed for a specific geographic area, a larger number of people need to be immunized, compared to the subsequent in-migration of people to that area. When immunization policies change, such as by expanding recommended age ranges for immunization, additional people suddenly need to be immunized. Compared to a routine immunization program or the previous policy, this situation is sometimes referred to as 'catch up' immunization. Mass immunization may be the technique used to get the new cohort caught up to the immunization level of the original cohorts.

Mass immunization is associated with certain occupational or clinical settings, such as training camps, schools, and municipal health clinics. Entering and exiting schools, job sites, refugee camps, and other recognized physical settings offer opportunities to screen immunization adequacy. Similarly, annual influenza immunization programs for the public or for employees can be used as a platform for assessing other immunization needs [18]. Most applications of mass immunization involve humans, but the same practices can be applied for veterinary and community health, such as prevention of rabies in dogs [20].

Immunizations administered via mass campaigns offer either prompt or long-term protection, or both. Prompt protection is needed against contagions that can spread rapidly within coming months (e.g., influenza, measles). Other immunizations can protect against environmental exposures expected to occur later in life (e.g., tetanus, hepatitis A).

3
Policy Making and Planning

Before considering how to implement a mass immunization strategy, policy makers and planners need to determine their public health goals and then decide whether mass immunization is the proper tool to achieve the goals.

Whether immunization is clinically appropriate for an individual is based on benefits expected from avoiding specific infections. Those infections have specific characteristics of incidence, prevalence, endemic level, transmissibility, and incubation period, as well as disease characteristics reflected by the clinical spectrum and duration of morbidity, the case-fatality ratio, availability and effectiveness of treatments, and other factors. The risks of adverse reactions to immunization similarly involve incidence, a clinical spectrum of severity, duration of impaired function, speed and probability of resolution, availability and effectiveness of treatments, and similar factors.

Then, to decide whether mass or routine immunization is the proper approach for a community or cohort, in contrast to sanitation or treatment [2, 9, 12, 16–19, 21–24] planners can model disease transmission dynamics. Such models take into account the degree of preexisting immunity in the population, their access to immunization services, and available resources. Policy makers will consider factors related to available infrastructure, the population's physical and psychological distance from it, the degree of antimicrobial resistance, and other factors. For developing countries, Foege and Eddins describe advantages and disadvantages of organizing mass immunizations based on house-to-house or collecting-point intervention [2]. And policymakers should consider how to sustain delivery of immunization services over sequential years [2].

In general, the cost per fully immunized child is higher in a mass immunization campaign than in a routine immunization program [2, 7, 25]. The cost of travel and the decreased efficiency of itinerant vaccinators contribute to this calculation. But in rural settings, a mobile immunization team may be one of the only effective ways to deliver immunization services [1, 2, 26]. If the people cannot or will not come to the immunization site, then the immunization team needs to do the traveling. In such cases, the travel cost is a required cost of achieving the public health goal, best amortized by delivering multiple immunizations and other services on the same trip [2].

In an acute outbreak, a limited window of opportunity to control the disease may tip the balance toward mass immunization. Examples include smallpox and meningitis, where promptly achieving herd immunity (i.e., community immunity) can slow disease transmission and bring an outbreak under control. Immunization policy making is situational. The factors that make mass immunization appropriate for one setting or region may differ from another setting, where a different policy would be appropriate [9]. In some cases, a mixed strategy of both routine and targeted mass immunization may be appropriate [11]. If an outbreak occurs where insufficient vaccine is available, planners may face difficult decisions on prioritizing access to the vaccine [27].

Unlike clinical prescribing decisions, where medication use is customized to individual patients, vaccine policies typically involve a few decisions that lead to medication administration to large populations of people. Vaccines are required to be among the safest of all categories of medications, because vaccines are given primarily to healthy people to keep them healthy. The acceptable side-effect profile of the average vaccine is milder than most other medications.

No medication, however, is 100% safe. So the standard of practice with vaccines is to screen everyone eligible for immunization, to identify the few individuals who should be exempted from that immunization [28]. Exemptions are granted based on medical contraindications or a history of serious adverse events after an earlier immunization. Some contraindications are absolute, but most are relative, where policy makers and clinicians need to weigh the individual benefit–risk ratio of immunization versus no immunization.

With the success of immunization in reducing the incidence of diseases such as poliomyelitis, measles, and rubella, the public-health sector faces increasing concerns about vaccine safety and adverse events experienced after immunization. Even one adverse reaction in thousands of vaccine recipients, if serious or with prolonged health impact, can cause concerns about the safety of an immunization program.

Administration of multiple immunizations on the same day has been practiced for decades in the EPI, as well as in civilian and military healthcare settings around the world. This approach mimics the natural experience of receiving multiple immunologic stimuli from viruses and bacteria in the natural environment. In a March 2004 report, the civilian physicians and scientists who comprise the US Armed Forces Epidemiological Board (AFEB) reviewed the scientific basis for the safety and effectiveness of simultaneous immunization [29]. Scientific panels consistently conclude that scientific studies have not documented any known serious health risk from simultaneous immunizations. To minimize discomfort to immunized personnel, the AFEB recommended strategies for US military personnel to decrease concurrent immunizations, without sacrificing the individual and population benefits of widespread immunization. These strategies included dispersing immunizations into clusters over time, increased use of serologic screening to eliminate redundant immunization, and increasing the frequency of individual immunization reviews. Naturally, discomfort from simultaneous immunizations is less influential in settings were the people have few contacts with organized healthcare [2].

4
Military Cohorts as Examples

High-density cohorts of military personnel have a long history of suffering from disease outbreaks and benefiting from mass immunization campaigns. Smallpox influenced the course of many wars, including the American Revolutionary War [1, 30]. Napoleon vaccinated his troops in 1805 [2], but the policy was later abandoned. By 1869, an estimated 200,000 Frenchmen died of smallpox [1]. During the Franco-Prussian War of 1870–1871, the Prussian Army of 800,000 men vaccinated and revaccinated their personnel and suffered 8,463 cases of smallpox, with a case-fatality ratio of 5.4%. In contrast, the French Army was unvaccinated and suffered 125,000 cases of smallpox, with a fatality rate if infected of 18.7%. Mass immunization programs eventually led to the eradication of natural smallpox from this planet [1, 2].

The first large-scale use of tetanus toxoid, mass administration for American military forces began in 1941. In this case, a change in policy led to the need for a mass immunization program. A record of tetanus toxoid doses administered was stamped on soldiers' identification tags, as well as in paper records. In contrast, the German Army relied on treatment with tetanus antitoxin, and suffered higher rates of morbidity and mortality from tetanus [3, 4].

Typhoid fever was a major scourge of the Spanish–American War of 1898 and the Boer War of 1899 [3–6]. Mass administration of various typhoid vaccine formulations during World War I and World War II decreased its toll substantially.

The devastating 1918–1919 influenza pandemic caused the greatest loss of life from any cause in a short period of time in history [3–6, 31]. The extraordinary loss of fighting strength led to the US Army's research program to develop viral influenza vaccines in the 1940s. Since then, US military forces are routinely immunized against influenza A and B using mass immunization techniques.

Meningococcal meningitis is a life-threatening bacterial infection that can spread rapidly in dense populations, including military training camps. In 1968, scientists at the Walter Reed Army Institute of Research (WRAIR) developed a successful meningococcal serogroup C vaccine and later a serogroup A vaccine. A few years later, colleagues at the Institut Mérieux in France manufactured similar vaccines using the WRAIR formulation [32]. The work of both teams permitted a massive response to meningococcal serogroup A epidemics that swept Finland and Saõ Paulo, Brazil. In 1973, the entire population of Finland, more than four million people, was immunized against group A at a series of mass immunization clinics to control an epidemic. The Brazilian epidemic of 1974 produced 150,000 cases of meningococcal disease and 11,000 deaths. In one of the most dramatic mass immunization efforts ever, 100 million doses of serogroup A vaccine were administered during the Brazilian epidemic. These and successor vaccines are now used to prevent disease outbreaks among military trainees and in other settings [3, 4, 6, 15, 33]. The military success with meningococcal immunization among repeated iterations of newly assembled cohorts was cited when recognition of elevated rates of meningococcal disease among college freshman and dormitory residents led to calls for immunization in those populations [34].

Today, military units in the US conduct mass immunization programs at training camps, before overseas deployments, and annually during influenza immunization campaigns. The vaccines selected for these programs protect against infections during training, as well as during later military service. The vaccines of most acute need during military training protect against pathogens that represent an imminent risk of contagious disease in settings of close contact: influenza, meningococcal, measles, mumps, rubella, and varicella. Other vaccines are given to prevent infections more likely to occur later, during international travel or during extended periods of military service. These immunizations include: hepatitis A, hepatitis B, influenza, poliovirus, and tetanus–diphtheria–pertussis.

One of the more remarkable instances of mass customized immunization occurred in early 2003, as more than 400,000 service members being deployed to southwest Asia were screened for smallpox immunization [35]. The mission to thoroughly educate both providers and recipients about the idiosyncrasies of smallpox vaccination, identify those with atopic dermatitis or other reasons not to be immunized, safely administer the vaccine, and care for the vaccination site was performed with standardized education materials, concise screening forms, bandages, and thoroughly prepared medical staff who performed vaccinations at hundreds of clinics on four continents and dozens of warships at sea.

5
Implementation Issues

The pragmatic aspects of implementing a mass immunization campaign can be grouped into a series of planning topics. The planning domains and quality standards are summarized in Tables 2 and 3.

Table 2 Planning domains for mass immunization

1. Identify campaign goals
2. Prepare facility and order supplies. Set up multiple lanes
3. Prepare staff
4. Issue information to vaccine candidates
5. Customize procedures to the session's unique circumstances
6. Educate vaccine candidates
7. Screen for contraindications
8. Double-check safeguards
9. Administer immunizations
10. Observe for anaphylaxis
11. Document immunizations
12. Evaluate and assess quality

Table 3 Standards for mass immunization

Inform and educate
  Train vaccine providers in vaccine administration, storage and handling, screening for contraindications, education of vaccinees, injection and related techniques, clinical ability to respond to adverse reactions

Vaccine storage and handling
  Maintain cold chain, refrigeration or freezing, as appropriate to the specific vaccine. Large stocks of vaccine inventories should be connected to recording thermometers and alarm systems

Assess immunization histories
  Identify earlier immunizations received and any adverse events to them

Assess contraindications
  Identify relevant contraindications that could make an immunization unsafe or unwarranted (e.g., relevant severe allergies, pregnancy, immune suppression)

Administer vaccine
  Administer the recommended dose by the proper route, observing safety and infection-control principles

Document
  Record the vaccinee's name, age, type of vaccine, dose, name of vaccine provider, date administered, manufacturer, and lot number

Monitor for adverse events
  Monitor patient for acute adverse reactions and treat appropriately. To improve knowledge about vaccine-associated adverse events, report adverse events to national authorities or program managers

5.1
Objectives and Standards

Before the details of a mass immunization campaign can be determined, the campaign's goals and purpose must be defined. Will the campaign deliver one vaccine or several? Who will be eligible or excluded? What facilities will be used, where, and when? Who will provide the services and with what quality standards? Will any nonimmunization services be provided [e.g., pregnancy testing, tuberculin skin testing, testing for human immunodeficiency virus (HIV), vitamin A supplementation, malaria prophylaxis, water purification measures]?

To facilitate logistical planning, planners must estimate the number of people to be educated, screened, immunized, and documented. They also must estimate the available labor supply, both professional and paraprofessional [2, 7], to perform these tasks. Budgets and job descriptions clarify constraints and roles. Complex programs may warrant exercises or mock scenarios to test contingency plans.

To properly deliver immunization services, each mass immunization site must adhere to high standards of excellence. These standards can be applied even in austere field environments, albeit with recognition of the circumstances.

5.2
Facility, Equipment, and Supplies

The logistical requirements for a mass immunization campaign can be daunting. Buildings, vehicles, tables, chairs, computers, syringes, needles, needle-disposal containers, bandages and more must be on-site, in sufficient quantity. Documents providing detailed logistical checklists appear in Table 4.

Room and furniture should be arranged to provide for a common education area. This allows one educator to orient and inform dozens or hundreds of people at the same time. After common educational sessions, the room arrangement or the time schedule should allow the speaker to answer personal questions not covered by the common briefing.

Evaluating the physical arrangement of the building or rooms available for the mass immunization program will allow a customized flow of people from reception through education, immunization, observation, and then exit. Recent documents developed by the Centers for Disease Control and Prevention (see Table 4) for mass smallpox vaccination clinics feature detailed depictions of room layout and patient flow.

Setting up multiple lanes allows the immunization process to relieve the rate-limiting steps (i.e., 'bottle necks') that slow throughput. After patients

Table 4 Core resources for mass immunization programs

Specific mass immunization resources

 WHO. Control of epidemic meningococcal disease, WHO practical guidelines, 2nd edn. WHO/EMC/BAC/98.3. Geneva: WHO, 1998. www.who.int/emc-documents/meningitis/whoemcbac983c.html

 WHO. Safety of mass immunization campaigns. Geneva: WHO, 2002. whqlibdoc.who.int/hq/2002/WHO_V&B_02.10.pdf

 WHO. Immunization, vaccines, and biologicals document centre. www.who.int/vaccines-documents/DoxGen/H3DoxList.htm

 CDC. CDC guidance for post-event smallpox planning. Atlanta: CDC, 29 Oct 2002. www.bt.cdc.gov/agent/smallpox/prep/post-event-guidance.asp

 CDC. Smallpox Response Plan and Guidelines. Annex 2. General guidelines for smallpox vaccination clinics. Atlanta: CDC, 29 Oct 2002. www.bt.cdc.gov/agent/smallpox/response-plan/files/annex-2.pdf

 CDC. Smallpox Response Plan and Guidelines. Annex 3. Guidelines for large scale smallpox vaccination clinics. Atlanta: CDC, 29 Oct 2002. www.bt.cdc.gov/agent/smallpox/response-plan/files/annex-3.pdf

General training resources

 CDC National Immunization Program Resources: www.cdc.gov/nip

 US Department of Defense (DoD) Vaccine Healthcare Centers Network: www.vhcinfo.org (includes 50 hours of internet-based training called "Project Immune Readiness")

 DoD Clinical Guidelines for Managing Adverse Events After Vaccination. Washington, DC: DoD, September 2004. www.vaccines.mil/documents/564acg040909.pdf

have started flowing through the steps, administrators should assess the process to find where patients back up. At those points, additional processing stations can be added to alleviate the delay. For examples, if people are waiting to have the vaccine injected, more immunization stations should be added. If people are accumulating in front of the station where contraindications are screened, more screeners should be added. When pressure is relieved at any point in the process, some other point may become the rate-limiting step, so the assessment process should be repeated iteratively.

Vaccine will typically be ordered from the regional health authority or directly from the manufacturer. Maintaining the cold chain at each step from manufacturer to clinic is essential to delivering potent immunizations. Other consumable supplies (e.g., syringes, needles, bandages, sharps containers) should also be ordered. Quantities should be neither so large that vaccine is wasted nor so small that people are turned away unimmunized.

Adhering to vaccine handling and storage recommendations is critical. Mishandling or inappropriate storage can render vaccines ineffective without anything appearing to be wrong. Vaccines either need to be refrigerated or frozen, in appliances where records of storage temperature are maintained. When vaccine supplies arrive, they need to be promptly moved to the appropriate storage conditions. Training all personnel who might receive a vaccine shipment is essential. Large stocks of vaccine inventories should be connected to recording thermometers and alarm systems that can call prompt attention to discrepancies 24 hours a day, 7 days a week.

Autodestruct or single-use syringes are preferred in most cases. Sterilizable syringes are neither practical nor economical for mass immunization settings and should not be used [36].

In the 1960s, needle-free multi-use-nozzle jet injectors (MUNJIs) capable of 600 or more injections per hour were used in the smallpox eradication campaign and other mass immunization settings [24]. Unfortunately, their use of the same unsterile nozzle and fluid pathway to inject consecutive patients could allow transmission of blood-borne pathogens (e.g., hepatitis B, HIV) [33]. In contrast, a new generation of needle-free disposable-cartridge jet injectors (DCJIs) avoid these safety concerns by using a disposable, sterile fluid pathway for each patient. Research is underway for automated prefilling and finger-free loading and ejecting of cartridges, to make future high-speed DCJIs suitable for mass immunization programs.

Computers can aid several elements of mass immunization campaigns. Electronic record-keeping is probably the most important one, as well as in educational presentations, supply reordering, and other forms of electronic communication [37]. In rural settings without reliable access to electricity, batteries and alternate energy supplies can be used to power computers.

5.3
Prepare Staff

As important as logistics is the quality of the education and preparation of the professional, paraprofessional, and clerical staff who will perform the steps in the immunization process. Vaccine providers must be appropriately trained in all aspects of their enterprise, including vaccine storage and handling, obtaining information from candidates before immunization, providing information before immunization, injection techniques, and the clinical ability to handle adverse reactions. The professional staff must be trained in the indications and the contraindications for vaccines given in the mass immunization campaign.

Training materials are available from a wide variety of national, international, professional, and other authorities. Several examples appear in Table 4.

For their own safety and the safety of vaccinees, all staff members need to be trained in appropriate infection-control procedures. This training should focus on blood-borne pathogens (e.g., hepatitis B, HIV) as well as hand washing and general hygiene. Avoiding needle sticks and other kinds of accidents should be emphasized [38]. Staff concerns about liability and worker compensation should be resolved before the campaign begins.

5.4
Invite Potential Vaccinees

When the timing and location of the mass immunization campaign sites is clear, it is appropriate to begin inviting people to come to be immunized. Culturally sensitive marketing and advertising materials should explain who is and is not eligible for immunization [2, 39]. People should be informed if they should bring anything (e.g., personal immunization records) to the campaign site or if specific types of clothing are encouraged (e.g., short sleeve length).

Public information about the mass immunization campaign should motivate those who would benefit from immunization to come to the clinic. It should also dissuade those for whom immunization is not recommended. Planners should be ready if concerns about disease outbreaks cause large numbers of people to seek immunization despite public-health recommendations to the contrary. For example, meningococcal outbreaks in several Canadian provinces in 1991–1992 and in Rhode Island in 1998 led to greater public demand for meningococcal immunization than public-health authorities recommended [39–42]. When mass immunization programs are assembled hurriedly to deal with an outbreak, the need for consistent communication with the public is essential [43].

5.5
Educate Vaccinees

As people arrive at the immunization site and complete any registration process, they should be educated about benefits and adverse effects of the immunizations to be delivered. To help with screening for contraindications, they should be told early of any health conditions that are exemptions from immunization. Written information summaries are useful for people to read while waiting. Audiovisual presentations can be used when planning allows. Whether or not literacy is a concern in a given community, vaccine candidates should be educated verbally, so that they are personally advised. The educational content should strike a balance between being thorough and succinct. The most important information for the most people should be featured in a way to make the primacy of the key information apparent. Then allow ample time for questions and answers. Vaccine providers need to be ready to accurately answer questions and concerns posed by the vaccinee, and point the way to more detailed information if needed.

For people with special circumstances or who have a long list of questions, individualized counseling should be provided. This allows the flow of people through the immunization site to continue without undue disruption. Appropriate counseling on deferring pregnancy after immunization should be discussed.

Few health problems are caused uniquely by immunization [44]. One of the few examples is paralytic poliomyelitis that rarely follows use of the live attenuated poliovirus vaccine. Instead, immunizations can be risk factors that increase the relative risk of an adverse event occurring. For example, Guillain–Barré syndrome has been more likely to occur among recipients of some annual formulations of influenza vaccine, but not others [45]. On the other hand, health conditions that occur in unimmunized people are fully expected to occur in immunized people, at the same background rates of incidence. Discerning when an adverse event that occurs after immunization is an adverse reaction causally attributable to immunization can be a clinical challenge. People should be given factual answers about vaccine safety, in the proper perspective for interpretation of those facts.

5.6
Customize Procedures

Although similar general principles apply to most mass immunization campaigns, each one is different. The people to be immunized differ, as well as their knowledge base, the outbreak or cultural situation, and other parameters. These differences will affect the style of educational programs and the information products to be used.

When possible, preexisting immunity of individuals appearing for immunization should be taken into account. For example, it may be appropriate in some settings to use serologic tests or documentation of prior immunizations to reduce the immunization workload on site and to reduce the administration of redundant immunizations to people who are already immune. When a substantial proportion of vaccine candidates is already immune, the cost of high-quality serologic testing will tend to be overshadowed by the product cost of the vaccine [46, 47].

Serologic screening adds additional delays and risks to mass immunization campaigns that need to be weighed against the potential for cost-savings. Due to the high specificity of modern serologic tests, missed immunizations due to false positive tests do not result in clinically significant numbers of nonimmunes. Missed immunizations caused by a proportion of the screened population failing to return once test results are available may reduce immunization coverage. Rapid point-of-care testing for pre-existing immunity, although not currently available, would eliminate this concern.

5.7
Screen for Contraindications

Vaccine providers should read the records of earlier immunizations received and should succinctly interview each candidate for immunization. The goals are to avoid duplicate or redundant immunization and to identify contraindications to immunization. At a minimum, the following information should be obtained from the vaccinee: vaccines previously received, pre-existing health conditions, allergies, and adverse events that occurred after previous immunizations. For women, ask about the possibility of pregnancy in a private, respectful way to elicit candid information. Consulting the vaccinee's medical record is the most reliable method of determining immunization status. Before applying tuberculosis skin tests, history of BCG immunization and positive tuberculosis tests should be assessed.

Even when hundreds of people appear for immunization within a short period of time, their immunization needs or contraindications can be assessed individually. Decades of experience show that customized immunization delivery with high throughput can be performed by breaking the tasks down to several stations, performing education in groups, setting up multiple lanes to overcome rate-limiting steps, and listening to individuals.

If a contraindication to immunization exists, this information should be provided to the clinic supervisor and the vaccine candidate, as well as documented in the medical record. Temporary and permanent contraindications should be annotated in (electronic) medical records, to avoid recalling someone for an immunization that should not be given or should be deferred. Vaccine providers should be aware of and avoid the most common misconceptions concerning contraindications [48]. Initial and update training for vaccine providers at all levels (e.g., medics, nurses, physicians) is important for quality immunization delivery.

5.8
Double-Check Safeguards

Before administering immunizations, assure that adequate preparations have been taken to cushion anyone who faints or to respond to anyone who develops an acute allergic reaction (e.g., anaphylaxis). For example, installing rubber mats on the floor and positioning furniture away from spaces where vaccinees are processed can help minimize injuries. Where syncope occurs without these measures, vaccinees can sustain injuries, ranging from simple contusions to dental trauma and facial or skull fractures. To further minimize these risks, those at greatest risk for syncope can be immunized while sitting in a chair.

5.9
Immunize

After all the preparatory steps described above, it is time to administer the immunizations. Vaccinees can assist with the procedure by swabbing their own arms with alcohol. For oral or nasal vaccines, it may be possible to observe them giving themselves the immunization. This is the point where it is essential to implement appropriate infection-control procedures. Discard used needles in rigid safety containers [38].

Specific information regarding the recommended route of administration and appropriate dose is included with each vaccine and summarized in various reference books. Most vaccines are administered intramuscularly or subcutaneously. The dose indicated should be the dose administered. Administering partial doses to potentially reduce the risk for adverse reaction is not an effective method and could result in inadequate protection against disease.

5.10
Observe

After immunization, observe vaccinees for a suitable period of time (e.g., 10–20 min), so that any acute allergic events can be properly treated. The risk of anaphylaxis is greatest within the first 10–20 min after immunization, but can occur as much as 1 h later. The interval of time to recommend should strike a balance between the safety benefits of observation and the more acute or practical uses of that time interval. The observation interval can serve a useful purpose if the time is spent in other educational or public-health activities. Making the interval an enjoyable experience will increase compliance.

Vaccine providers must be trained to recognize and treat adverse reactions. The supplies and equipment needed to do so must be readily available on site. Although severe systemic reactions are rare, they can be life threatening. Vaccine providers should be trained to use medications (e.g., epinephrine) and conduct procedures necessary to maintain the airway and manage cardiovascular collapse (e.g., cardiopulmonary resuscitation, use of a self-reinflating ventilating bag to provide positive-pressure ventilation during resuscitation).

Vaccine providers should be in close proximity to a telephone or radio, so that emergency medical personnel can be summoned immediately, if necessary.

To improve knowledge about vaccine-associated adverse events, all serious adverse events should be reported to national authorities or program managers. Reporting adverse events after immunization that involve hospitalization, a life-threatening event (e.g., anaphylaxis), or an event related to suspected contamination of a vaccine vial are especially important.

When vaccines are administered to groups, the physical responses of the recipients may be similar. The mechanism is the same as that for mass reactions in other circumstances. These phenomena have been categorized as mass psychogenic illness (MPI) [49]. MPI is the collective occurrence of symptoms (e.g., headache, dizziness, weakness, loss of consciousness) suggesting organic illness in a group with shared beliefs about the cause of the symptoms. Outbreaks have been reported in various cultural and environmental settings, including developing and industrialized countries, in the work place, in public settings, in schools, and in military cohorts. The perceived threats have involved food, fire, toxic gases, and vaccines. Immunization managers should be aware that mass immunization events can generate MPI reactions.

5.11
Document

All immunizations should be documented in the designated paper or electronic immunization tracking system promptly after immunization. Electronic records offer advantages in terms of data searching and sharing [37].

Planners should set minimum expectations for data elements to record, such as the vaccinee's name, age, type of vaccine, dose, site and route of administration, name of the vaccine provider, date vaccine was administered, manufacturer and lot number. For multi-dose vaccines, the date the next dose is due should be communicated to the vaccinee. Electronic immunization tracking systems can calculate these dates automatically. Transferring electronic immunization records to central repositories reduces the needless duplication of immunizations related to lost paper records.

5.12
Check Quality

All immunization programs should adopt principles of continuous quality improvement. Planners should evaluate implementation early after mass immunization begins, and periodically thereafter. Evaluation parameters should include proper implementation of education and screening efforts, safe administration of immunizations, and the degree of the population that achieves immunity [2, 12, 20, 39, 50, 51]. For example, knowing that mass immunization against diphtheria in the Ukraine reached 92% of the rural population and 58% of the urban population, and why, allowed improvements to educational messages [13].

Conduct quality-improvement programs, to identify and respond to medication errors [52, 53], accidents [38], or other untoward incidents. Some of the most common errors involve selecting the wrong product or the wrong diluent. Logistical problems related to vaccine resupply and maintenance of the cold chain should be routinely reviewed [2].

6
Conclusion

Successful mass immunization programs require early planning that builds on existing competencies. These programs are best implemented with a deliberate timeline by experienced immunization staff supplemented by locally trained support personnel. Complex programs can benefit from exercises and mock scenarios. Mass immunization programs underway should be evaluated early and repeatedly to identify opportunities for improving the process. Good mass immunization programs share information with the public and the news media, fostering open lines of communication with all who have a stake in the program's success or failure [14].

In the twenty-first century, the quality of immunization delivery has taken on increased importance. People have more knowledge and inquisitiveness about the safety of vaccines than in years passed. Healthcare workers need to be able to answer questions about vaccinology and offer support services essential to the continued success of immunization for a population.

As the number of available vaccines increases, prioritizing which vaccines to administer during mass campaigns requires consideration of effectiveness, safety, and a cost–benefit equation from both the individual and the community perspectives. Extensive efforts have been made to evaluate and re-evaluate specific vaccine safety questions, including comprehensive analyses by the US National Academy of Sciences, the WHO, and other expert bodies.

Mass immunization campaigns aim to maximize immunization to maintain the health of a population, but the campaigns need to be customized based on individual contraindications to immunization. Mass immunization programs need to be conducted ethically, with considerations of benefit versus risk and the need for detailed education of healthcare workers and vaccinees.

References

1. Fenner F, Henderson DA, Arita I, Jezek Z, Ladnyi ID (1988) Smallpox and Its Eradication. World Health Organization, Geneva
2. Foege WH, Eddins DL (1973). Mass vaccination programs in developing countries. Prog Med Virol 15:205–243
3. Benenson AS (1984) Immunization and military medicine. Rev Infect Dis 6:1–12
4. Parish HJ (1965) A History of Immunizations. E & S Livingstone Ltd., London
5. Plotkin SL, Plotkin SA (2003) A short history of vaccination. In: Plotkin SA, Orenstein WB (eds). Vaccines, 4th edn. Elsevier, Philadelphia, pp 1–12
6. Woodward TE (1981) The public's debt to military medicine. Mil Med 146:168–173
7. Jajoo UN, Chhabra S, Gupta OP, Jain AP (1985) Annual cluster (pulse) immunization experience in villages near Sevagram, India. J Trop Med Hyp 88:277–280
8. Hinman AR (1960) Mass vaccination against polio. JAMA 173:1521–1526
9. McLean AR, Anderson RM (1988) Measles in developing countries. Part II. The predicted impact of mass vaccination. Epidemiol Infect 100:419–442
10. Bushra HE, Mawlawi MY, Fontaine RE, Afif H (1995) Meningococcal meningitis group A: A successful control of an outbreak by mass vaccination. East Afr Med J 72:715–718
11. Robbins JB, Schneerson R, Gotschlich EC, Mohammed I, Nasidi A, Chippaux JP, Bernardino L, Maige MA (2003) Meningococcal meningitis in sub-Saharan Africa: The case for mass and routine vaccination with available polysaccharide vaccines. Bull WHO 81:745–750
12. Richardson G, Linkins RW, Eames MA, Wood DJ, Campbell PJ, Ankers E, Deniel M, Kabbaj A, Magrath DI, Minor PD, et al. (1995) Immunogenicity of oral poliovirus vaccine administered in mass campaigns versus routine immunization programmes. Bull WHO 73:769–777
13. Lewis LS, Hardy I, Strebel P, Tyshchenko DK, Sevalnyev A, Kozlova I (2000) Assessment of vaccination coverage among adults 30–49 years of age following a mass diphtheria vaccination campaign: Ukraine, April 1995. J Infect Dis 181 (Suppl. 1):S232–S236
14. Plaitano S, Sagliocca L, Mele A, Bove C, Protano D, Adamo B, Palumbo F, Cauletti M, Franco E, Pasquini P (1993) Hepatitis B mass immunization of adolescents: A pilot study in a community. Eur J Epidemiol 9:307–310
15. Monath TP, Craven RB, Adjukiewicz A, Germain M, Francy DB, Ferrara L, Samba EM, N'Jie H, Cham K, Fitzgerald SA, Crippen PH, Simpson DI, Bowen ET, Fabiyi A, Salaun JJ (1980) Yellow fever in the Gambia, 1978–1979: Epidemiologic aspects with observations on the occurrence of orungo virus infections. Am J Trop Med Hyg 29:912–928
16. Legros D, Paquet C, Perea W, Marty I, Mugisha NK, Royer H, Neira M, Ivanoff R (1999) Mass vaccination with a two-dose oral cholera vaccine in a refugee camp. Bull WHO 77:837–842
17. Tarr PE, Kuppens L, Jones TC, Ivanoff B, Aparin PG, Heymann DL (1999) Considerations regarding mass vaccination against typhoid fever as an adjunct to sanitation and public health measures: Potential use in an epidemic in Tajikistan. Am J Trop Med Hyg 61:163–170

18. Grabenstein JD, Smith LJ, Watson RR, Summers RJ (1990) Immunization outreach using individual need assessments of adults at an army hospital. Public Health Rep. 105:311–316
19. Veeken H, Ritmeijer K, Hausman B (1998) Priority during a meningitis epidemic: Vaccination or treatment? Bull WHO 76:135–141
20. Seghaier C, Cliquet F, Hammami S, Aouina T, Tlatli A, Aubert M (1999) Rabies mass vaccination campaigns in Tunisia: Are vaccinated dogs correctly immunized? Am J Trop Med Hyg 61:879–884
21. Barlow R (1976) Applications of a health planning model in Morocco. Int J Health Serv 6:103–122
22. Grenfell BT, Anderson RM (1989) Pertussis in England and Wales: An investigation of transmission dynamics and control by mass vaccination. Proc R Soc Lond B Biol Sci 236:213–252
23. Scherer A, McLean A (2002) Mathematical models of vaccination. Br Med Bull 62:187–199
24. Centers for Disease Control & Prevention (1986) Hepatitis B associated with jet gun injection—California. MMWR 35:272–276
25. World Health Organization (2004) Economics of immunization: Guide to the literature and other resources. WHO/V&B/04.02. Geneva: WHO www.who.int/vaccines-documents/DocsPDF04/www769.pdf
26. Loevinsohn BP, Loevinsohn ME (1987) Well child clinics and mass vaccination campaigns: An evaluation of strategies for improving the coverage of primary health care in a developing country. Am J Public Health 77:1407–1411
27. Silverman RD, May T (2003) Terror and triage: Prioritizing access to mass smallpox vaccination. Creighton Law Rev 36:359–374
28. National Vaccine Advisory Committee (2000) Adult immunization programs in nontraditional settings: Quality standards and guidance for program evaluation. MMWR 49(RR-1):1–13
29. Armed Forces Epidemiological Board. Recommendation 2004–04 (2004) Multiple concurrent immunizations and safety concerns. Falls Church, VA: 16 April 2004 www.vaccines.mil/documents/477AFEB2004.pdf
30. Fenn EA (2001) Pox Americana: The Great Smallpox Epidemic of 1775–82. Hill & Wang, New York
31. Kolata G (1999) Flu: The Story of the Great Influenza Pandemic of 1918 and the search for the virus that caused it. Farrar Straus Giroux, New York
32. Chase A (1982) Magic Shots. William Morrow, New York
33. Brundage JF, Ryan MA, Feighner BH, Erdtmann FJ (2002) Meningococcal disease among United States military service members in relation to routine uses of vaccines with different serogroup-specific components, 1964–1998. Clin Infect Dis 35:1376–1381
34. Advisory Committee on Immunization Practices (2000) Prevention & control of meningococcal disease; Meningococcal disease and college students. MMWR 49(RR-7):1–20
35. Grabenstein JD, Winkenwerder W Jr (2003) US military smallpox vaccination program experience. JAMA 289:3278–3282

36. World Health Organization (2000) Sustainable outreach services (SOS): A strategy for reaching the unreached with immunization and other services. V&B/00.37. Geneva: WHO www.who.int/vaccines-documents/DocsPDF00/www555.pdf
37. Billittier AJ 4th, Lupiani P, Masterson G, Masterson T, Zak C (2003) Electronic patient registration and tracking at mass vaccination clinics: A clinical study. J Public Health Manag Pract 9:401–410
38. Abraham E, Middleton D (1997) Needlestick injuries during a mass vaccination campaign. Can J Public Health 88:38–39
39. Nolan P (2004) The Rhode Island meningitis vaccine experience—Mass vaccination campaigns, politics and health policy. Med Health R I 87:65–67
40. Gold R. Meningococcal disease in Canada: 1991–92 (1992) Can J Public Health 83:5–6
41. Gray C (1992) Meningococcal disease: Was Ottawa's mass-vaccination program necessary? CMAJ 146:1033, 1036–1037.
42. Hume SE (1992) Mass voluntary immunization campaigns for meningococcal disease in Canada: Media hysteria. JAMA 267:1833–34, 1837–1838
43. Ward JD, McCall BD, Cherian SG (2001) An exercise in communication: Analysis of calls to a meningococcal disease hotline. Commun Dis Intell 25:281–282
44. Advisory Committee on Immunization Practices (1996) Update: Vaccine side effects, adverse reactions, contraindications, and precautions. MMWR 45(RR-12):1–35, errata 227
45. Lasky T, Terracciano GJ, Magder L, Koski CL, Ballesteros M, Nash D, Clark S, Haber P, Stolley PD, Schonberger LB, Chen RT (1998) The Guillain-Barre syndrome and the 1992–1993 and 1993–1994 influenza vaccines. N Engl J Med 339:1797–1802
46. Howell MR, Lee T, Gaydos CA, Nang RN (2000) The cost-effectiveness of varicella screening and vaccination in US Army recruits. Mil Med 165:309–315
47. Jacobs RJ, Saab S, Meyerhoff AS, Koff RS (2003) An economic assessment of pre-vaccination screening for hepatitis A and B. Public Health Rep 118:550–558
48. Grabenstein JD (1998) Vaccine misconceptions and inappropriate contraindications lead to preventable illness and death. Hosp Pharm 33:1557–1558, 1561–1564, 1567
49. Clements CJ (2003). Mass psychogenic illness after vaccination. Drug Safety 26:599–604
50. Centers for Disease Control & Prevention (1994) Assessment of undervaccinated children following a mass vaccination campaign—Kansas, 1993. MMWR 43:572–573
51. Paneth N, Kort EJ, Jurczak D, Havlichek DA Jr., Braunlich K, Moorer G, Vanderjagt D, Sienko D, Lieby P, Gibbons C (2000) Predictors of vaccination rates during a mass meningococcal vaccination program on a college campus. J Am Coll Health 49:7–11
52. Grabenstein JD, Proulx SM, Cohen MR (1996) Recognizing and preventing errors with immunologic drugs. Hosp Pharm 31:791–794, 799, 803–804
53. World Health Organization (2000) Supplementary information on vaccine safety. Part 2: Background rate of adverse events following immunization. V&B/00.36. Geneva, WHO. www.who.int/vaccines-documents/DocsPDF00/www562.pdf

Immunization Campaigns in the UK

K. Noakes · D. Salisbury (✉)

Department of Health, London UK
david.salisbury@dh.gsi.gov.uk

1	Introduction	54
1.1	Strategic Planning for Implementation	55
1.2	Vaccine Supply	55
1.3	Communication	56
1.4	Surveillance	57
2	UK Activities	57
3	Immunization Campaigns in the UK	58
3.1	Polio (1956 and 1962)	58
3.2	MMR (1988)	59
3.3	*Haemophilus influenzae* b (1992)	61
3.4	Measles Rubella (1994)	62
3.5	Meningitis C (1999)	64
3.6	Hib Booster (2003)	65
4	Annual Influenza Campaigns	67
5	Conclusion	68
References		69

Abstract A mass immunization campaign is a rapid vaccination intervention across age groups as opposed to provision through routine vaccination at a specified age attainment. Some countries use campaigns routinely as they have experience that shows that in their health systems higher coverage can be reached through campaigns than by routine service provision. Whilst many industrialized and non-industrialized countries have introduced new vaccines into their routine programme, the UK is unusual in deliberately doing this via campaigns. A number of mass immunization campaigns have been implemented in the UK, either integrated into the routine immunization programme such as the annual influenza immunization campaign; as a catch-up campaign alongside the introduction of a new vaccine into the routine vaccination schedule (MMR, *Haemophilus influenzae* b, Meningococcal C conjugate vaccine); or as a one-off campaign, to boost immunity in a particular age group, without introducing the vaccination into the schedule routinely at that age (*Haemophilus influenzae* b). Campaigns require intense planning at national and local level with leadership to achieve proper management. Although the components of an immunization campaign can be described separately—strategic planning, vaccine supply, communication and surveillance; for a programme to be successful integrated planning is essential.

1
Introduction

A mass immunization campaign is a rapid vaccination intervention across age groups as opposed to provision through routine vaccination at a specified age attainment. The age range targeted in a campaign is defined by a specific risk factor relevant to that age group. Such mass vaccination programmes are carried out to halt an observed or predicted increase in disease, rapidly interrupt the spread of an infectious disease or contribute to global eradication programmes. Some countries use campaigns routinely as they have experience that shows that in their health systems higher coverage can be reached than through routine service provision [1]. Whilst many industrialized and non-industrialized countries have introduced new vaccines into their routine programme, the UK is unusual in deliberately doing this via campaigns.

The implementation of mass immunization programmes requires complex planning and coordination in order to ensure that high levels of vaccine coverage are achieved in the shortest length of time. A number of mass immunization campaigns have been implemented in the UK, either integrated into the routine immunization programme such as the annual influenza immunization campaign; as a catch-up campaign alongside the introduction of a new vaccine into the routine vaccination schedule (MMR, *Haemophilus influenzae* b, Meningococcal C conjugate vaccine); or as a one-off campaign, to boost immunity in a particular age group, without introducing the vaccination into the schedule routinely at that age (*Haemophilus influenzae* b). The impact that these campaigns have had on disease levels, including the effect of herd immunity and duration of impact has been measured through surveillance and modelling [2–4]. A campaign can have a greater overall effect on disease levels than if it had just been introduced as part of the routine programme. For instance, the impact of Hib vaccine introduction in the UK, which included a catch-up campaign, was particularly effective, and the impact was faster than when the same vaccine was introduced in the Netherlands without a catch up.

Figure 1 compares the decline in cases of invasive Hib disease in the UK and the Netherlands; the decline in the UK was faster than that in the Netherlands, where a catch-up campaign was not used.

The key elements of implementing a mass immunization campaign are described below.

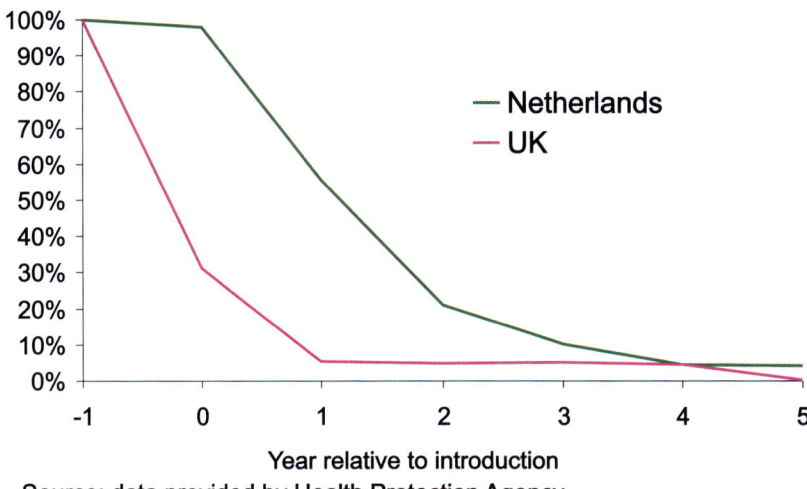

Fig. 1 Comparison of the decline in cases of invasive Hib disease in the UK and The Netherlands relative to year of introduction

1.1
Strategic Planning for Implementation

A well implemented introduction of a mass immunization programme requires the matching of availability of large quantities of vaccine without interruption but at the same time avoiding unnecessary wastage. Within the planning processes, policy-makers have to decide the priorities for which cohorts should be immunized first, based on those most at risk and vaccine availability.

1.2
Vaccine Supply

The Department of Health (London), in conjunction with two governmental agencies [the NHS Purchase and Supply Agency (contract expertise) and NHS Logistics (finance and logistical expertise)] oversees vaccine procurement and supply management for the UK. All procurement exercises are undertaken in line with EU procurement directives. The vaccines are centrally purchased and provided free of charge for administration to children and adolescents.

Monthly forecasts for vaccine supplies are calculated using the birth cohort for the UK and previous annual monthly usage. Forecasts are done more than a year in advance together with budget forecasts and take into account possible changes to the programme. Planning for supply provision for campaigns usually requires at least 1 year advance purchase arrangements in view of the large quantities of vaccine that may be needed. During this time, manufacturers must prepare stocks of country-specific vaccine, this must be batch-released, and if the campaign is to be run over a short period of time, must all be in place before the campaign start date.

In the UK, when there are multiple vaccine suppliers, a minimum of 3 months worth of stock is held as a buffer in case of an unforeseen problem with supply or rising demand. Slightly higher amounts of vaccines such as MMR are held in case of local outbreaks, allowing for implementation of local level campaigns at short notice. When there is a sole vaccine supplier, a 6-months buffer stock is held.

A contracted distributor that specializes in storage and distribution of refrigerated pharmaceutical products takes orders for, stores and distributes all the vaccines in the childhood programme throughout the UK. The UK increasingly uses a system of vaccine allocation rather than *ad libitem* ordering so that advanced ordering by general practitioners (GPs) is not needed, deliveries are matched to availability and specific cohorts are called for vaccination according to epidemiological risk and operational constraints. There is an amount of flexibility in the allocation system to ensure that sufficient vaccines are received and children are vaccinated when required. This degree of control of the supply chain favours the application of vaccination campaigns—not permissible when there is an extensive private sector involvement in immunization, or widespread decentralization of immunization programme responsibility.

Manufacturers deliver stock directly to the one appointed distributor who is responsible for ensuring the cold-chain from receipt to the final delivery point. For primary care based campaigns, the distributor delivers the required vaccines to each general practice; for school-based campaigns, the vaccine is delivered to community service pharmacists. The latter work in conjunction with local immunization coordinators to ensure that vaccines are delivered to schools where and when immunization is being undertaken.

1.3
Communication

Public acceptance of vaccine is influenced by many factors in the UK. For a vaccination programme to be successful in industrialized countries, parental attitudes to the introduction of a new vaccine need to be taken into account. Prior to the introduction of MMR vaccine nationally in 1988, this was achieved by undertaking pilot campaigns in three health districts in advance of the national programme [5].

Since 1991, twice-yearly surveys of parents have been run in the UK, exploring attitudes to vaccinations and the diseases they prevent. The surveys have provided a means by which parents' attitudes towards new and existing vaccines and the perception of the seriousness of the diseases they prevent can be evaluated in advance of the introduction of the vaccine programme [6]. This survey and others have shown that parents accept a new vaccine if they perceive the disease it protects against to be severe [7] and if they think the vaccine is safe [8].

In addition to this quantitative work, qualitative studies are undertaken through focus groups. These also provide opportunities to pre-test and refine communication materials such as leaflets, posters, television and radio advertising for comprehensibility, clarity and acceptability that will support a new campaign. Together, this information forms the basis of a communication strategy, which will both address the fears that parents may have been shown to have over the introduction of the new vaccine, and answer key questions.

This research has also shown the importance of providing parents with the same information that health professionals receive. The immunization information materials produced in the UK, including the website www.immunisation.nhs.uk, have thus been written for both parents and health professionals alike.

1.4
Surveillance

With the introduction of any new initiative into the routine immunization programme a comprehensive surveillance strategy should be established to monitor all of its impacts. This includes vaccine coverage, disease levels, seroepidemiology, and effects of advertising, as well as operational aspects of the campaign such as vaccine supplies.

Thus campaign planning must include a range of activities from the strategic overview needed for resource mobilization at a national level to microplanning at a local level. Surveillance of adverse events is also essential as adverse events in a campaign may take on heightened prominence: although the frequency of adverse events, relative to the number of doses applied, may not change, the perception of the absolute number of adverse events detected may attract concern, calling into question the safety of the vaccine [9, 10].

2
UK Activities

A number of key structural changes have been made to the delivery of the UK immunization programme in the last 25 years. All of these have been pivotal in the ability to deliver immunization campaigns within an industrialized country health system.

Key changes to the implementation of the immunization programme are:

- Since the 1980s, children have been enrolled on a national computerized database from birth, run by the Child Health Computer System (CHCS). This database automatically schedules immunizations, calculates local coverage and can arrange payments for GPs. It is used to actively identify children to call up for campaign immunizations.

- Twice yearly surveys of parental attitudes have been run in the UK, investigating mothers' attitudes to vaccinations and the diseases they prevent. The survey has provided a means by which parents' attitudes towards a new vaccine or a campaign can be sought in advance and information materials produced to suit the needs of parents.

- Since 1992, vaccines for the childhood immunization programme have been centrally purchased and managed, and delivered to primary care from one central distribution company. In planning national campaigns, such a process is essential to assure adequate vaccine supplies.

3
Immunization Campaigns in the UK

3.1
Polio (1956 and 1962)

The polio immunization campaign, which started in 1956, targeted all individuals under 40 years of age initially with monovalent inactivated polio vaccine. Vaccine supplies in the first 2 years of the programme were limited. Children over the age of 1 and under the age of 10 years were the first age groups to be offered polio immunization in 1956 and 1957. Local authorities were asked to arrange for the registration of children born in the relevant years for whom vaccination was desired. The percentage of eligible children registered for polio vaccination then varied widely between local health authorities (between 5% and 55%) depending on the amount of local publicity given to the scheme [11]. The selection for children to receive vaccine was made on the month of birth. Initially children were given two doses of the vaccine. Field trials carried out in the UK involving those children initially registered to receive polio vaccine showed the following year that three doses were required to mount a full response. The cohorts to be immunized were

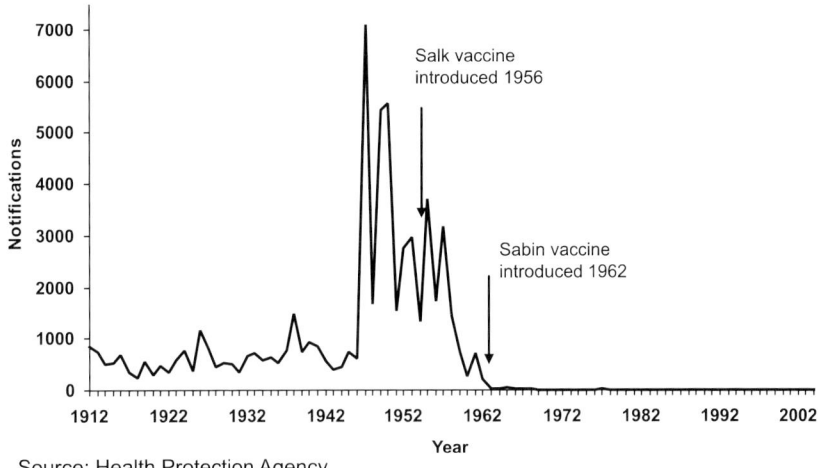

Fig. 2 Polio notifications for England and Wales (1912–2004)

widened as vaccine availability increased. The immunization campaigns were carried out in schools, cinemas, theatres, places of work as well as at GP surgeries. This campaign was later repeated starting in 1962 with live attenuated oral vaccine (OPV-Sabin).

Figure 2 shows the impact of the IPV and subsequent OPV campaigns in England and Wales. The greatest impact came from the introduction of IPV.

3.2
MMR (1988)

The next major immunization campaign was the introduction of Measles, Mumps, and Rubella (MMR) vaccine in October 1988 replacing single measles vaccination. This involved the introduction of routine MMR immunization of children at 13 months, and a catch-up programme of all children under 5 years of age. The purpose of the catch-up programme was to speed up the interruption of rubella transmission in primary school children and thereby prevent cases of congenital rubella syndrome (CRS).

Table 1 shows the effect of the MMR campaign. Rubella infections, especially in parous women, have declined as a consequence of the prevention of their exposure to rubella from their own or their friends' children.

Prior to the national introduction of MMR vaccine, three health districts (Somerset, Fife and North Hertfordshire) had run pilot programmes. Adverse events were monitored by asking parents of every child to complete a daily

Table 1 Risk of laboratory-confirmed rubella infection according to parity in susceptible pregnant women (source: Health Protection Agency)

Year	Nulliparous			Parous			Total		
	Susceptible	Infected	Risk/1,000	Susceptible	Infected	Risk/1,000	Susceptible	Infected	Risk/1,000
1987	1,150	11	9.6	636	17	26.7	1,786	28	15.7
1988/89	1,163	7	4.2	691	4	5.8	2,354	11	4.7
1990/91	1,192	4	3.4	662	1	1.5	1,854	5	2.7

diary for 3 weeks recording any symptoms following the vaccine [12]. In an analysis of more than 7,000 records for children aged 1–2 years, the incidence of adverse reactions (fever, rash and malaise) were similar to that for children previously given measles vaccine and monitored in the same way. The introduction of the vaccine was positively received by over 90% of parents. Both the information on adverse event reporting and parent acceptability were included with the information materials produced for health professionals and parents prior to the launch of the national campaign [13].

At national level, the campaign publicity materials were researched with parents of children in the target age groups. An extensive advertising programme was put in place, with articles placed in the press and magazines and radio advertising. Special consideration was made to areas of the country with previously low measles vaccination uptake. In such areas there was a heightening of the exposure to advertising materials. The Department of Health worked with vaccine manufacturers and voluntary sector groups such as Sense (The National Deaf-Blind and Rubella Association) to ensure that information materials (printed materials and videos) were complementary to those produced by the Department of Health.

Regional meetings were organized many months in advance of the introduction of the new vaccine to explain the changes to health professionals. Immunization coordinators (one in each district health authority) played an important role in informing other health professionals, and slide sets were prepared for them by the Department of Health so that uniform training presentations could be made locally.

Because demand for the vaccine was expected to be high, a national price was negotiated by the Department of Health and financial allocations made to each health district based on estimated target populations. This system was difficult to implement because of disagreements over the target population size, affected by children moving between health districts.

A new national surveillance system was put in place in advance of the campaign to monitor the effectiveness of the MMR vaccination programme. Local vaccine uptake data were collected, rubella and mumps were made notifiable diseases (measles had been a notifiable disease since 1940) and disease incidence recorded. Rubella infections in pregnancy continued to be monitored, including laboratory-confirmed infections, terminations of pregnancy due to rubella infection and cases of CRS. Serological surveillance was also put in place. Antibody levels to measles, mumps and rubella following immunization were checked in successive cohorts and rubella susceptibility in pregnant women continued to be measured. It was the implementation of this 'warning system' which later alerted policy makers to the emergence of a susceptible cohort of children and the potential for a measles epidemic [14].

3.3
Haemophilus influenzae b (1992)

Haemophilus influenzae b vaccine was added to the routine childhood programme in October 1992, as a separate injection given at the same visit as the routine diphtheria, tetanus, pertussis (DTP) and oral polio vaccine at 2, 3 and 4 months of age. In the campaign, children who had already started their primary immunizations were called back for additional visits to complete a course of three doses of *Haemophilus influenzae* b vaccine. Children over 1 year and under the age of 4 years were recalled through the national computer scheme for a single dose of vaccine. Appointments for the catch-up programme for older children were scheduled over the first year of the programme so that priority was given to children under 12 months of age, at the greatest risk from *Haemophilus influenzae* b disease. Wherever possible, appointments were made through the computerized registers to coincide with other scheduled visits, such as MMR.

A notable change to the childhood immunization programme at the time of the *Haemophilus influenzae* b campaign was the central purchase and supply of all routine vaccines. Prior to this, local health authorities were responsible for ordering and distributing the childhood vaccine to GPs. From October 1992, the NHS Supplies Authority became responsible for negotiating national contracts for the supply of all routine childhood vaccines. It was particularly important to have this control over vaccine supplies at the start of the *Haemophilus influenzae* b campaign: there were two *Haemophilus influenzae* b vaccines on the UK market and at the time there was not information that they could be used interchangeably. This central management permitted tight control of which children received which vaccine and at which time. Because of the intense public interest in availability of a vaccine to prevent

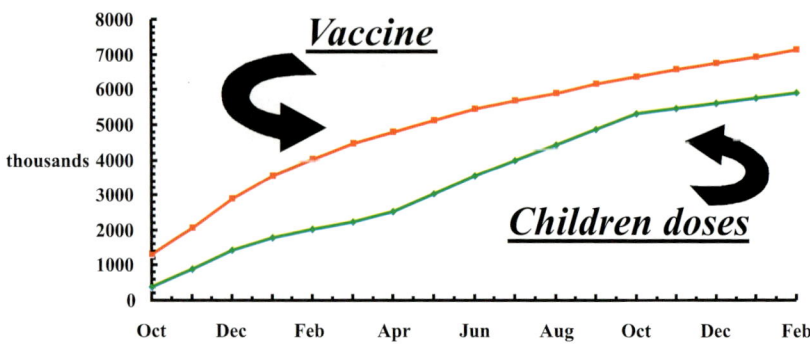

Source: Department of Health

Fig. 3 Cumulative Hib vaccine supplies and calculated demand

meningitis, in part driven by the Department of Health advertising, there was a huge pressure on supplies. Despite stock being distributed in excess of the calculated requirements, shortages occurred and these led to much dissatisfaction and critical media reporting.

Figure 3 compares the quantities of *Haemophilus influenzae* b vaccine provided for the campaign with the calculated requirement for vaccine, based on the scheduling of children through the campaign. Despite the surplus of vaccine over calculated demand, there were vaccine shortages, in part because of insufficient 'front-loading' of supplies, and because of lack of management of the demand and the supply.

3.4
Measles Rubella (1994)

A one-off Measles Rubella (MR) catch-up campaign was carried out in 1994. This followed the availability of date from serological surveillance which identified high probabilities of an imminent measles epidemic. Although uptake of MMR vaccine since its introduction in 1988 had been high, measles vaccine coverage in young children had been low previously and there was now a considerable number of school age children who had never been immunized and who had never caught measles. Mathematical modelling predicted that the UK could expect an epidemic of between 100,000 and 200,000 cases in 1995 [15] and an epidemic had already started in Scotland [16]. International experience showed that the most effective way to prevent such epidemics was through mass immunizations campaigns carried out over a short period of time [17]. If high coverage is achieved then transmission is prevented.

The campaign was implemented in November 1994. As a result of this programme, seven million children aged 5–16 years were vaccinated with MR vaccine, 92% of all children in this age group. MR vaccine was used to provide protection against measles and to accelerate population immunity against rubella, permitting the subsequent discontinuation of rubella immunization of teenage girls.

Although the ideal would have been to use MMR vaccine, MR vaccine was used because at the time there was intense pressure worldwide on MMR vaccine supplies. With the anticipated measles epidemic, delaying any intervention to wait for MMR vaccine in order to include mumps vaccine in the campaign could not be justified.

The impact on immunity to measles and rubella in the target populations was confirmed by sero-epidemiology surveys using samples taken before and after the campaign.

Figure 4 compares susceptibility to measles, by age, before the MR catch-up campaign and subsequently. The pre-campaign susceptibility in school-aged children, sufficient to sustain measles transmission, has been reduced considerably.

In the event, a measles epidemic was averted. Some critics of this campaign failed to understand the scientific basis on which the prediction and modelling had been made, and appeared to have preferred to wait for the prediction to have been validated by an epidemic. Great care was taken to investigate and review adverse events [18].

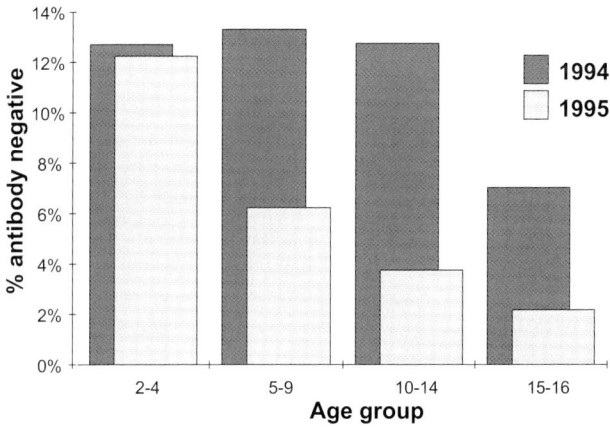

Fig. 4 Measles susceptibility in England and Wales, before and after MR campaign

3.5
Meningitis C (1999)

A vaccine against meningococcal group C disease (Meningitis C vaccine) was introduced in 1999, following an intensive 5-year clinical trials research programme sponsored by the Department of Health. The Department of Health-funded trial programme together with complementary manufacturer-sponsored studies resulted in the licensure of the world's first meningococcal group C conjugate vaccine. The implementation of the immunization programme was brought forward by a year (it was originally planned for October 2000) due to the continuing increase in meningococcal C infections seen in the winter 'meningococcal season' of 1998/1999.

Vaccine supplies were initially limited and had to be provided first to those most at risk. The vaccine was introduced as a rolling campaign, immunizing particular age groups during different phases. Organizing the cohorts for immunization was a challenge because there were two age groups most at risk—young babies and young people 15–17 years of age. Those aged 5–17 years were vaccinated through schools and those aged less than 5 years through general practice. Local immunization coordinators were briefed on the campaign and asked to provide estimates of the numbers of children in each age group in order to plan vaccine allocation for the schools' based activities. Estimates on the number of children under 5 years cared for by each GP were based on the number of doses of diphtheria/tetanus/pertussis/Hib (DTP/Hib) vaccine that they had ordered over the previous 2 years.

Meningococcal C conjugate vaccine was issued to GP practices either weekly or fortnightly—no ordering was necessary. The projected dates of vaccine delivery to GP practices were given to the Child Health System (national computer registry) who sent out invitations for immunization through the automated immunization schedule database.

The advertising strategy for the Meningitis C campaign was unusual because rather than creating a demand for vaccination it was needed to control demand. The key message was not to rush to get the vaccine but to wait until children were invited and every child would be invited for the new immunization in turn.

The rollout of the programme began in November 1999 starting with young people aged 15–17 years. The second phase of the programme started a few weeks later with the routine immunization of babies at 2, 3 and 4 months and with the catch-up campaign for infants. The programmes were phased in locally, as vaccine became available. During 2000, children aged 11–14 years and children under 5 years were called up for their vaccination, and in 2002 onwards the programme was extended to all those under 25 years of age, with special attention paid to those attending university or colleges.

Immunization Campaigns in the UK

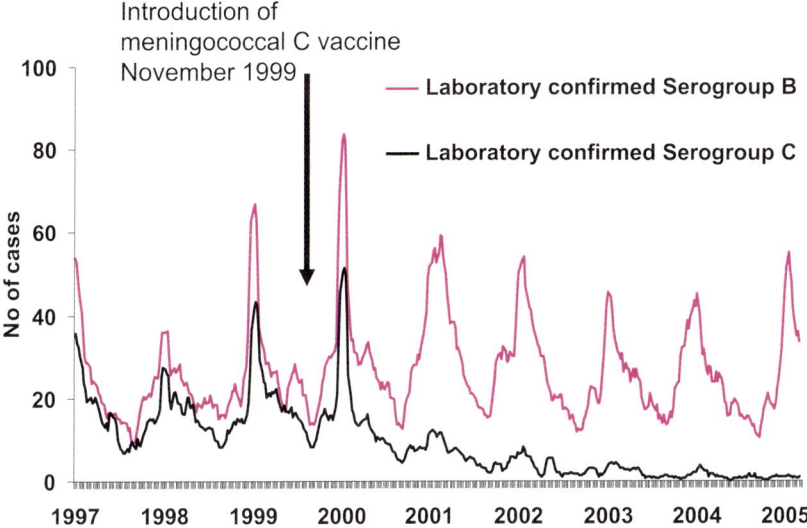

Source Health Protection Agency

Fig. 5 Laboratory-confirmed cases of meningococcal disease England and Wales (five weekly moving averages): 1997–2005

Figure 5 shows the impact of the 1999 and subsequent immunization campaign and compares the changes in prevalence of Group C meningococcal disease with those for Group B meningococcal disease, for which there is no vaccine available.

3.6
Hib Booster (2003)

The introduction of Hib vaccine into the routine immunization programme in 1992, along with a catch-up programme for children aged under 4 years had proved very successful and by 1998, laboratory confirmed cases of Hib disease in children under 5 years had fallen by 98%. However, since 1998 national enhanced surveillance of Hib disease had identified a gradual increase in cases especially in this age group [19]. At the end of 2002 the Joint Committee on Vaccination and Immunisation (JCVI) agreed that action should be taken immediately to halt this increase in cases. A one-off Hib booster campaign was carried out from May 2003 [20]. All children between 6 months and 5 years of age on 1st April 2003 were recalled and immunized with an additional dose of Hib vaccine.

The campaign was implemented over a short period of time (6 months) in order to obtain immediate high levels of vaccine coverage and to restore herd immunity to halt and reverse the increase in Hib cases. It was also important to complete this 'one-off' programme before the start of the annual influenza vaccination campaign when general practices (primary care providers) would be busy. Information from direct feedback from local immunization coordinators and by means of annual telephone surveys with health professionals have informed the Department of Health's communication strategy on changes to the immunization programme. Health professionals prefer to have early warning of proposed changes to the programme albeit at a stage where not all the details of the change may have been finalized as long as they receive further information later. Rather than finding this confusing, health professionals can start to plan for any increased immunization workload and rearrange other activities. To this effect, health professionals were immediately warned of the forthcoming campaign by a letter from the Chief Medical Officer in February 2003 outlining the rationale for the one-off immunization programme. More specific details of the campaign were then provided in a further letter to health professionals in April 2003, 1 month before the start of the campaign.

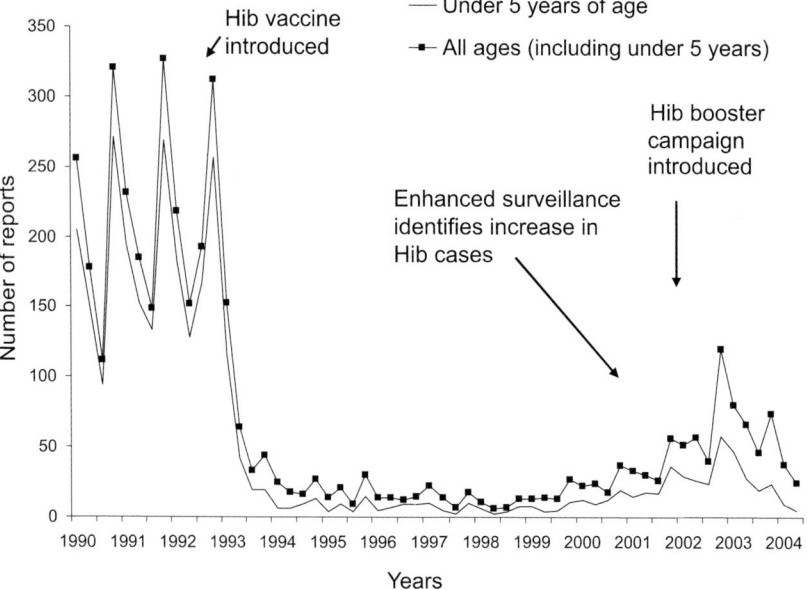

Fig. 6 Laboratory reports of Hib disease in England and Wales (1990–2004)

The results of the campaign were impressive. Disease levels were halted in those younger age groups who were immunized and dropped to their lowest ever levels. The campaign also had an impact on older age groups, first of all in older children and by 2004 disease levels had also declined in adults.

Figure 6 shows the impact of the 2003 Hib catch-up campaign with cases of invasive Hib disease falling back to extremely low levels. It is notable that cases had also risen in older individuals, including adults, and these also declined after the campaign—in the absence of immunization.

4
Annual Influenza Campaigns

As well as the one-off immunization campaigns that are periodically undertaken in the UK, annual influenza vaccination campaigns are carried out. Since 2000 the programme has included the immunization of all those aged 65 years and over as well as those aged over 6 months in the clinical risk groups, notably: chronic respiratory, heart, renal or liver disease, diabetes or lowered immunity due to disease or treatment. Since 2000, vaccine uptake during the campaign has been collected monthly (from October to December). The communication strategy for promoting annual vaccination campaigns must ensure that people continue to return for their annual vaccination and that high vaccine coverage levels are maintained every year. The communications for the campaign start with a letter sent out by the Chief Medical Officer to health professionals in early summer, with details of vaccine supplies and policy recommendations for the forthcoming 'flu season. This is followed by a comprehensive advertising and PR campaign that includes TV, radio, Internet and press coverage. The public relations programme works locally to support areas where vaccine uptake is low and also targets particular risk groups. A range of information materials is produced including leaflets (in English and ethnic minority languages, audio tape and Braille), fact sheets and posters. As well as using standard distribution routes such as GP practices and pharmacies, the Department of Health also works with voluntary sector groups and supermarkets in order to distribute bulk supplies of leaflets and posters.

In the UK, pharmacists are playing an increasingly important role in providing customers with advice and information on immunization issues. During the annual 'flu campaign, pharmacists play an active part in distributing information materials to customers. Pharmacy prescription bags are also produced by the Department carrying the message 'Get your jab'.

Table 2 shows the progressive increases in coverage of influenza vaccine in individuals aged 65 years and over.

Table 2 Vaccine uptake in the UK since the start of the influenza immunization programme for those aged 65 years and over (source: UK Health Departments)

Year	England (%)	Scotland (%)	Wales (%)	Northern Ireland (%)
2000/01	65.4	65	39	68
2001/02	67.5	65	59	72
2002/03	68.6	69	54[a]	72.1
2003/04	71.0	72.5	63	73.4
2004/05	71.5	71.7	63	72.7

[a] Some GP practices experienced problems in collating and reporting data

5
Conclusion

Campaigns require intense planning at national and local level with leadership to achieve proper management. Although the components of an immunization campaign can be described separately—strategic planning, vaccine supply, communication and surveillance, for a programme to be successful integrated planning is essential.

It is important to capitalize on investments such as advertising. Advertising can be used to raise awareness of a new vaccine and the seriousness of the disease it protects against, promote the vaccine's benefits or simply used to direct parents to sources of information.

However, following the initial launch of any campaign, there is still much continuing work to do—ensuring timely completion of the campaign, monitoring of adverse reactions and carrying out surveillance during campaign implementation and thereafter.

At a time when countries have undertaken preparations in case of bioterrorism attacks, for which vaccination against agents such as smallpox may be essential, experience of campaign implementation is imperative. In the case of a need for a mass smallpox vaccination campaign, the UK had benefited from its previous immunization campaigns and had developed smallpox campaign plans that included nationwide vaccination in 5 days [21]. Similarly, in the event of an emergence of an influenza pandemic, not only will vaccines need to be introduced on a campaign basis, but so may provision of antivirals. Vaccination campaign experience is proving invaluable.

References

1. Pan American Health Organization (http://www.paho.org)
2. Miller E, Waight P, Gay N, Ramsay M, Vurdien J, Morgan-Capner P, Hesketh L, Brown D, Tookey P, Peckham C (1997) The epidemiology of rubella in England and Wales before and after the 1994 measles and rubella vaccination campaign: fourth joint report from the PHLS and the National Congenital Rubella Surveillance Programme, Commun Dis Rep CDR Rev 7(2):R26–R32
3. Gay N, Miller E, Hesketh L, Morgan-Capner P, Ramsay M, Cohen B, Brown D (1997) Mumps surveillance in England and Wales supports introduction of two dose vaccination schedule. Commun Dis Rep CDR Rev7(2):R21–R26
4. Trotter CL, Ramsay ME, Slack MP (2003) Rising incidence of Haemophilus influenzae type b disease in England and Wales indicates a need for a second catch-up vaccination campaign. Commun Dis Public Health 6:55–58
5. Miller C, Miller E, Rowe K, Bowie C, Judd M, Walker D (1989) Surveillance of symptoms following MMR vaccine in children.Practitioner. 233:69–73
6. Yarwood J, Noakes K, Kennedy D, Campbell H, Salisbury D (2005) Tracking mothers attitudes to childhood immunisation 1991–2001. Vaccine 2005, in press
7. Keane V (1993) et al. Perceptions of vaccine efficacy, illness and health among inner city parents. Clinical Pediatrics 1993:2–7
8. Chen RT, Davis RL, Sheedy KM (2004) Safety of Immunizations. In: Plotkin SA, Orenstein WA (eds). Vaccines, 4th edn. W.B. Saunders Company, p1557
9. da Silveira CM, Kmetzsch CI, Mohrdieck R, Sperb AF, Prevots DR (2002) The risk of aseptic meningitis associated with the Leningrad-Zagreb mumps vaccine strain following mass vaccination with measles-mumps-rubella vaccine, Rio Grande do Sul, Brazil, 1997. Int J Epidemiol 5:978–982
10. da Cunha SS, Rodrigues LC, Barreto ML, Dourado I (2002) Outbreak of aseptic meningitis and mumps after mass vaccination with MMR vaccine using the Leningrad-Zagreb mumps strain. Vaccine 20:1106–1112
11. HM Stationery Office, Chief Medical Officer, Annual Report, 1957
12. Miller C, Miller E, Rowe K, Bowie C, Judd M, Walker D (1989) Surveillance of symptoms following MMR vaccine in children. Practitioner. 233(1461):69–73
13. MMR Three way protection for your child, Question and Answer paper
14. HM Stationery Office, 1988
15. Ramsay M, Gay N, Miller E, Rush M, White J, Morgan-Capner P, Brown D (1994) The epidemiology of measles in England and Wales: rationale for the 1994 national vaccination campaign. Commun Dis Rep CDR Rev 11(4):R141–R146
16. Ramsay M, Gay N, Miller E, Rush M, White J, Morgan-Capner P, Brown D (1994) The epidemiology of measles in England and Wales: rationale for the 1994 national vaccination campaign. Commun Dis Rep CDR Rev 11(4):R141–R146
17. Carter H, Gorman D (1993) Measles outbreak in Fife: which MMR policy? Public Health 107:25–30
18. Progress toward interrupting indigenous measles transmission–Region of the Americas, January 1999-September 2000. MMWR Morb Mortal Wkly Rep 2000 3(49):986–990
19. Medicines Control Agency (1995) Adverse reactions to measles and rubella vaccine. 21:9–10

20. Trotter CL, Ramsay ME, Slack MP (2003) Rising incidence of Haemophilus influenzae type b disease in England and Wales indicates a need for a second catch-up vaccination campaign. Commun Dis Public Health 6:55–58
21. http://www.dh.gov.uk/assetRoot/04/11/40/18/04114018.pdf

Diphtheria

C. R. Vitek (✉)

MS E-45, 1600 Clifton Road, Atlanta, GA, USA
cxv3@cdc.gov

1	Clinical Picture and Pathophysiology of Diphtheria	72
2	Diphtheria Immunization	74
2.1	Development of Diphtheria Vaccines	74
2.2	Diphtheria Immunization Schedules	75
3	Epidemiology	75
4	Diphtheria Outbreaks and Control	77
5	Diphtheria Epidemic in the Countries of the Former Soviet Union	81
5.1	Diphtheria Control and Resurgence	81
5.1.1	Pre-1980	81
5.1.2	The 1980s	81
5.1.3	The 1990s	82
5.2	Response to the Diphtheria Epidemic in the Former Soviet Union	82
5.3	Implementation of the Mass Immunization Strategy and Results	83
5.3.1	Western	86
5.3.2	Southern	87
5.4	Reasons for the Reemergence of Epidemic Diphtheria	87
5.5	Lessons Learned and Future Needs	89
5.6	Epidemic Control: Case-Centered Control Measures and Mass Immunization	89
5.7	Prevention	91
	References	92

Abstract Diphtheria is a contagious upper respiratory illness that was a major cause of childhood mortality in the prevaccine era. In the early twentieth century, an effective toxoid vaccine was developed. Implementation of childhood vaccination virtually eliminated diphtheria from developed countries after the Second World War and implementation of the Expanded Program on Immunization in developing countries led to rapid declines in diphtheria globally in the 1980s. However, in the 1990s, a massive epidemic of diphtheria spread throughout the countries of the former Soviet Union. Unlike the prevaccine era, most cases of severe disease and deaths were reported among adults. Multiple factors contributed to the epidemic, including increased susceptibility among both adults and children; suboptimal socioeconomic conditions;

high population movement; and delay in implementing appropriate control measures. Mass immunization was the key element in the epidemic control strategy developed and implemented in a well-coordinated response by an international public health coalition. This strategy focused on rapidly raising population immunity of both adults and children; the immunization of more than 140,000,000 adults and adolescents and millions of children successfully controlled the epidemic. While improved coverage of children in developing countries with diphtheria toxoid has led to progressive decreases in diphtheria; eradication is unlikely in the foreseeable future and gaps in immunity among adult population exist or are developing in many other countries. Routine childhood immunization with diphtheria toxoid is the key to controlling diphtheria while the role of routine adult reimmunization is less established; mass immunization will remain an important control measure for widespread diphtheria outbreaks.

1
Clinical Picture and Pathophysiology of Diphtheria

Diphtheria is an acute infectious upper respiratory illness caused by the gram-positive bacillus *Corynebacterium diphtheriae*. The disease is characterized by a membranous inflammation of the upper respiratory tract and by damage to other organs, most commonly the myocardium and peripheral nerves. These primary manifestations of diphtheria are caused by the local and systemic action of a potent exotoxin produced by strains of *C. diphtheriae* containing the *tox* phage.

Diphtheria typically has an insidious onset after an incubation period of 1–5 days. The initial symptoms of diphtheria are nonspecific and include sore throat, fatigue, and low-grade fever associated with mild injection of the pharyngeal mucosa. Progressive damage to the pharyngeal mucosa by diphtheria toxin and other bacterial factors results in the appearance of membranes, initially in patches but then becoming increasingly confluent over 2–3 days. These membranes can spread to the tonsillar areas, soft palate, and uvula and less commonly to the posterior nasal passages, larynx, and trachea. The fully developed membrane is usually thick, grayish colored, and firmly adherent. In some patients, cervical lymphadenopathy and edema of the surrounding soft tissues produce marked neck swelling ('bull-neck'); this appearance is a hallmark of severe disease and is associated with higher morbidity and mortality. In untreated patients without complications, systemic symptoms improve approximately 1 week after onset of symptoms, coincident with softening and sloughing of the membrane.

The main clinical impact of diphtheria is caused by complications of the local membranes and by the effects of absorbed toxin on other organs. Laryngeal diphtheria is more common in young children and laryngeal membranes frequently cause respiratory obstruction and death from asphyxiation. Extension of the membrane into the tracheobronchial tree can produce pneumonia or respiratory obstruction. In the upper respiratory tract, the membrane and surrounding swelling can result in secondary otitis media and sinusitis.

Most deaths from diphtheria are due to the effects of absorbed diphtheria toxin on the heart and peripheral nerves. The most common severe complications are acute systemic toxicity, myocarditis, and peripheral neuritis. The extent of local disease correlates with the risk of complications due to increased production and absorption of the toxin from larger membranes.

Myocardial involvement appearing in the first week of the illness is usually part of a syndrome of severe acute systemic toxicity and is usually fatal. Myocarditis can also present, most frequently with arrhythmias, in the second week or third week of illness when the patient is otherwise improving. The neurological complications associated with diphtheria occur in approximately 15%–20% of cases and usually begin 2–8 weeks after the onset of illness. The primary manifestations are peripheral neuropathies from which functional recovery almost always occurs.

Production of the exotoxin coded for by the *tox* gene is overwhelmingly the most important factor associated with the development of diphtheria. The biology of diphtheria toxin has been extensively studied (Collier 2001; Holmes 2000). Infection of *C. diphtheriae* by a bacteriophage containing the *tox* gene gives the bacteria the ability to produce diphtheria toxin. Diphtheria toxin is a polypeptide with a molecular weight of about 58,000. The toxin is a highly potent inhibitor of protein synthesis which results in cell death; the susceptibility of different human cell types may represent variation in the presence of receptors for the toxin. On mucous membranes, the toxin causes local cellular destruction, and the cellular debris, fibrin, and bacteria form the characteristic membrane. Toxin can then be absorbed across the membrane and circulate to cause damage to the myocardium, nervous system, and kidneys.

Several other bacterial components are known to contribute to the local damage and to invasiveness. The recent sequencing of the *C. diphtheriae* genome may aid in the identification of other virulence and colonization factors (Cerdeño-Tárraga 2003). A better understanding of the interaction of pathogenic strains of *C. diphtheriae* and the human host may help to develop improved methods of immunization and treatment and improve our understanding of why certain toxigenic strains appear to have more potential to cause large-scale epidemics.

2
Diphtheria Immunization

2.1
Development of Diphtheria Vaccines

The discovery of diphtheria toxin in the late nineteenth century was followed by the use of toxin to immunize animals and produce sera ('antitoxin'). Antitoxin proved to be capable of neutralizing the effects of diphtheria toxin when administered to other animals or humans and clinical use in the 1890s demonstrated that antitoxin treatment profoundly lowered the mortality from diphtheria (Hróbjartsson 1998). Contemporary scientists then turned their attention to developing safe immunizing agents for humans. By 1913, it was demonstrated that injections of balanced mixtures of toxin and antitoxin successfully immunized humans. Toxin–antitoxin preparations were rapidly adopted for use in some cities in the US and Europe. Although effective, these preparations occasionally produced serious adverse events due to inadequate neutralization of the toxin in certain batches. In 1923, Ramon reported that small amounts of formaldehyde caused diphtheria toxin to lose its toxic properties while retaining its immunogenicity, thus becoming a toxoid (Ramon 1923).

Diphtheria toxoid gradually replaced toxin–antitoxin preparations for immunization and remains the basis of current diphtheria vaccines. Improvements have included increasing immunogenicity with alum adjuvants since the 1920s and producing a combined vaccine against diphtheria, tetanus, and pertussis [diphtheria and tetanus toxoids and whole-cell pertussis vaccine (DTP)] beginning in the 1940s. Diphtheria toxoid is also available combined with tetanus toxoid in both a higher diphtheria antigen preparation used for immunizing children (DT) and a lower diphtheria antigen preparation used for immunizing adolescents and adults (Td).

Beginning in the 1990s, combinations of diphtheria and tetanus toxoids with acellular pertussis components (DTaP) have replaced DTP for routine childhood use in many developed countries due to their lower reactogenicity; other combinations of DTaP with *Haemophilus influenzae* b (Hib) vaccine, inactivated poliovirus vaccine, and hepatitis B vaccine are also in use. Combination vaccine products with reduced antigen content of diphtheria toxoid (Tdap) have been licensed for use in adolescent and adult populations in some countries and are under consideration for licensure in the US.

Three doses of diphtheria toxoid vaccines will produce minimally protective levels of antibodies [>0.01 international units (IU) per ml] in almost all vaccinees and highly protective levels (>0.1 IU/ml) in most. The levels of these antibodies fall and substantial proportions of individuals will lose immunity over several years; booster doses of diphtheria toxoid will rapidly produce protective levels of antibodies again.

A series of epidemiologic investigations of diphtheria outbreaks have evaluated the effectiveness of diphtheria toxoid in preventing diphtheria. Most estimates of the effectiveness of three doses have ranged from 70% to 93%. Among those immunized individuals who develop diphtheria, the disease is likely to be milder and less likely to be fatal than diphtheria disease among unimmunized individuals.

2.2
Diphtheria Immunization Schedules

Currently, in the US, five doses of DTaP are recommended (at 2, 4, 6, and 15–18 months and at school entry before the seventh birthday) for routine immunization of children followed by booster doses of Td approximately every 10 years. In other countries, the recommended immunization schedules for diphtheria toxoid vary; the number of doses recommended tends to be lower in less developed countries (WHO Vaccine Preventable Diseases Monitoring System). Those countries classified by the World Health Organization (WHO) as 'least developed' frequently use the schedule recommended by the WHO Expanded Programme on Immunization (EPI): three doses of DTP in infancy with no routine additional doses. Many developing countries recommend one or two additional childhood doses while developed countries frequently also recommend an adolescent booster. Most countries do not currently recommend routine adult immunization with diphtheria toxoid although several countries began to recommend adult booster doses after the epidemic in the former Soviet Union.

3
Epidemiology

Humans are the only natural host for *C. diphtheriae*, although the organism has also been isolated from the environment of persons infected with *C. diphtheriae*. Transmission is person-to-person, primarily by intimate respiratory and physical contact. The epidemiology of the circulation of toxigenic *C. diphtheriae* has been profoundly affected by immunization. In unimmunized populations, toxigenic strains circulated widely, especially in urban populations; most infections resulted in asymptomatic carriage. In temperate climates, diphtheria occurred year-round but most often during colder months, probably because of the close contact of children indoors. In tropical climates and under conditions of poor hygiene, cutaneous diphtheria is more common than respiratory diphtheria and is unrelated to season.

In unimmunized populations, maternally derived antibodies were present in infants at birth but were lost by the end of the first year of life. Thereafter, the proportion of immune children gradually increased to 75% or more presumably due to repeated subclinical infections. However, preschool and school-aged children were also the group most often affected by clinically manifest respiratory diphtheria. Diphtheria was rare among urban adults in unimmunized populations due to acquired immunity. Natural immunity is not always lifelong but is long-lasting and was reinforced by periodic natural boosting in unimmunized populations.

In immunized populations, circulation of toxigenic strains of *C. diphtheriae* drops dramatically once high levels of immunity to diphtheria are achieved, although nontoxigenic strains of *C. diphtheriae* continue to circulate widely as part of normal human respiratory tract flora (Pappenheimer 1982). Although no animal or persistent environmental reservoir exists for *C. diphtheriae*, disappearance of the toxigenic phage is unlikely because a related bacterial species *C. ulcerans* may carry the phage and an animal reservoir does exist for this bacteria. Given the worldwide ubiquity of carriage of *C. diphtheriae* and the persistence of bacteriophages that can produce toxin, eradication of diphtheria does not currently seem achievable.

The drop in circulation of toxigenic strains in highly immunized populations contributes to herd immunity by protecting unimmunized persons but also leads to profound changes in the immune structure of the population (Galazka 1995). Childhood populations are highly immune due to vaccination but more adults are susceptible because of incomplete vaccination coverage and waning immunity among vaccinated persons in the absence of boosting from natural circulation or repeat immunization. Increased proportions of adults without protective antibody levels have been documented in many countries in the vaccine era (Galazka 1995). The most susceptible cohorts of adults will vary in age in different countries depending on when routine childhood immunization was implemented. In general, these cohorts will include those age groups which include many individuals who were: (1) young children or adolescents when immunization began; (2) missed by the early immunization program; and () escaped natural infection due to rapidly falling rates of disease once immunization started. Additional nonimmune adults will include individuals who were immunized but have lost protective antibody levels. Despite these populations of susceptible adults, diphtheria outbreaks involving susceptible adults have been rare as long as childhood immunity remains very high.

4
Diphtheria Outbreaks and Control

Although descriptions of diphtheria appear beginning in ancient Egyptian and Greek times, diphtheria became a devastating public health problem in large population centers in the Industrial Age. Beginning in the seventeenth century, severe outbreaks occurred in Spain and recurred periodically thereafter; severe outbreaks also were reported in the American colonies in the eighteenth century. In the nineteenth century, persistent outbreaks of diphtheria caused extremely high morbidity and mortality among children in urban centers in Europe and North American. The best data from North America comes from Massachusetts and Ontario (U.S. Bureau of the Census 1975; McKinnon 1942). In these areas, the death rate from diphtheria exceeded 50 per 100,000 annually in most years in the late 1800s. The discovery and introduction of diphtheria antitoxin treatment in the 1890s led to a decline in the death rate in both areas to 15 per 100,000 over the next 20 years but diphtheria remained a leading killer of children until diphtheria immunization became commonplace.

After the development of toxin–antitoxin preparations, immunization campaigns began rapidly in some North American cities. In 1914, the New York City Department of Health began immunizing children in schools and orphanages (Zingher 1921). By 1933, more than a million children had been immunized in New York; diphtheria cases had declined by more than 70% and deaths by 80% (Griffith 1979). The introduction of safer diphtheria toxoid in the 1920s led to wider adoption of diphtheria immunization. A campaign targeting Toronto schoolchildren in 1926–1929 produced major declines in cases (75%) and deaths (80%) (McKinnon 1931). Immunization campaigns were extended to pre-school aged children in some cities by the mid 1930s (Craster 1941).

The availability of DTP led to further increases in immunization; by the late 1950s, diphtheria was markedly reduced in the US and increasingly concentrated in a limited number of states. In the 1960s and 1970s, a progressive decline in nonoutbreak cases occurred throughout the country with diphtheria disappearing from most areas. A series of outbreaks were reported, primarily in the Southwestern states, in the late 1960s and early 1970s. Molecular epidemiology analyses suggested clonality of the intermedius strains responsible for most of these outbreaks (McCloskey 1972) and those responsible for last large outbreak of diphtheria in the US in Seattle (Coyle 1989). The Seattle outbreak occurred from 1972 to 1982, primarily among socio-economically disadvantaged adults.

Beginning in 1980, reported diphtheria cases abruptly declined in the US. Part of the decline was due to the exclusion of cutaneous diphtheria cases from national reporting beginning in 1980. However, improved childhood immunization in Mexico and other developing countries due to the implementation of the EPI in the late 1970s is likely to have reduced importations of toxigenic strains. By the mid-1990s, many experts felt that toxigenic strains of *C. diphtheriae* were no longer circulating in the US. However, in the 1990s, surveillance revealed circulation of toxigenic strains in a northern Plains Indian community and in some native communities in Canada. Molecular epidemiology linked the recently identified strains to strains collected from the same areas during the 1970s and 1980s, suggesting ongoing endemic circulation (Marston 2001). Circulation has also been reported among the aboriginal population in central Australia (Patel 1999). The common denominator in these communities is likely to be poverty, crowding, poor hygiene, and suboptimal immunization rates.

In Europe, immunization with toxin–antitoxin preparations was also implemented in parts of Germany as early as 1914. Limited immunization programs with diphtheria toxoid began in several European countries in the 1920s and 1930s, although the disease remained highly endemic in many countries. In Great Britain, the coverage and disease impact of routine diphtheria immunization remained modest until 1942 when a national mass immunization campaign targeting children 6 months to 15 years of age rapidly led to a marked and sustained decline in diphtheria incidence (Griffith 1979). This campaign helped Great Britain avoid the a major outbreak of diphtheria that spread throughout Europe during World War II; more than one million cases were estimated to have occurred in 1943 alone (Stowman 1945). In some areas, adults were the primary age group affected. In response, mass immunization campaigns were conducted in some areas; routine immunization and living conditions also improved after the war ended. The incidence of diphtheria declined rapidly in most affected countries.

In developing countries, the implementation of the EPI program in the 1970s led to dramatic increases in childhood immunization and falls in reported diphtheria cases (Fig. 1). In 2003, it was estimated that the proportion of infants worldwide who had received three doses of diphtheria toxoid in combination with tetanus toxoid and pertussis vaccine had risen from ~20% in 1980 to 78% worldwide; infant coverage is lowest in Southeast Asia (~70%) and sub-Saharan Africa (~55%) (Fig. 2). Before the EPI program began, it was estimated that close to a million cases of diphtheria occurred annually in the Third World with 50,000 to 60,000 deaths. From 1980 to 2003, reported cases of diphtheria globally decreased from 97,427 to 6,654; in 2003, two-thirds of

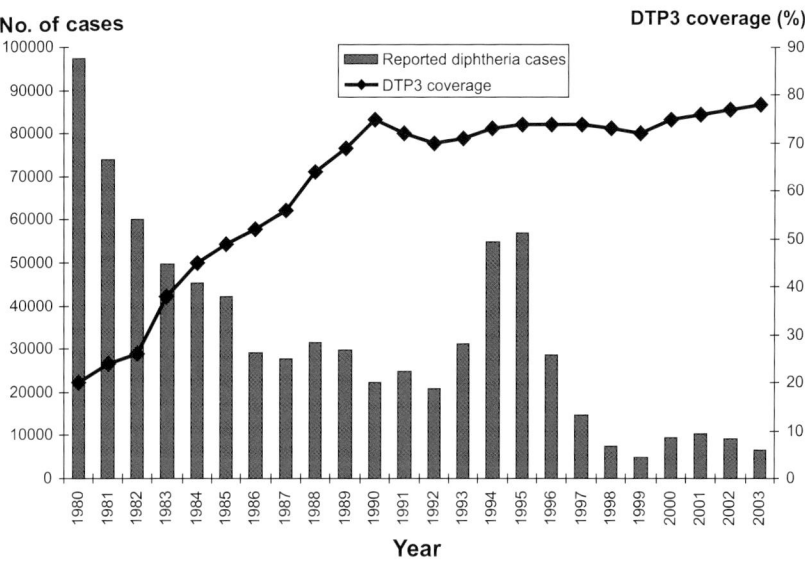

Fig. 1 Global reported diphtheria cases (all ages) and estimated DTP3 coverage among infants, 1980–2003

cases were reported from the Southeast Asian region (Department of Vaccines and Biologicals 2004).

Despite the overall improvement, large differences exist between developing countries in the degree of control of diphtheria. Some countries such as Malaysia, Singapore, and South Korea now have high living standards and immunization coverage; these countries have achieved success in controlling diphtheria similar to highly industrialized countries. Many other developing countries, such as Thailand, achieved marked reductions in diphtheria but continue to report sporadic cases and outbreaks (Tharmaphornpilas 2001). In those countries that have largely controlled diphtheria, increased proportions of adults are susceptible, as documented in recent serosurveys in Thailand (Tharmaphornpilas 2001) and Taiwan (Lee 1999).

In the least developed countries, the available data are limited but suggest that diphtheria remains highly endemic although decreased because of EPI. Frequently only large outbreaks or exported cases are detected and reported as illustrated by the recent reports of a large outbreak in a refugee camp in Afghanistan (Anonymous 2003) and a fatal case in a US traveler to Haiti (CDC 2004). Although data are lacking, it is likely that adult population immunity remains high in these least developed countries.

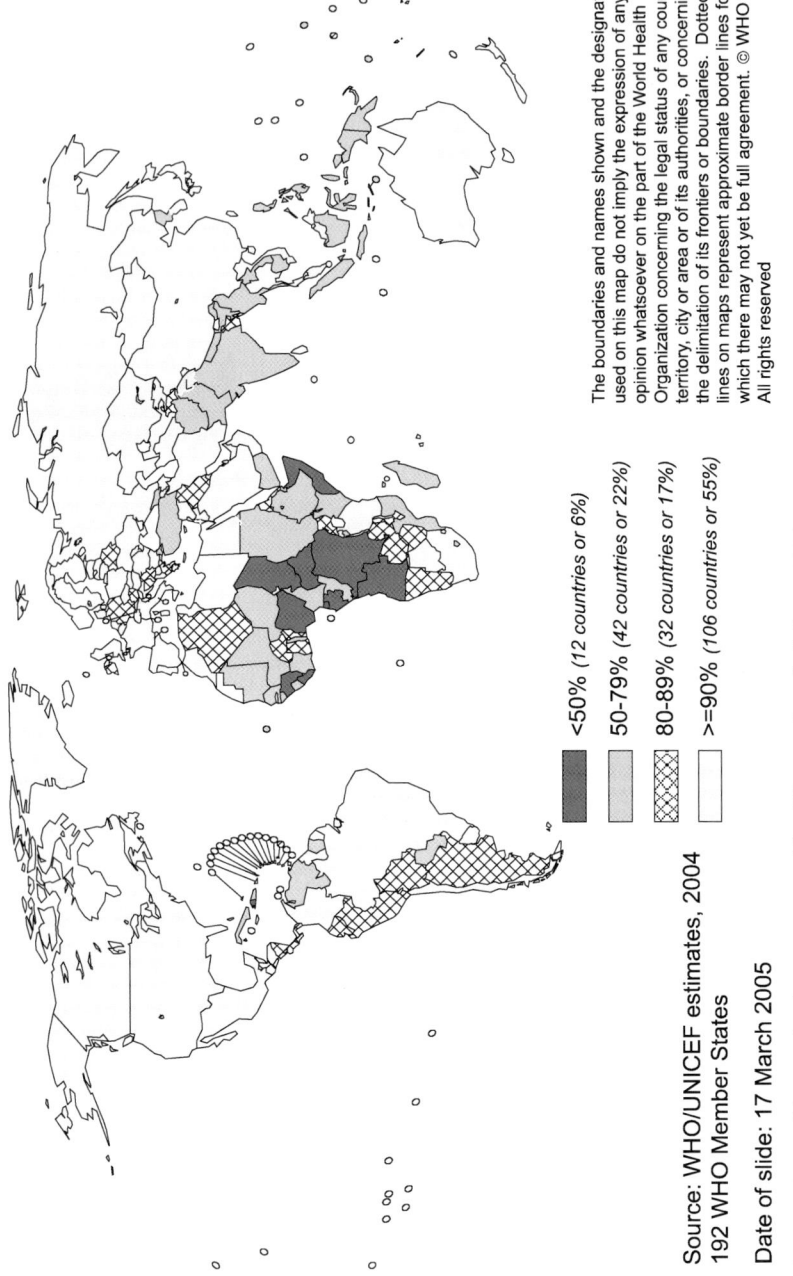

Fig. 2 Estimated immunization coverage with DTP3 vaccines in infants, 2003

5
Diphtheria Epidemic in the Countries of the Former Soviet Union

5.1
Diphtheria Control and Resurgence

5.1.1
Pre-1980

In the late 1920s, some Soviet cities began immunization programs using diphtheria toxoid. After World War II, immunization programs spread and diphtheria mortality fell in many urban areas (Markina 2000). However, diphtheria rates continued to be extremely high in many areas until universal childhood immunization was instituted throughout the Soviet Union in 1958–1959. By 1963, the incidence of diphtheria had decreased by >90% and in 1976, only 198 cases were reported.

5.1.2
The 1980s

In the 1980s, an upsurge in diphtheria cases was reported that peaked in 1984 with 1609 cases; adults were primarily involved for the first time. Diphtheria control measures were modified to include limited immunization for adults; reported cases subsequently gradually declined to 839 cases in 1989. In the 1980s, significant gaps in population immunity to diphtheria developed among both children and adults. Changes in Soviet immunization policy, medical practice, and public acceptance led to less intensive immunization of children against diphtheria. Among the policy changes were increased contraindications to vaccination, the allowance of the use of lower antigen content Td for primary vaccination, and delaying the booster dose formerly given at school-entry. Public support for mandatory immunization programs also declined as the perceived benefits appeared modest due to successful control of many childhood diseases. Reported coverage of infants with a primary series of diphtheria toxoid containing vaccines dropped to <80% in some Soviet republics (Dittmann 2000). In addition, serologic studies found that cohorts of adults born in the 1940s and 1950s had high levels of susceptibility. As in other countries, individuals in the most susceptible age-cohorts in the Soviet Union had been children and adolescents when diphtheria incidence had began to fall as immunization programs were being implemented.

5.1.3
The 1990s

In 1990, multiple diphtheria outbreaks, primarily involving adult cases, were reported in and around Moscow, accounting for more than one-third of the Soviet total of 1431 cases. In 1991, outbreaks of diphtheria increased in Moscow and spread to other major cities in Russia; 3,167 cases were reported from what had now become the Newly Independent States (NIS) and Baltic States after the Soviet Union officially dissolved. In 1992, the epidemic spread within Russia and the Ukraine and extended into Belarus; the NIS and Baltic States reported a total of 5,749 cases. Despite the worsening situation, these countries continued to use the case-centered control measures modified during the 1980s; these measures included case and carrier identification and isolation, improving routine childhood coverage rates, and immunizing case-contacts and adults in occupational groups at perceived increased risk. In 1993, the Russian Federation alone reported 15,209 diphtheria cases, while Ukraine reported 2,982 and the other NIS and Baltic States reported 1,293 cases. By the end of 1994, diphtheria had spread throughout the former Soviet Union with sharp outbreaks or country-wide epidemics being reported from all countries except Turkmenistan. In 1995, which represented the peak year of the epidemic, 50,425 diphtheria cases were reported from the NIS and Baltic States. In many countries the epidemic was made worse by large numbers of refugees, severe economic declines, and shortages of energy; armed conflict worsened the situation in Moldova, the Caucasus, and Tajikistan.

5.2
Response to the Diphtheria Epidemic in the Former Soviet Union

After the breakup of the Soviet Union, the international community's response to assist the NIS and Baltic States included both general support of immunization programs and focused coordinated effort to stop the diphtheria epidemic. Although Russia remained self-sufficient, the other NIS and Baltic States had little, if any, vaccine production and no systems to procure these items from the international market. Beginning in 1992, multiple bilateral and multilateral efforts provided assistance to strengthen immunization programs throughout the region. WHO began providing technical assistance on the diphtheria epidemic in 1991. In 1994, multiple national governments and international organizations, including WHO, formed an Interagency Immunization Coordinating Committee (IICC). The IICC focused on efforts to control the diphtheria epidemic, to ensure the eradication of poliomyelitis, and to improve primary childhood immunization in the NIS and Baltic States.

With the input and approval of the NIS and Baltic States, the international organizations developed a strategy to control the diphtheria epidemic that focused on three main components: (1) rapid initiation of mass immunization of all age groups in the population with at least one dose of diphtheria toxoid; (2) ensuring the rapid detection and proper management of diphtheria cases; and (3) ensuring the rapid identification and proper management of close contacts of diphtheria cases, including antibiotic prophylaxis (WHO/UNICEF 1995). This strategy was based on the available epidemiologic and laboratory data; however, several immunogenicity studies using booster doses of diphtheria and tetanus toxoids were conducted in the NIS in 1994–1996 to further inform the strategy (Sutter 2000; Golaz 2000; Khetsuriani 2000; Ronne 2000). These studies, conducted among >3300 adults in the Ukraine, Georgia, and all three Baltic States, showed a high degree of consistency in their findings. A single dose of diphtheria toxoid produced high levels of immunity to diphtheria among almost all age groups, frequently in excess of 90% of individuals achieved titers >0.1 IU. However, this level of immunity was achieved by only 62%–79% of individuals in the highest risk age group (40–49 years of age). One study that looked at multiple doses found that a significant proportion of these individuals would require three doses for high-level protection (Sutter 2000). The data from these studies led to a modification of the strategy that recommended two additional diphtheria toxoid doses for age groups at increased risk, e.g., persons 30–50 years of age.

5.3
Implementation of the Mass Immunization Strategy and Results

The implementation of the strategy was made possible by the combination of international assistance and the efforts of the thousands of well-trained health care workers in the networks of primary health care and public health centers established in the Soviet period. These networks continued to function despite severe economic strains. International assistance helped to provide vaccine, supplies, antitoxin, and antibiotics, and to strengthen the areas where equipment and expertise were lacking such as cold chain and modern methods of social mobilization.

Responding to the failure of existing control methods to slow the epidemic, the Russian government issued orders in late 1993 to vaccinate all Russian adults (>120 million) against diphtheria. This effort was rapidly organized and implemented without large-scale international assistance; however, the resulting demand for Td vaccine initially outstripped supply. Domestic production of Td vaccine greatly increased during 1994, allowing nearly 70 million older adolescents and adults to be vaccinated between January 1993 and December

1995. Elsewhere in the NIS and Baltic States, implementation of the mass immunization strategy required massive international assistance in close collaboration with the national health authorities; the international agencies provided large-scale assistance with material supplies, logistics, cold-chain establishment, immunization policy, campaign planning, and social mobilization.

Challenge of mass immunization of essentially the entire adult population led to the development of similar strategies throughout the NIS and Baltic States building on Soviet social mobilization methods. Implementation initially focused on immunizing adults at work sites followed by additional intensified efforts to reach adults who were unemployed or working in nontraditional venues. These efforts included campaigns that vaccinated house-to-house, and in jails, markets, and transportation centers. Childhood coverage was improved by reducing contraindications, using only full-strength vaccine preparations, reinstating school-entry booster doses, and in some countries such as Azerbaijan, through mass immunization campaigns targeting children.

The mass immunization efforts began in some countries in 1994 and were conducted throughout the NIS and Baltic States in 1995–1996. In countries that quickly implemented national mass immunization and achieved high levels of coverage among all age groups, diphtheria incidence rates fell rapidly. In Moldova, a rapidly implemented population-wide immunization campaign in 1995 achieved high coverage among both children (>96%) and adults (>92%) and quickly achieved control of the epidemic (Fig. 3) (Magdei 2000). In Russia, high on-time childhood coverage with all doses and 67% adult coverage with more than one dose was reached by December 1994; diphtheria incidence began to fall in early 1995 and the decline in incidence accelerated as coverage continued to rise (Markina 2000; Vitek 1999). In Mongolia, an outbreak linked to importation from the NIS was rapidly brought under control by a mass immunization campaign (WHO 1997). In some countries, implementation of the mass campaigns took longer to reach high coverage, especially among adults, and control of the epidemics also took longer to achieve.

In 1996, reported diphtheria cases declined in all of the NIS and Baltic States and continued to decline in subsequent years. By 1999, the epidemic had been controlled albeit after more than >157,000 reported cases and 5,000 deaths. Based on the reported results of the immunization campaigns, more than 140,000,000 older adolescents and adults were immunized with one or more doses of diphtheria toxoid, representing one of the largest mass immunizations of adults in history (Wharton 2000). Control of the epidemic is estimated to have prevented an additional 560,000 cases and 15,000 deaths. However, circulation of toxigenic *C. diphtheriae* continues in the NIS and Baltic States

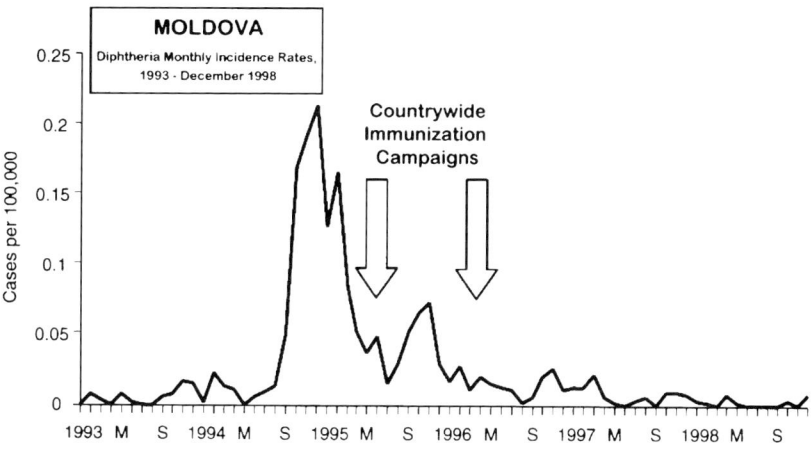

Figure from Dittmann 2003.

Fig. 3 Reported incidence of diphtheria by month, Moldova, 1993–1998

despite the massive amount of adult and childhood immunization; 1,177 cases were reported in 2002, primarily from Russia and the Ukraine.

The mass immunization campaigns among adults in the NIS outbreak proved to be highly safe. Few adverse events were reported in the national campaigns, regardless of whether diphtheria toxoid vaccines produced by Western or by Russian suppliers were used; the events reported were primarily local soreness or redness. In the Ukrainian immunogenicity studies where surveillance for adverse events was enhanced, the most frequent local reaction noted was pain among 18%–33% of vaccinees while 5% or less reported fever. No reaction was severe enough to result in missed work (Sutter 2000; Golaz 2000). Similarly, few reactions were reported during an adult immunization campaign conducted in Stockholm in 1995–1996 to raise population immunity during the epidemic in the former Soviet Union. Almost 100,000 adults were immunized with one to three doses of highly purified diphtheria toxoid vaccines and enhanced passive surveillance was conducted for adverse events. Only 1.8%–5.4% of vaccinees reported local reactions, and systemic reactions, primarily fever, were reported by less than 1% (Christenson 2001).

The NIS epidemic demonstrated conclusively the potential susceptibility of adults to epidemic diphtheria in the vaccine era. Adults and older adolescents made up a majority of reported cases in the epidemic; outbreaks and clusters of cases were reported among adults in enclosed civilian or military institutions. Within the NIS countries, there were two general patterns of

Table 1 Diphtheria cases and deaths by age group, Russia (1990–1997) and Azerbaijan (1990–1996) (from Markina 2000 and Vitek 2000)

Age group	Russia (population 148.1 million) 'Western' pattern			Azerbaijan (population 7.3 million) 'Southern' pattern		
	Cases (% total)	Deaths (% total)	Case fatality ratio	Cases (% total)	Deaths (% total)	Case fatality ratio
0–14 years	31,985 (32)	759 (26)	2.4%	1,140 (53)	213 (75)	18.7%
15–29 years	24,358 (24)	138 (5)	0.6%	690 (32)	58 (20)	8.4%
30–49 years	34,794 (35)	1,467 (49)	4.2%	324 (15)	15 (5)	4.6%
50 years and older	8,819 (9)	603 (20)	6.8%	16 (1)	0	0.0%
Total	99,956	2,967	3.0%	2,170	286	13.2%

age distribution, roughly defined by geographic location into 'western' and 'southern' patterns (Table 1). These patterns are likely to reflect several factors in the southern former NIS countries including larger proportions of children in the population; lower coverage with primary immunization of school-aged children, greater immunity among adults 40 years of age or older due to greater circulation of toxigenic *C. diphtheriae* prior to the initiation of Soviet mass immunization in the 1950s; possibly greater immunity among young adults due to continued circulation in the 1960s and 1970s; lower socio-economic levels; and regional differences in surveillance (Dittmann 2000).

5.3.1
Western

In the Baltic States and western NIS, the proportion of cases reported among adults was higher (64%–82%) and adults 40–49 years old had extremely high incidence and death rates; in some countries, this age group accounted for nearly half of all deaths. Older adults (>50 years of age) had relatively few cases. In the western NIS and Baltic States, the childhood age groups had low death rates with fatalities primarily occurring among children who had not received a primary vaccination series (Markina 2000).

5.3.2
Southern

In Moldova and the Caucasus and Central Asian countries, the proportion of cases reported among adults was lower (38%–59%); in most of these countries, adults less than 40 years of age had a higher incidence of diphtheria than older adults. Incidence in populations of children was high, especially in the initial phases of the epidemic. In many of the countries such as Georgia, Azerbaijan, and Tajikistan, the death rate was much higher among children, consistent with inadequate previous coverage with primary immunization.

While a high rate of adult susceptibility to diphtheria is critical, other factors appear to also be needed to produce widespread epidemic diphtheria among adults; data from the epidemic in the NIS and Baltic States supports the continued importance of populations of susceptible children in generating widespread epidemics. Russian data found that among the general civilian population, adult cases were frequently linked to child carriers, clusters of adult cases in routine work settings were rare, and the carriage rate among adult contacts of cases in routine settings were low. School-age children and adolescents had high reported incidence rates of diphtheria, primarily mild, as well as high rates of carriage of toxigenic *C. diphtheriae* (Fig. 4) (Dittmann 2000). The differing epidemiology of cases and contacts among school-aged children as compared to noninstitutionalized adults suggests that children remained a critical population for amplification of the epidemic in the general civilian population, probably due to their high contact rates in schools and day-care settings. This is also suggested by the disproportionate proportion of cases among school-aged children in Azerbaijan and some of the Central Asian countries early in the epidemic, followed by increasing cases in the adult population. Importations of diphtheria from the NIS outbreak to other highly industrialized countries (Germany, Finland, and Poland) with high rates of adult susceptibility but very high childhood immunization coverage led to either small numbers of secondary cases or to no spread at all (Galazka 1997; Anonymous 1997).

5.4
Reasons for the Reemergence of Epidemic Diphtheria

The Soviet epidemic can provide an important guide for assessing the risks of future major diphtheria epidemics. While the reasons for the epidemic remain incompletely understood, at a minimum, they appear to include the introduction of toxigenic strains into the general population, the less intense immunization and low coverage with diphtheria toxoid containing vaccines

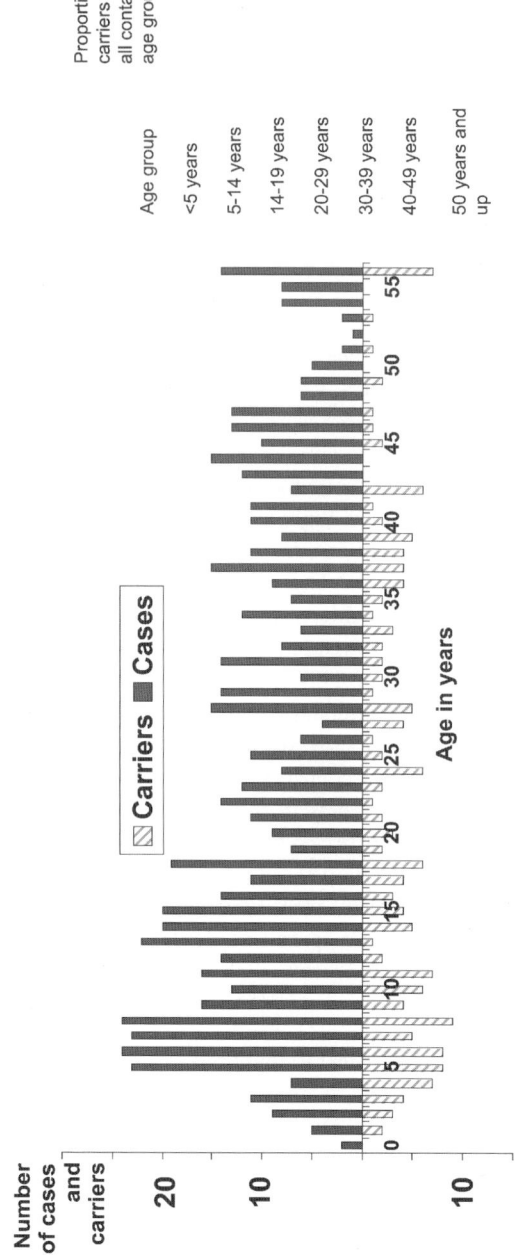

Fig. 4 Diphtheria cases and carriers among their close contacts by age (1994–1996) and proportion of carriers among close contacts by age group

among children in the 1980s and early 1990s, and a large gap of immunity among adults (Dittmann 2000). In addition, the spread of the epidemic was facilitated by several factors including: (1) large-scale population movements as ethnic Slavs emigrated from Central Asian and Caucasian countries to Russia and the Ukraine and as refugees fled conflict in the Caucasus, Tajikistan, and Moldova; (2) rapid socioeconomic decline; (3) deterioration of the health infrastructure; (4) delay in implementing aggressive measures to control the epidemic; (5) inadequate information for physicians and the public; and (6) inadequate supplies of diphtheria vaccines and therapeutics. The quality of Russian-manufactured diphtheria toxoid vaccine does not appear to have contributed to the epidemic; this vaccine was highly effective in the Russian mass immunization campaign as well as in epidemiologic and serologic studies conducted in the Ukraine and Russia.

5.5
Lessons Learned and Future Needs

The struggle to control epidemic diphtheria in the NIS and Baltic States provided important lessons. The experience of what was successful supports that the most important goal of control measures in a widespread diphtheria epidemic is achieving the highest possible immunization coverage for the whole population and that the needed levels of population immunity needed for epidemic control can most quickly be achieved by a mass immunization campaign. Maintenance of population immunity should be accomplished by routine immunization. There is incomplete agreement on the appropriate target levels for adult population immunity in the absence of a widespread diphtheria outbreak, reflecting limitations on the ability to predict the risk of future diphtheria outbreaks.

5.6
Epidemic Control: Case-Centered Control Measures and Mass Immunization

The primary lesson in epidemic control learned from the NIS and Baltic States was that case-centered control efforts are likely to be ineffective if large population immunity gaps exist while rapidly raising immunity to high levels among all age groups will be effective in controlling even a widespread diphtheria epidemic. Recommended case-centered diphtheria control measures include the isolation and antibiotic treatment of cases, and antibiotic prophylaxis and full immunization of contacts (Farizo 1993). Case-centered control efforts failed to stop the spread of diphtheria in any of the affected countries in 1990–1994; this widespread failure suggests that case-centered control measures could similarly fail in future outbreak situations where substantial child and adult population immunity gaps exist. However, case-centered control measures will facilitate rapid control of an epidemic and need to be fully implemented; incomplete implementation of some measures, especially the antibiotic prophylaxis of contacts, in the NIS epidemic may have facilitated spread of the epidemic.

In contrast, the mass immunization campaigns that reached nearly the entire population were highly effective in the NIS epidemic, especially when carried out quickly. While one to three doses of diphtheria toxoid are needed to induce diphtheria immunity in an individual depending on their prior immunization, a rapid 'one-dose for all' strategy worked extremely well in the NIS. This strategy aimed to rapidly deliver one dose of diphtheria toxoid containing vaccine (at least 2 Lf diphtheria toxoid per dose) to virtually the entire adult population while ensuring full age-appropriate immunization for children. The NIS experience also suggests that a rapid one-dose strategy has great logistic advantages in diphtheria epidemics involving large populations. The amount of vaccine needed in a multi-dose strategy for large populations can be difficult to procure and transport; despite heroic efforts by national and international partners, limitations on vaccine supply slowed implementation of the NIS mass immunization strategy.

A similar 'one-dose for all' strategy will be appropriate during future epidemics in populations where the majority of the population has been immunologically primed. However, certain distinct age groups of adults, such as the 30–50-year-old adults in the NIS epidemic, are likely to have larger numbers of individuals who have not been immunologically primed against diphtheria due to incomplete initial implementation of immunization programs and decreasing exposure to diphtheria over time. It is likely that these cohorts can be identified by epidemiologic analysis of the outbreak cases; supplemental serologic studies can be conducted for confirmation. The epidemic control strategy should ensure that these most-susceptible age cohorts receive a full primary series and could later provide a three-dose primary series to all other adult age groups, if warranted. Successful implementation of a multiple dose strategy will require special measures for tracking adult immunization since routine immunization monitoring systems are exclusively focused on childhood immunization in almost all countries. In the implementation of the mass campaigns during the NIS epidemic, some countries exempted children who had recently completed full immunization from mass campaigns; although no adverse effect on the results of the mass campaigns is discernable, such a practice is highly dependent on the availability of reliable childhood immunization records.

A higher susceptibility among rural residents was observed previously in unvaccinated populations and in some parts of the NIS and Baltic States during the epidemic. No strategy adjustment for rural–urban differences proved necessary in the NIS epidemic; however, these differences may be more important in future large-scale diphtheria epidemics as immunization programs in some developing countries may be less effective in reaching rural areas than was the case in the Soviet Union.

A further lesson in epidemic control from the NIS and Baltic States epidemic outbreak was in how to develop an effective international response. During the epidemic, an international coalition with close collaboration between international partners and national health authorities of the affected countries was developed; this coalition generated the guiding strategy and sufficient resources to implement that strategy. The coalition required coordination by a body with sufficient personnel and financial resources.

5.7
Prevention

A primary lesson learned from the diphtheria epidemic in the NIS and Baltic States is that large numbers of susceptible children coupled with an immunity gap in adults creates the potential for an extensive epidemic. In 1996, the Advisory Group on Immunization for the WHO European Region recommended steps in routine immunization policy to eliminate these gaps by focusing on the following three areas: (1) achieving very high coverage with primary immunization with DTP vaccine in infancy and ensuring booster doses of diphtheria toxoid containing vaccines at 16–36 months of age, school entry, and school exit; (2) including an additional booster dose during school years in countries with ongoing or recent diphtheria epidemics; and (3) implementing periodic booster doses for adults in high-diphtheria risk countries and considering booster doses in other countries depending on the degree of risk, the ability to provide boosters, and the quality of diphtheria surveillance.

Broad consensus in all countries exists for improving coverage with primary immunization for preschool aged children; there is less agreement on immunization of older age groups with booster doses of diphtheria toxoid. In 1998, the Scientific Advisory Group of Experts (SAGE) for immunization policy for WHO recommended a gradual phase-in of Td to replace monovalent tetanus toxoid for use in school-based booster dose programs (beginning in countries with high DTP coverage) and for immunizing women of child-bearing age (WHO 1998). Countries in Europe and the Americas have added additional booster doses of diphtheria toxoid for older children, adolescents, and at least some populations of adults such as women of child-bearing age; however, few countries in other regions have intensified immunization of older children and adults against diphtheria. A subsequent WHO advisory group noted that due to concerns that the global tetanus vaccine supply could be adversely affected, optimal vaccine policymaking would require an improved understanding of the epidemic risk related to the build-up of diphtheria susceptible persons (WHO 2004).

There are numerous areas where better data could lead to an improved understanding of the risk for future outbreaks of diphtheria. Although the NIS epidemic illustrates that there is a danger posed by immunity gaps in children and adults, it remains unclear what level of population immunity in these groups is needed to prevent epidemic spread and whether immunity gaps isolated to adult groups pose any significant increased risk. There may be differences in the risk of epidemic spread associated with different strains of toxigenic *C. diphtheriae* and with different levels of socioeconomic development. In addition to our imperfect understanding of the theoretical framework of epidemic spread of diphtheria, the ability to predict diphtheria risk is hampered by extremely limited data for most developing countries on levels of population immunity and the prevalence of diphtheria. Even fewer data are available on the circulation of toxigenic *C. diphtheriae* in these countries.

With the low likelihood of eradication of toxigenic *C. diphtheriae* and our imperfect understanding of future risk, the current priority for improved control of diphtheria should remain improving coverage with diphtheria toxoid containing vaccines among children in developing countries. In the longer term, diphtheria control and immunization policy would benefit from improved quality and availability of epidemiologic data and improvements in diphtheria vaccines that could result in improved duration or quality of immunity while reducing the frequency of adverse events.

References

Anonymous (1997) Diphtheria cases notified in the European Union. Eurosurveillance 2:63–64
Anonymous (2003) Diphtheria, Afghanistan. Weekly Epidemiological Record 78:314.
Centers for Disease Control and Prevention (2004) Fatal respiratory diphtheria in a U.S. traveler to Haiti–Pennsylvania, 2003. Morbid Mortal Weekly Rep 52:1285–1286
Cerdeño-Tárraga AM, Efstratiou A, Dover LG, Holden MTG, Pallen M, et al. (2003) The complete genome sequence and analysis of *Corynebacterium diphtheriae* NCTC13129. Nucl Acids Res 31:6515–6523
Christenson B, Hellström U, Sylvan SPE, Henriksson L, Granström M (2001) Impact of a vaccination campaign on adult immunity to diphtheria. Vaccine 19:1133–1140
Collier RJ (2001) Understanding the mode of action of diphtheria toxin: a perspective on progress during the 20th century. Toxicon 39:1793–1803

Coyle MD, Groman NB, Russell JQ, Harnisch JP, Rabin M, et al. (1989) The molecular epidemiology of three biotypes of *Corynebacterium diphtheriae* in the Seattle outbreak, 1972–1982. J Infect Dis159:670–679

Craster CV (1941) The mass immunization of pre-school children. J Med Soc New Jersey 38:39–41

Department of Vaccines and Biologicals (2004) WHO Vaccine-Preventable Diseases: Monitoring System. 2004 Global Summary. World Health Organization, Geneva

Dittmann S, Wharton M, Vitek, C, Ciotti M, Galazka A, et al. (2000) Successful control of epidemic diphtheria in the states of the former Soviet Union of Soviet Socialist Republics: lessons learned. J Infect Dis 181 (Suppl. 1):S10–S22

Farizo KM, Strebel PM, Chen RT, Kimbler A, Cleary TJ, et al. (1993) Fatal respiratory disease due to *Corynebacterium diphtheriae*: case report and review of guidelines for management, investigation, and control. Clin Infect Dis 16:59–68

Galazka AM, Robertson SE (1995) Diphtheria: Changing patterns in the developing world and the industrialized world. Eur J Epidemiol 11:107–117

Galazka A, Tomaszunas-Blszczyk J (1997) Why do adults contract diphtheria? Eurosurveillance 2:60–63

Golaz A, Hardy IR, Glushkevich TG, Areytchiuk EK, Deforest A, et al. (2000) Evaluation of a single dose of diphtheria-tetanus toxoids among adults in Odessa, Ukraine, 1995: immunogenicity and adverse reactions. J Infect Dis 181 (Suppl. 1):S203–S207

Griffith AH (1979) The role of immunization in the control of diphtheria. Developments in Biological Standardization 43:3–13

Hróbjartsson A, Gøtzche PC, Gluud C (1998) The controlled clinical trial turns 100 years: Fibiger's trial of serum treatment of diphtheria. Br Med J 317:1243–1245

Holmes RK (2000) Biology and molecular epidemiology of diphtheria toxin and the *tox* gene. J Infect Dis 181 (Suppl. 1):S156–S167

Khetsuriani N, Music S, Deforest A, Sutter RW (2000) Evaluation of a single dose of diphtheria toxoid among adults in the Republic of Georgia, 1995: immunogenicity and adverse reactions. J Infect Dis 181 (Suppl. 1):S208–S212

Lee HF, Tseng LR, Yueh YY, Wu UC (1999) Immunity against diphtheria in Taiwan (Chinese). J Microbiol, Immunol, Infect32:206–212

Magdei M, Melnic A, Benes O, Bukova V, Chicu V, et al. Epidemiology and control of diphtheria in the Republic of Moldova, 1946–1996. J Infect Dis 181 (Suppl. 1):S47–S54

Markina SS, Maksimova NM, Vitek CR, Bogatyreva EY, Monisov AA (2000) Diphtheria in the Russian Federation in the 1990 s. J Infect Dis 181 (Suppl. 1):S27–S34

Marston CK, Jamieson F, Cahoon F, Lesiak G, Golaz A. et al. (2001) Persistence of a distinct *Corynebacterium diphtheriae* clonal group within two communities in the United States and Canada where diphtheria is endemic. J Clin Microbiol 39:1586–1590

McCloskey RV, Saragea A, Maximescu P (1972) Phage typing in diphtheria outbreaks in the southwestern United States, 1968 – 1971. J Infect Dis 126:196–199

McKinnon NE, Ross MA, Defries RD (1931) Reduction in diphtheria in 36,000 Toronto school children as a result of an immunization campaign. Can Public Health J 22:217–223

McKinnon NE (1942) Diphtheria prevented. In Cruickshank R (ed). Control of the Common Fevers. The Lancet Ltd, London, 1942, pp 41 56

Pappenheimer AM Jr. (1980) Diphtheria: studies on the biology of an infectious disease. Harvey Lectures 1980–81 76:45–73

Patel M, Morey F, Butcher A, Moore C, Brennan R, Mollison L (1994) The frequent isolation of toxigenic and non-toxigenic *C. diphtheriae* at Alice Springs Hospital. Commun Dis Intel 18:310–311

Ramon G (1923) Sur le pouvoir floculant ct sur les proprietes immunisantes d'une toxin diphterique rendue anatoxique (anatoxine). C. R Acad Sci 177:1338–1440.

Ronne T, Valentelis R, Tarum S, Griskevica A, Wachmann CH, et al. (2000) Immune response to diphtheria booster vaccine in the Baltic States. J Infect Dis 181 (Suppl. 1):S213–S219

Stowman K (1945) The epidemic outlook in Europe. Br Med J 1:72–74

Sutter RW, Hardy IR, Kozlova IA, et al. (2000) Immunogenicity of tetanus-diphtheria toxoids (Td) among Ukrainian adults: implications for diphtheria control in the Newly Independent States of the former Soviet Union. J Infect Dis 181 (Suppl. 1):S197–S203

Tharmaphornpilas P, Yoocharoan P, Prempree P, Youngpairoj S, Sriprasert P, et al. (2001) Diphtheria in Thailand in the 1990s. J Infect Dis 184:1035–1040

US Bureau of the Census (1975) Historical Statistics of the United States, Colonial Times to 1970, Bicentennial Edition, Part 1. US Department of Congress, Washington, DC, pp 58, 63

Vitek CR, Brisgalov SP, Bragina VY, Zhilyakov AM, Bisgard KM, et al. (1999) Epidemiology of epidemic diphtheria in three regions, Russia, 1994–1996. Eur J Epidemiol 15:75–83

Vitek CR, Velibekov AS (2000) Epidemic diphtheria in the 1990s: Azerbaijan. J Infect Dis 181 (Suppl. 1):S73–S79

Wharton M, Dittmann S, Strebel PM, Mortimer EA (eds) (2000) Control of epidemic diphtheria in the Newly Independent States of the former Soviet Union. J Infect Dis 181 (Suppl. 1):S1–S248

WHO (1995) WHO/UNICEF strategy for diphtheria control in the Newly Independent States. World Health Organization, Regional Office for Europe, Copenhagen

WHO Vaccine Preventable Diseases Monitoring System. Antigen schedule selection centre: accessed on January 30, 2005 at
http://www.who.int/vaccines/globalsummary/immunization/scheduleselect.cfm

WHO (1997) Expanded programme on immunization (EPI): Diphtheria control. Weekly Epidemiological Record 72:128–130

WHO (1998) The Children's Vaccine Initiative (CVI) and WHO's global programme for vaccines and immunization (GPV) - Recommendations from the Strategic Advisory Group of Experts (SAGE). Weekly Epidemiol Rec73:281–284

WHO (2004) Recommendations from the Strategic Advisory Group of Experts to the Department of Immunization, Vaccines, and Biologicals. Weekly Epidemiol Rec79:43–52

Zingher A (1921) Diphtheria preventive work in the public schools of New York City. Arch Pediatr 38:336–359

Universal Mass Vaccination Against Hepatitis A

F. E. André (✉)

23 Rue du Moulin, 1330 Rixensart, Belgium
feandre@yahoo.com

1	Introduction	96
2	Virology and Epidemiology of HAV	97
3	Disease Burden	99
4	Vaccine Properties and Vaccination Policies	100
5	Early Demonstration Projects	102
6	Planned Mass Prevention Programmes Carried Out	102
6.1	Puglia, Italy	102
6.2	Catalonia, Spain	103
6.3	North Queensland, Australia	104
6.4	Israel	105
6.5	USA (11 States Routine Vaccination "Recommended" and in Six "for Consideration")	106
6.6	Other Pioneers	108
7	Is Elimination or Even Eradication Possible?	108
	References	110

Abstract When first introduced in 1992 the hepatitis A vaccine was recommended for individuals at high risk of exposure. This policy was not expected to have a significant impact on disease incidence at population level in view of the epidemiology of the hepatitis A virus (HAV). More recently two countries, Israel and Bahrain, and regions or subpopulations in others (Australia, China, Byelorussia, Italy, Spain, US) have embarked upon more ambitious vaccination programmes that aim to immunize whole birth cohorts. After a brief survey of the virology and epidemiology of HAV, the disease burden it inflicts and a short history of the development of HAV vaccines – both live (in China) and killed vaccines are available – the vaccination programmes introduced in the countries mentioned above are described. The results have been spectacular: disease incidence, not only in the vaccinated cohorts but also in the whole population, have plummeted within a few years of the start of mass vaccination. There is now convincing evidence that the vaccine confers herd immunity if the main spreaders of the virus are targeted for immunization. This finding should encourage other countries to start mass vaccination programmes against HAV, particularly as pharmacoeconomic studies are beginning to show that such a strategy could be a cost-effective way of controlling the disease. It is now even conceivable to eradicate HAV. In fact, this should be easier to achieve than polio eradication as HAV vaccines confer more durable immunity than polio vaccines. However, the global disease burden of HAV is generally thought not to be high enough to justify such an undertaking in the foreseeable future.

1
Introduction

The successful outcome of the long search for a vaccine against hepatitis A [1, 2] was celebrated and discussed at an international symposium, held in Vienna, Austria, in January 1992. The symposium was attended by most of the researchers who had made the major scientific and technical breakthroughs that made possible its development. It provided the occasion to present Havrix – an inactivated (killed) alum-adsorbed whole-virion vaccine – to the scientific community [3]. It was the first hepatitis A vaccine to be licensed. Since then, three similar vaccines – two alum-adsorbed (Avaxim and Vaqta) and one (Epaxal) formulated in 'immunostimulating reconstituted influenza virosomes' – have been made available [4]. These vaccines are now on the market in most developed and many developing countries. They are essentially interchangeable. Any difference between the inactivated vaccines produced by reputable manufacturers in developed countries are probably not of clinical importance [5]. Therefore, the vaccine used in the vaccination programmes described hereafter will not be mentioned. A bivalent hepatitis A and B vaccine (Twinrix) has also been introduced. In China, a live attenuated vaccine has been developed [6]. It is now in routine use there. Since this vaccine is not efficacious orally and must therefore, like the killed vaccines, be injected, it has no medical advantage over them. Because of the theoretical advantages of killed vaccines, and their outstanding safety and efficacy, the development of a live vaccine has been stopped in Western countries [7]. When the vaccine was first introduced, the recommendations of the public health authorities in all countries, no doubt because of economic considerations, were to vaccinate only individuals belonging to high-risk groups. This was a policy doomed to have a limited impact on disease incidence in the general population as was predicted from the known epidemiology of the infection [8]. A gradual shift to more effective strategies occurred when, with increasing use, it became clear that hepatitis A vaccines are safe and highly efficacious [4, 9, 10, 11]. At the end of the twentieth century, several countries (or regions of some countries) have embarked upon more ambitious immunization programmes to control the disease on a population-wide basis. Pharmacoeconomic studies are increasingly demonstrating the socioeconomic wisdom of this approach not only for hepatitis A [12, 13] but also for all prevalent vaccine-preventable diseases since "for most childhood vaccination programs......every dollar invested leads to significant savings to the society" [14].

In this chapter, the spectacular results obtained recently in some countries by mass vaccination against hepatitis A will be summarized. The possibility, in the future, of national, regional or even global control of disease caused by the hepatitis A virus (HAV) will also be examined. Before that, a brief description of the relevant virological and epidemiological characteristics of HAV and the disease burden that it inflicts will be given.

2
Virology and Epidemiology of HAV

Human HAV is a picornavirus with several unique properties that justify its classification in its own genus, named hepatovirus [15]. Although HAV may replicate in a variety of human cells – including intestinal cells that are an inescapable passage to the liver through the blood stream – and other primate cells it naturally grows to any extent only in human hepatocytes. From there, it gains entry, through the bile duct, to the gut and is then shed in faeces. Human faeces constitutes the sole reservoir that is epidemiologically relevant, in spite of the fact that HAV has occasionally been isolated in other primates [16]. It is remarkably resistant to physicochemical inactivation. It can survive for many weeks in the environment under what might seem unfavourable conditions, such as in sea water. There, it can be concentrated in shellfish [17]. The catastrophic epidemic that occurred in Shanghai during the Chinese New Year of 1988 was caused by the widespread consumption of raw or inadequately cooked contaminated hairy clams [18].To be inactivated HAV must be exposed to a temperature of 85 C for at least 1 min [19] and it will survive for weeks in dried faeces [20]. Although genetic heterogeneity, that has allowed delineation of four distinct genotypes, has been demonstrated, only one serotype is recognized. This is the reason that a vaccine for worldwide use need contain only one strain of the virus [21].

Infection with HAV occurs when a nonimmune individual ingests food, water or fomites contaminated by faeces from a person in the shedding phase of a HAV infection. Very rarely, it can also be transmitted iatrogenically through inoculation of blood products during blood transfusions, therapy of clotting disorders or medical procedures with unsterilized equipment since there is a viraemic phase of the infection [22]. However, spread of the virus in a population is essentially by the faecal – oral route since the main natural source of the virus is human faecal matter [23]. The endemicity of this virus has been abundantly documented under different societal conditions, including times of warfare [24–26].

Throughout history, what we now call hepatitis A was known as the jaundice of military campaigns and it has influenced the outcome of many battles. Virus transmission is facilitated by poor sanitation and unhygienic practices and is therefore rampant in socioeconomically underprivileged nations, communities, and situations where human faeces is disposed in ways that allow contamination of food and drinking water. In such environments exposure to the virus is almost inevitable and most children are infected, in most cases subclinically, before they reach the age of 5 years and thus become naturally immune, as evidenced by the appearance of serum HAV antibodies that persist for life. Naturally-acquired – and probably also vaccine-induced immunity (see later) – against re-infection and, certainly, disease is lifelong. Populations with a high level of natural immunity in all age groups live under circumstances where infection is highly endemic. In communities with very good sanitation and hygienic habits – like the unfailing provision of safe drinking water, hygienic methods of preparing and distributing food and good personal habits (such as scrupulous handwashing after defecation)–exposure to the virus may not happen until adult life. At that stage, exposure and infection may occur when a nonimmune individual travels to a highly endemic area for pleasure or business [27] and because of the adoption of unsafe personal lifestyles, like promiscuous sexuality or behaviour associated with drug addiction [28, 29]. In populations with low levels of natural immunity until early or late adult life (which usually reflects infection in a distant less affluent past) the endemicity of infection is low or very low.

There, the main route of infection is through close direct or indirect contact with an infected person and not by consumption of contaminated food or water. In the rest of the world, where infection occurs gradually with increasing age through both ingestion of contaminated food and water and close personal contact with persons excreting infectious virus the endemicity is described as being intermediate. On the basis of this classification, global maps have been produced, showing, in different colours, areas of the world with "very low", "low", "intermediate" and "high" endemicities. However, this is an oversimplification of the real world where low and high endemicities may coexist next to each other in different communities of the same country. Furthermore, the situation has been changing rapidly in the last few decades and, because of improving socioeconomic conditions, many less developed countries are shifting from "high" to "intermediate" endemicities. A recent review of global anti-HAV seroprevalence shows that, apart from the poorest countries in Africa, levels of natural immunity are declining in all parts of the world [30]. The socioeconomically privileged in many developing countries are already experiencing "intermediate" or even "low" endemicities. This trend, paradoxically, is bringing with it new dangers (which will be discussed later) that plead in favour of more extensive immunization programmes in countries or communities that can afford it, particularly when cost – effectiveness analysis shows that they are more efficient than many generally accepted health care interventions [31].

3
Disease Burden

From seroprevalence surveys of anti-HAV [30] it can be deduced that hepatitis A is one of the most prevalent viral infections in the world. On average, about 1.5 million cases are estimated by the World Health Organization to occur annually [32]. However, because of under-reporting, the true disease incidence is undoubtedly very much higher. In the US a thorough study, that used a sophisticated mathematical model to estimate case incidence from observed age-adjusted seroprevalence rates, came to the conclusion that between 1980 and 1999 the true case incidence was 10.4 times that actually reported [33]. In other parts of the world the degree of under-reporting is unlikely to be lower. Estimation of global disease incidence is rendered difficult by the fact that infection results in clinical disease at very different frequencies depending upon age at infection. In early life infection generally is asymptomatic, subclinical or mild. With advancing age infection more frequently causes disease of increasing severity, and even death, from fulminant hepatitis or complications, is no longer exceptional. The case-fatality rate for those above 40 years of age was ~1% in 1995 in the US [34]. Clinical hepatitis A typically manifests itself 28 days (range, 15–50 days) after infection. It is an acute disease, characterized by the rapid onset of increasing fatigue, malaise, nausea, anorexia, vomiting, fever, myalgia and diffuse abdominal pain and – in children – diarrhoea. This may be followed, within a few days to a week, by the appearance of dark urine, pale stools and jaundice. This symptomatology is no different from that experienced by patients suffering from other forms of hepatitis (B, C, D, E, etc.) and a specific laboratory diagnosis (detection of serum anti-HAV IgM) is necessary; a requirement not fulfilled in most parts of the world. The natural course of the disease varies but most patients start feeling better within a few weeks. Most will recover fully, although sometimes after a convalescence of many months. In the 1988 epidemic in Shanghai only 47 deaths occurred among 310,746 reported cases in mainly adolescents and young adults [35].

Hepatitis A infection never leads to a chronic state but can progress to usually benign complications such as cholestatic jaundice, relapsing hepatitis and other rare exta-hepatic disorders. The most dreaded complication, with a high case-fatality rate, is fulminant hepatitis (which develops at an average rate of 1 per 10,000; with a wide range depending upon age in different series) that often requires liver transplantation to save life. Hepatitis A has been identified as "the predominant aetiology of acute hepatitis and fulminant hepatic failure in Argentina and probably in the world" [36]. In Latin America, hepatitis A is recognized as a major cause of acute liver failure [37]. A trustworthy estimate of deaths caused worldwide by HAV is not available.

Another way of measuring the burden of hepatitis A is its economic impact. It has been estimated that it drains 1.5–3 billion $US per year from the world economy. For example, in 1997 the total cost to society in the US was put at $488 million [38]. The impact of the disease on a national economy will vary tremendously depending upon local variables like inflicted morbidity, mortality and cost of health care delivery. Countries in the high endemicity category, that are usually economically weak, are less affected than rich countries because infection occurs asymptomatically in early life and treatment costs for the relatively few clinical cases are low. When endemicity moves into the intermediate category, due to socioeconomic improvements, the economic drain may be much higher since infection will occur later in life (and will therefore be more serious) and health care becomes more expensive. In future, the ongoing improvements of sanitation and hygiene in most parts of the world, will, paradoxically, result in a greater disease burden as past experience in Greece [39] among many other countries – has clearly shown. Disease burden, measured by morbidity, mortality, economic costs and – as is often forgotten – psychological distress, must be assessed locally and be continuously updated due to rapidly changing conditions.

4
Vaccine Properties and Vaccination Policies

Protection conferred against infection by killed hepatitis A vaccine, is mainly mediated by neutralizing antibodies [40]. It is expected to last at least 25 years because of the slow decline of vaccine-induced antibodies [41] and probably much longer – possibly for life – due to the induction of immunological memory and the long incubation period of the disease.

Booster doses are thought to be unnecessary to maintain disease immunity [42]. The response to the vaccine is blunted by the presence of pre-existing serum antibodies acquired from passive immunization with immunoglobulin [43] or through the placenta [44]. Consequently, the vaccine is licensed only after 1 year of age (2 years in the US) when maternally acquired antibody has largely disappeared. However, immunological memory is elicited even in the presence of maternal antibodies [45] and the vaccine would, no doubt, be efficacious in infancy in environments where natural immunity is rare in women of child-bearing age.

Vaccination policies can range from banning vaccine use to mandatory inoculation of everybody. The efficient strategy is to aim for maximal disease reduction with a minimum financial outlay. Any policy must also take into consideration other perceived needs, available resources and other possible beneficial interventions. However, given the availability of a safe and efficacious vaccine, it is obvious that reason dictates that it should be used as effectively as possible. In order to maximize the efficiency of a vaccination programme, it is important to know the predominant ways in which the pathogen is spread within and between age groups and other subsections in a population, the period during which a pathogen is transmissible and its infectiousness. Age-related disease burden and peak incidence are also relevant parameters that influence what constitutes the most efficient policy [46, 47]. Characteristics of the vaccine that are critical include the duration of vaccine-induced protection, the earliest age at which it is efficacious and practical considerations like ease of administration and cost of delivery. Clearly it is not easy to choose an "optimal" policy. Computer-assisted modelling of epidemiological and economic parameters should, in defined situations, help to make an objective choice between possible policies [48]. In the end, any recommended policy is a sociopolitical decision informed by economic considerations. As mentioned earlier, economic reasons were, no doubt, at the root of the timid policy of all public health authorities of restricting vaccine use to some population groups (like presumed nonimmune travellers to high endemicity regions, men who have sex with men, drug addicts, food-handlers who may spread the virus to their clients and individuals – such as patients with chronic liver disease – who may suffer more severe illness) in spite of the fact that such high risk groups were known to contribute, in total, only a minority of the cases in the general population [49]. It took some time and well-conducted epidemiological studies to establish the now generally accepted message that "sustained nationwide reductions in incidence are more likely to result from routine childhood vaccination than from targeted vaccination of high-risk groups" [50] a simple truth that was also learned slowly in the case of hepatitis B [51]. In the case of hepatitis A, this conclusion is even more justified since the evidence that children are the main spreaders of the virus in the general population has gradually become more persuasive [52, 53]. An obvious hypothesis that begged to be tested is that interruption of virus circulation, through vaccination as early as possible in childhood, would result in a major reduction of virus transmission – and thus disease incidence – in the whole population, not by producing classical herd immunity [54] but rather through the mechanism of community immunity [47].

5
Early Demonstration Projects

The protective efficacy of inactivated hepatitis A vaccine was clearly demonstrated in two randomized double-blind field trials [55, 56]. The first hint that vaccine-induced community immunity could play a major role in overall reduction of hepatitis A disease incidence came in the demonstration project in Slovakia where a large community-wide outbreak, that started in two villages in December 1991, was terminated by vaccination – in December 1992 – of pupils attending the common school [57]. A more extensive proof of the effectiveness of vaccination was provided by the rapid state-wide elimination of shepatitis A in Alaska by the inoculation – between April and May 1993 – of only a single dose of vaccine.

Evidence that vaccination of at least 70% of the targeted population (the presumed nonimmune) resulted in herd immunity was obtained. The results were so impressive that the editor of the journal that published the findings felt it was appropriate to state that she was "proud to publish proof that prevention practices produce profound performances" [58]. Other projects have further demonstrated the perspicacity of this pronouncement [59, 60].

6
Planned Mass Prevention Programmes Carried Out

After the scientific proof of the wisdom of mass vaccination against hepatitis A was provided, several jurisdictions realized it was their sociopolitical duty to implement that strategy of control where local epidemiological and economical data – not to mention political motives – justified it. What follows is a chronological record of what has been done and achieved in the recent past.

6.1
Puglia, Italy

Puglia, a region in the southeast of Italy with a population of four million, experienced intermediate HAV endemicity until the 1990s. The main mode of transmission was identified as the consumption of shellfish [61]. In interepidemic periods the annual incidence was 20–30/100,000. There were large epidemics in 1992 and 1996–1997. In 1995, a computerized system of infectious disease notification was instituted which allowed a fairly accurate estimate of the number of cases that occurred in 1996 and 1997. The numbers reported were respectively, 5673 (138.8/100,000) and 5389 (131.8/100,000) cases; mainly in the 11–30 year-old group. A pharmacoeconomic study of the 1996 epidemic showed that it had cost over 40 million $US to society as a whole [62]. This finding, coupled with strong epidemiological arguments, prompted the local government to administer, as from the end of 1997, a dose of hepatitis A vaccine at 15–18 months (simultaneously with MMR vaccine) and to replace the monovalent hepatitis B vaccine given in three doses at 12 years in the national hepatitis B programme mandated by law since 1991 [63] with the bivalent hepatitis A+B vaccine. This policy was expected to bring "important economic savings" [64] which, no doubt, (actual figures are not yet available), have been realized in view of the fact that HAV epidemics have not occurred since and cases are now rare in the region. On the other hand, in a neighbouring region, Campania, where routine vaccination was not performed, an outbreak with 615 cases occurred in 2004 [65].

6.2
Catalonia, Spain

Catalonia, an autonomous province of Spain with 6 million inhabitants, started a programme of vaccination against hepatitis B in schools in 1990. This programme proved very successful since the coverage rate attained was >90% and it resulted in a reduction of ~80% in the incidence of hepatitis B in the 10–19 year age group over an 8-year follow-up [66, 67]. In Catalonia, the main mode of HAV transmission that has been identified in reported cases is person-to-person contact (31%) and ~50% of the cases were of unidentified source. As the main brunt of the HAV disease burden is borne by adolescent and young adults and the initial recommendation of vaccinating only those individuals in high-risk groups (travellers, day-centre staff, male homosexuals and others) would prevent at most 16% of cases, it was obvious to think of replacing the monovalent hepatitis B vaccine with the bivalent A+B vaccine. This idea was particularly attractive as, in view of the existing infrastructure to deliver hepatitis B vaccine, it would entail an incremental cost of only 1.98€ per vaccinated child. In September 1998, the switch was made, at first in pilot mode and later throughout the province. The outcome of this initiative has been shown to be highly beneficial.

The reduction in disease incidence observed in the 3 years before (1996–1998) and after (1999–2001) the programme started was statistically significant in all age groups of the population except the >60 year olds. The effectiveness of the programme in the vaccinated cohorts was estimated at 97.0 (95% confidence interval, 78.5–99.6). In the <5, 5–9, 10–14, 15–19, 20–29, 30–39, 40–49, 50–59 year age groups the fold-reductions in disease incidence were respectively 1.7, 2.4, 5.9, 2.6, 2.5, 2.1, 3.6, and 2.4 being only 1.6 (not significant) in the >60 year age group. Although, as clearly stated by the authors reporting these spectacular results [68], the cyclical nature of hepatitis A disease incidence could explain these findings, the most likely explanation remains that the vaccination programme was the cause. Recently, the Cataluyan group presented data to show that the programme "is a very efficient intervention programme that saves money for the health system" [69]. Can any Minister of Health ask for more?

6.3
North Queensland, Australia

In the 1990s, hepatitis A reached the status of a "major public health problem" [70] in North Queensland because two large epidemics occurred during the decade [71]. It was only from 1996 that an enhanced surveillance system allowed the clear demonstration that Indigenous people had a much higher incidence of disease than the non-Indigenous (110 versus 25 per 100,000 in 1996–1999). Three Indigenous children aged under 5 years had died of fulminant hepatitis A between 1993 and 1998 [72]. This situation demanded action. Starting in February 1999, free hepatitis A vaccine was offered at 18 and 24 months of age to Indigenous children and a catch-up vaccination, up to their sixth birthday was carried out. In 2000–2003 the incidence rate dropped to 4.0 and 2.5 per 100,000 respectively in the Indigenous and non-Indigenous populations of the region. The conclusion was that "a hepatitis A vaccination programme targeting a high-risk population within a community can reduce disease incidence in the broader community" [70]. Figure 1 illustrates this beautifully. A subsidiary – but necessary – postulate for this hypothesis to be correct is that the targeted high-risk group must be the main spreaders of the virus in the whole community. This method of conferring population immunity (i.e., breaking the chain of transmission by immunizing the transmitters) – that could be described as "transmitter-targeted-vaccination"–would be a very efficient elimination strategy.

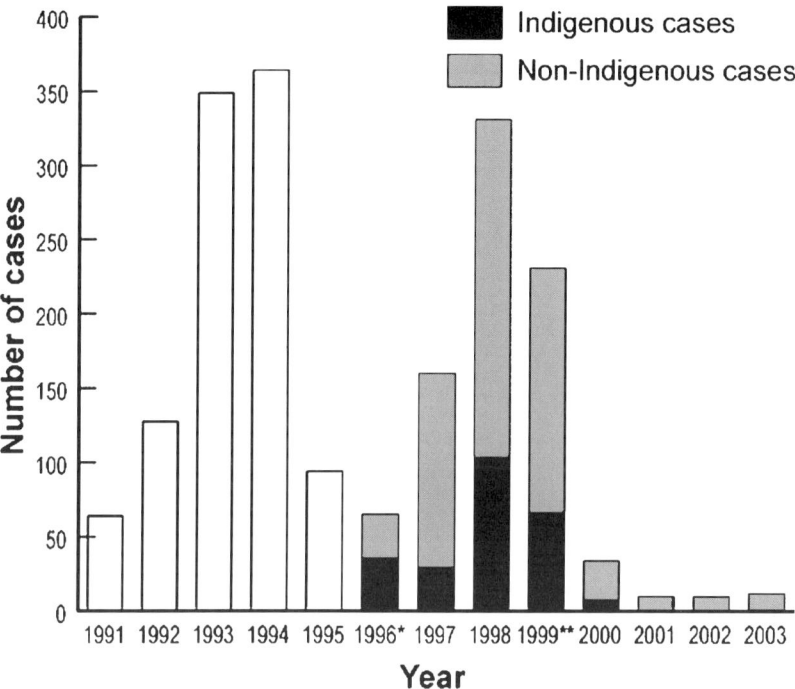

Fig. 1 Hepatitis A in North Queensland 1991–2003. Note: enhanced surveillance, with recording of ethnicity of cases, started in 1996 and the vaccination program began in February 1999. (The original of this figure was kindly supplied by Dr. Jeffrey Hanna and is reproduced with permission)

6.4
Israel

In that country, epidemiologists convinced themselves that toddlers, most of whom attend day-care centres, were not only the nursery of HAV but were also the main direct or indirect source of the virus for others in the whole population. Stopping virus transmission in that group could have a major impact on disease incidence in the country. In late 1996, an extended epidemic of hepatitis A had been halted by the vaccination of children aged 1–6 years [73]. The government therefore decided to embark upon a national programme to test the validity of the hypothesis since, furthermore, a pharmacoecomic study had highlighted its financial advantages [13]. On 1 July 1999, a free-of-charge programme of mass vaccination for all toddlers aged 18 months – with a second dose scheduled at 24 months – started in the whole country. No vaccine was offered to the rest of the population who were therefore faced with

Table 1 Reduction in reported age-specific hepatitis A disease incidence (per 100,100) in Israel in 1993–1998, 2002, 2003, 2002–2003

Age group	1993–1998	2002	2003	2002–2003	Reduction (95%CI)
<1 year	18.28	1.42	1.39	1.40	92% (79–97)
1–4 years	123.60	0.92	1.62	1.28	99% (98–99)
5–9 years	186.13	6.50	4.93	5.70	97% (96–98)
10–14 years	81.91	3.29	3.07	3.18	96% (95,97)
15–44 years	22.57	2.08	2.47	2.27	90% (88–92)
45–64 years	7.80	0.82	0.71	0.77	90% (84–94)
>65 years	3.74	1.09	1.22	1.15	69% (47–82)
All	47.98	2.16	2.21	2.18	95.4% (95–96)

% Routine vaccination of 18-month-olds with a second dose at 24 months started on 1 July 1999. (Data supplied by R. Dagan and N. Givon)

having to pay privately for protection; a prospect that only a few relished. The implementation of the programme was exemplary since the coverage attained in the target group was ~90%. Less than 10% of individuals in the rest of the population received vaccine.

The outfall was stupendous. Three years after the start of the programme disease incidence had fallen to less than less than 5/100,000 in the whole population whereas before the programme it had been at an average of 37.2 and 57.8 per 100,000 in respectively the Jewish and non-Jewish communities. The drastic disease reduction occurred not only in the vaccinated cohort but also in all age groups supporting the hypothesis that toddlers were the major transmitters of HAV in Israel (Table 1). This dramatic achievement in such a short time puts in doubt the need for routine vaccination in older age groups [74, 75]. A full account of this latest triumph of mass immunization has recently been published [76].

6.5
USA (11 States Routine Vaccination "Recommended" and in Six "for Consideration")

Inactivated hepatitis A vaccine became available in 1995 in the US. In 1996, the Advisory Committee on Immunization Practices (ACIP) recommended that it should preferentially be given to individuals at high risk of infection (travellers to countries with high or intermediate endemicity, men who have sex with men, injecting-drug users, patients with clotting-factor disorders) and patients with chronic liver disease who are prone to develop fulminant hepatitis A. It was also recommended to vaccinate children in communities with high rates of disease (Alaska Natives, American Indians, selected Hispanic and religious communities) [77]. This policy – even if fully implemented – was expected, from the known epidemiology of the virus, to have a limited impact on overall disease incidence. On 1 October 1999 updated recommendations of ACIP were published [78]. In addition to the 1996 recommendations it was stated that "children in states, counties, and communities with rates twice the 1987–1997 national average (20 per 100,000) or greater" should be vaccinated routinely – 11 states fell in that category – whereas for those living where rates are between 10 and 20 per 100,000 – six states – routine vaccination should be "considered". The impact of these two successive ACIP recommendations on disease incidence in children and their communities has been well documented. First, among American Indians and Alaska Natives the hepatitis A rates "declined dramatically coincident with implementation of routine hepatitis A vaccination" [79]. Nationally, hepatitis A has declined to "historically low rates" and a thorough analysis of the vaccine coverage and disease notification data from vaccinating and nonvaccinating areas in the US have supported the conclusion that "much of the recent reduction of hepatitis A rates is attributable to immunization and that immunization has been associated with a strong herd immunity effect" [80]. A mathematical dynamic model of hepatitis A in the US has also demonstrated that vaccination can induce strong herd immunity by targeting infants [81]. Now that pharmacoeconomic studies are demonstrating that "childhood hepatitis A vaccination is most cost-effective in areas with the highest incidence rates but would also meet accepted standards of economic efficiency in most of the US" [31] and that even assuming that "adults at high HA risk can be identified and vaccinated, the cost of targeted vaccination would exceed that of universal childhood vaccination" [82] it is only a matter of time before routine childhood vaccination is adopted nationwide [83]. In the US, the reduction in disease incidence in the vaccinating states, counties and communities – as well as in the nonvaccinating regions – has been most encouraging as shown in Table 2. In 2002, disease incidence was only 2.9 per 100,000 [84]. The latest situation analysis in the US regarding hepatitis A, showing that the disease is being brought under control by vaccination, was published very recently [85]. Elimination, in the mid-term future, is even conceivable in a country the size of the US. Also elsewhere – in Puglia, Catalonia, North Queensland and in Israel – where, in the last few years mass vaccination of well-chosen cohorts have been carried out in an exemplary fashion the results have been spectacular (Table 3). These have, no doubt, been obtained due to the "community immunity" conferred by targeting the most important virus transmitters in the population.

Table 2 Incidence of Hepatitis A by US region, 1990–2002

US region	Vaccination policy	Incidence (per 100,000) in 1987–1997	Coverage rate in 2003 [% (95%CI)]	Disease reduction in 2000–2002 (%)
11 states	Recommended statewide	>20	50.9 (47.6–54.2)	86
6 states	Consider vaccination	>10 to <20	25.0 (21.8–28.2)	89
33 states	No statewide vaccination	<20	1.4 (1.0–1.8)	50

Coverage data were obtained from [83] and disease reduction from [84]

6.6
Other Pioneers

Not many have, so far, followed the trail blazed by Puglia, Catalonia, North Queensland, Israel and some US states. Only one other country – Bahrain in late 2003 – has included hepatitis A vaccine in their national childhood vaccination programme. As yet, the author is not aware of the impact. In China, vaccination against hepatitis A is gaining favour among the well-to-do but only the richest province – Guanzhou – has formally made the recommendation, at the end of 2003, of universal vaccination; at the expense of the parents. However the successes of the trailblazers are attracting more and more interest. Some are already beginning to follow. For example, the Minsk district in Belarus started routine vaccination of 6-year-old children in 2003. The coverage rate is now ~95% [86].

7
Is Elimination or Even Eradication Possible?

This possibility was discussed at the Vienna symposium in 1992 but, at the time, all participants felt it was too early to consider it seriously [87]. Elimination has probably been achieved already in Alaska and is within sight in some other parts of the world. Although it could be argued that elimination worldwide or even eradication is possible – this should be not more and may even be less difficult than for polio (since hepatitis A vaccine gives more durable immunity than polio vaccines – both OPV and IPV – against infection) the sensible position to take is not to "dream the impossible dream" and only hope that the disease will be gradually controlled "by improving living

Table 3 Summary of hepatitis A mass vaccination programmes

Region and country	Start date	Vaccine(s) used, ages and doses	Coverage rate (%)	Period and incidence (per 100,000)	Period and incidence (per 100,000)	Disease reduction (%)	Reference
Puglia, Italy	12/1997	Monovalent A: 15–18 months (1 dose) Bivalent A+B: 12 years (3 doses)	? (~90)	1996–1997 (~135)	1999 (very low)	(~100)	[64]
Catalonia, Spain	10/1998	Bivalent A+B: preadolescents (3 doses)	>90	1996–1998 (6.2)	1999–2001 (2.6)	Overall (2.4-fold) but (97.0) in vaccinated	[68]
North Queensland, Australia	2/1999	Monovalent A: dose 1: 18 months Dose 2: 24 months Catch-up: <6 years (only Indigenous) Whole population	104 (!) 77 ? ?(low)	1996–1998 Indigenous: (110) Non-Indigenous: (25) All	2000–2003 Indigenous: (4) Non-Indigenous: (2.5) All	96.4 90.0 '12-fold'	[70]
Whole of Israel	7/1999	Monovalent A: Dose 1:18 months Dose 2:24 months	~90	1993–1998 (48.0)	2002–2003 (2.2)	95.4	[73, 74] [75]
AIAN and selected US communities	12/1996	Monovalent A: (2 doses) Children >2 years	2000 (42–71) 2003 (25.0-50.9)	1985–1989 (25.3–69.8) 1987–1997 (~20)	2000 (1.8) 2002 (2.9)	'>20-fold' Overall (~86)	[79] [83, 84]
11 US states, counties and communities with high rates in 6 states	10/1999	Catch-up: 10–12 years Children >2 years					

AIAN, American Indian and Alaska Natives

conditions in the developing world and the wise application of the existing vaccines in other areas" as a masterful treatise on the subject concluded [88]. In such areas, wisdom increasingly indicates the need for mass vaccination of children [89]. However, unfortunately, implementation of this wisdom will be dictated more by politico-economical than scientific, technical, rational and humanitarian considerations.

References

1. Deinhardt F (1992) Prevention of hepatitis A: past, present and future. Vaccine 10(Suppl.1):S10–S14
2. Hilleman MR (1993) Hepatitis and hepatitis A vaccine: a glimpse of history. J Hepatol 18(Suppl. 2):S5–S10
3. Hollinger FB, André FE, Melnick J (eds) (1992) Proceedings of International Symposium on active immunization against hepatitis A. Vaccine 10 (Suppl.1):S1–S176
4. André FE (1997) Hepatitis A vaccine: current status and future use. In: Proceedings of IX Triennial International Symposium on Viral Hepatis and Liver Disease. Rizetto M, Purcell RH, Gerin JL, Verne G (eds.).Minerva Medica, Rome, Italy, pp 624–626
5. André FE (2002) Randomised, cross-over controlled comparison of two inactivated hepatitis A vaccines. Vaccine 20:292–293
6. Mao JS, Dong DX, Zhang HY, et al. (1989) Primary study of attenuated live hepatitis A vaccine (H2 strain) in humans. J Infect Dis 159:621–624
7. André FE (1995) Approaches to a vaccine against hepatitis A: development and manufacture of an inactivated vaccine. J Infect Dis 171(Suppl.1):S33–S39
8. Margolis HS, Shapiro CN (1992) Who should receive hepatitis A vaccine? Considerations for the development of an immunization strategy. Vaccine 10(Suppl.1):S85–S87
9. Committee for Safety of Medicines (1994) Hepatitis A vaccination (Havrix). Curr Prob Pharmacovigilance 20:16
10. Niu MT, Salive M, Krueger C, Ellenberg SS (1998) Two-year review of hepatitis A vaccine safety: data from the Vaccine Adverse Event Reporting System (VAERS). Clin Infect Dis 26:1475–1476
11. André FE, Van Damme P, Safary A, Banatvala J (2002) Inactivated hepatitis A vaccine: immunogenicity, efficacy, safety and review of official recommendations for use. Exp Rev Vaccines 1(1):9–23
12. Jacobs RJ, Margolis HS, Coleman PJ (2000) The cost-effectiveness of adolescent hepatitis A vaccination in states with the highest disease rates. Arch Pediatr Adolesc Med 154(8):763–770
13. Ginsberg GM, Slater PE, Shouval D (2001) Cost-benefit of a nationwide infant immunization programme against hepatitis A in an area of intermediate endemicity. J Hepatol 34:92–99
14. Chabot I, Goetghebeur MM, Grégoire J-P (2004) The societal value of childhood immunization. Vaccine 22:1992–2005

15. Melnick JL (1992) Properties and classification of hepatitis A virus. Vaccine 10 (Suppl.1):S24–S26
16. Balayan MS (1992) Natural hosts of hepatitis A virus. Vaccine 10(Suppl.1):S27–S31
17. Garin D, Biziagos E, Crance JM et al. (1996) Survival of infectious hepatitis A virus in mineral water and seawater. In: Proceedings of the International Symposium on enterically-transmitted hepatitis viruses. Buisson Y, Coursaget P, Kane M (eds). La Simarre, Tours, France pp 48–49
18. Halliday ML, Kang LY, Zhou TK, et al. (1991) An epidemic of hepatitis A attributable to the ingestion of raw clams in Shanghai, China. J Infect Dis 164:852–859
19. Favero MS, Bond WW (1998) Disinfection and sterilization. In:Zuckerman AJ, Thomas HC (eds)Viral Hepatitis: Scientific Basis and Clinical Management. New York, Alan R. Liss, pp 565–575
20. McCaustland GL, Bond WW, Bradley DW, et al. (1982) Survival of hepatitis A in feces after drying and storage for 1 month. J Clin Microbiol 16:957–958
21. Lemon SM, Jansen RW, Brown EA (1992) Genetic, antigenic and biological differences between strains of hepatitis A virus. Vaccine 10(Suppl.1):S40–S44
22. Lemon SM (1994) The natural history of hepatitis A: the potential for transmission by transfusion of blood and blood products. Vox Sang 67(Suppl.4):19–23
23. Tassapoulos NC, Papaevangelou GL, Ticehurst JR, et al. (1986) Fecal excretion of Greek strains of hepatitis A virus in patients with hepatitis A and in experimentally infected chimpanzees. J Infect Dis 154:231–237
24. Zuckerman AJ (1983) The history of viral hepatitis from antiquity to the present. In: Deinhardt F, Deinhardt J (eds.). Viral Hepatitis: Laboratory and Clinical Science. Marcel Decker, New York, pp 2–32
25. Gust IG (1992) Epidemiological patterns of hepatitis A in different parts of the world. Vaccine 10(Suppl.1):S56–S58
26. Banatvala J (1996) Epidemiology of hepatitis A (HAV) in Europe and its relationship to immunisation. In: Proceedings of the International Symposium on enterically-transmitted hepatitis viruses. Buisson Y, Coursaget P, Kane M (eds), La Simarre, Tours, France pp 72–77
27. Steffen R, Kane MA, Shapiro CN, et al. (1994) Epidemiology and prevention of hepatitis A in travelers. JAMA 272:885–889
28. Friedman MS, Blake PA, Koehler JE et al. (2000) Factors influencing a communitywide campaign to administer hepatitis A vaccine to men who have sex with men. Am J Public Health 90:1942–1946
29. Harkness J, Gildon B, Istre GR (1989) Outbreaks of hepatitis A among illicit drug users, Oklahoma, 1984–1987. Am J Public Health 79:463–466
30. Jacobson KH, Koopman JS. (2004) Declining hepatitis A seroprevalence: a global review and analysis. Epidemiol Infect 132:1005–1022
31. Jacobs RJ, Greenberg DP, Koff RS, Saab S, Meyerhoff AS (2003) Regional variation in the cost-effectiveness of chilhood hepatitis A immunization. Pediatr Infect Dis J 22:904–914
32. WHO (2000) Weekly Epidemiol Rec 75:38–44
33. Armstrong GL, Bell BP (2002)Hepatitis A virus infection in the United States: model-based estimates and implications for childhood immunization. Pediatrics 209:839–845

34. CDC (2000) Hepatitis Surveillance Report No.57 38:1–31
35. Yao G (1991) Clinical spectrum and natural history of viral hepatitis A in a 1988 Shanghai epidemic. In:Hollinger FB, Lemon SM, Margolis HS (eds).Viral Hepatitis and Liver Disease. Williams & Wilkins, Baltimore, pp 76–78
36. Ciocca M (2000) Clinical course and consequences of hepatitis A infection. Vaccine 18(Suppl.1):S71–S74
37. Reverbel da Silveira T, Ciocca M, Moreira-Silva SF et al. (2002) Hepatitis A as an etiological agent of acute liver failure in six Latin American countries. Presentation at 3rd World Congress of Pediatric Infectious Diseases, Santiogo, Chile, November 19–23, 2002
38. CDC (1999) MMWR 48:1–37
39. Kremastinou L, Kalapothaki V, Trichopoulos D (1984) The changing epidemiology of hepatitis A in urban Greece. Am J Epidemiol 120:703–706
40. André FE, D'Hondt E, Delem A, Safary A (1992) Clinical assessment of the safety and efficacy of an inactivated vaccine: rationale and summary of findings. Vaccine 10(Suppl.1):S160–S168
41. Van Herck K, Beutels P, Van Damme P et al. (2000) Mathematical models for assessment of long-term persistence of antibodies after vaccination with two inactivated hepatitis A vaccines. J Med Virol 60(1):1–7
42. Van Damme P, Banatvala J, Fay O et al. (2003) Hepatitis A booster vaccination: is there a need? Lancet 362:1065–1071
43. Leentvaar-Kuijpers A, Coutinho RA, Brulein V, Safary A (1992) Simultaneous passive and active immunization against hepatitis A. Vaccine 10(Suppl.1):S138–S141
44. Piazza M, Safary A, Vengente A et al. (1999) Safety and immunogenicity of hepatitis A vaccine in infants: a candidate for inclusion in the childhood vaccination programme. Vaccine 17:585–588
45. Dagan R, Amir J, Mijalovsky A et al. (2000) Immunization against hepatitis A in the first year of life: priming despite the presence of maternal antibodies. Pediatr infect Dis J 19:1045–1052
46. Anderson RM, May RM (1985) Age-related changes in the rate of disease transmission: implications for the design of vaccination programme. J Hyg (Camb) 94:365–436
47. Fine PEM (2004) Community immunity. In: Vaccines, 4th ed. Plotkin SA, Orenstein WA (eds.) Elsevier, Philadelphia, pp 1443–1461
48. Miller M, Hinman AR (2004) Economic analyses of vaccine policies. In: Vaccines, 4th ed. Plotkin SA, Orenstein WA (eds.) Elsevier Inc., pp 1463–1490
49. Shapiro CN, Coleman PJ, McQuillan GM, Alter MJ, Margolis HS (1992) Epidemiology of hepatitis A: seroepidemiology and risk groups in the USA. Vaccine 10(Suppl.1) S59–S62
50. Bell BP, Shapiro CN, Alter MJ et al. (1998) The diverse patterns of hepatitis A in the United States—implications for vaccination strategies. J Infect Dis 178:1579–1584
51. World Health Organization (1992) Expanded Programme on Immunization global advisory group. Weekly Epidemiol Rec 3:11–16
52. Smith PF, Grabau JC, Wertzberger A, et al. (1997) The role of young children in a community-wide outbreak of hepatitis A. Epidemiol Infect 118:243–252
53. Gorkum J, Leenvaar-Kuijpers A, Kool JL, Coutinho RA (1998) Association between the yearly hepatitis A epidemic and travel behavior of children of immigrants in the four major cities of The Netherlands. Ned Tijdschr Geneesk 34:1919–1923

54. Fine PEM (1993) Herd immunity: history, theory, practice. Epidemiol Rev 15:265–302
55. Wertzberger A, Mench B, Kuter B et al. (1992) A controlled trial of a formalin-inactivated hepatitis A vaccine in healthy children. N Eng J Med 327:453–457
56. Innis BL, Snitbhan R, Kunasol P et al. (1994) Protection against hepatitis A by an inactivated vaccine. JAMA 271:28–34
57. Prikazsky V, Olear A, Cernoch A, Safary A, André FE. (1994) Interruption of an outbreak of hepatitis A in two villages by vaccination. J Med Virol 44:457–459
58. McMahon BJ, Beller M, Williams J et al. (1996) A program to control an outbreak of hepatitis A by using an inactivated hepatitis A vaccine. Arch Pediatr Adolesc Med 150:733–739
59. Averhoff F, Shapiro C Hyams I et al. (1996) The use of inactivated hepatitis A vaccine to interrupt a communitywide hepatitis A outbreak. Interscience Conference on Antimicrobial Agents and Chemotherapy (ICAAC) Washington DC: American Society for Microbiogy 176: [Abstract H73].
60. Craig AS, Sockwell DC, Schaffner W et al. (1998) Use of hepatitis A vaccine in a communitywide outbreak of hepatitis A. Clin Infect Dis 27:531–535
61. Mele A, Stroffolini T, Palumbo F et al. (1997) Incidence of and risk for hepatitis A in Italy: Public health indications from a 10-year surveillance. J Hepatol 26:743–747
62. Lucioni C, Cipriani V, Mazzi S, Panunzio M (1998) Cost of an outbreak of hepatitis A in Puglia, Italy. Pharmacoeconomics 13:257–266
63. Mele A, Stroffolini T, Sagliocca L et al. (1997) Control of hepatitis B in Italy. In: Proceedings of IX Triennial International Symposium on Viral Hepatitis and Liver Disease. Rizetto M, Purcell RH, Gerin JL, Verne G (eds.).Minerva Medica, Rome, Italy pp 675–677
64. Lopalco PL, Salleras L, Barbuti S et al. (2001) Hepatitis A and B in children and adolescents – what can we learn from Puglia (Italy) and Catalonia (Spain)? Vaccine 19:470–474
65. Boccia D (2004) Community outbreak of hepatitis A in southern Italy-Campania, January-May 2004. Eurosurveillance Weekly 8(23): http://www.eurosurveillance.org/ew/2004/040603.asp
66. de la Torre J, Esteban R (1995) Implementing universal vaccination programmes: Spain. Vaccine 13(Suppl.1):S72–S74
67. Salleras L, Brugera M, Buti M, Dominguez A (2000) Prospects for vaccination against hepatitis A and B in Catalonia (Spain). Vaccine 18(Suppl.1):S80–S82
68. Dominguez A, Salleras L, Carmona G, Batalla J (2003) Effectiveness of a mass hepatitis A vaccination program in preadolescents. Vaccine 21:698–701
69. Navas E,Salleras l,Gisbert R, Dominguez A, Prat A (2004) Economic evaluation of the incorporation of the hepatitis A vaccine as a combined A+B vaccine to the universal hepatitis B vaccination programme of preadolescents in schools. Fourth World Congress on Vaccines and Immunization in Tokyo, Japan, September 30-October 3 2004 [Abstract S1–S10]
70. Hanna JN, Hills SL, Humphreys JL (2004) Impact of hepatitis A vaccination of Indigenous Children on notifications of hepatitis A in North Queensland. Med J Aus 181:482–485
71. Merritt A, Symons D, Griffiths M (1999) The epidemiology of acute hepatitis A in North Queensland, 1996–1997. Commun Dis Intell 23:120–124

72. Hanna JN, Warnock TH, Shepherd RW, Selvey LA (2000) Fulminant hepatitis A in Indigenous children in North Queensland. Med J Aus 172:19–21
73. Zamir C, Rishpon D, Zamir D, Leventhal A, Rimon N, Ben-Porath E (2001) Control of a community-wide outbreak of hepatitis A by mass vaccination with inactivated hepatitis A vaccine. Eur J Clin Microbiol Infect Dis 20:185–187
74. Dagan R, Leventhal A, Anis E, Slater P, Shouval D (2002) National hepatitis A virus (HAV) immunization program aimed exclusively at toddlers in an endemic country resulting in >90% reduction in morbidity rate in all ages. 40th Annual Meeting of Infectious Diseases Society of America [Abstract 825]
75. Shouval D (2004) Universal immunization against hepatitis A to toddlers in Israel is leading to disappearance of HAV infection – The Jerusalem experience. Proceedings Biennial Scientific Meeting of International Association for Study of the Liver, Bahia, Brazil 4;4–5
76. Dagan R, Leventhal A, Anis E, Slater P, Ashur Y, Shouval D (2005) Incidence of hepatitis A in Israel following universal immunization of toddlers. JAMA 294:202–210
77. CDC (1996) Prevention of hepatitis A through active or passive immunization. Recommendations of the Advisory Committee on Immunization Practices (ACIP). MMWR 45(RR-15):1–30
78. CDC (1999) Prevention of hepatitis A through active or passive immunization. Recommendations of the Advisory Committee on Immunization Practices (ACIP). MMWR 48(RR-12):1–37
79. Bialek SR, Thoroughman DA, Hu D et al. (2004) Hepatitis A incidence and hepatitis A vaccination among American Indians and Alaska Natives, 1990–2001. Am J Public Health 94:996–1001
80. Samandari T, Bell BP, Armstrong GL (2004) Quantifying the impact of hepatitis A immunization in the United States, 1995–2001. Vaccine 22:4342–4350
81. Van Effelterre T, Zink TK, Rosenthal P (2005) A model of hepatitis A transmission in the US. Poster 19 at Conference of American College of Preventive Medicine held on February, 16–20, Washington DC
82. Jacobs RJ, Zink T, Meyerhoff AS (2004) Hepatitis A immunization strategies: universal versus targeted approaches. Proceedings annual Meeting of Pediatric Academic Societies, San Francisco, May 1–4
83. CDC (2005) Hepatitis A vaccination coverage among children aged 24–35 months, United States, 2003. MMWR 54:141–144
84. CDC hepatitis A slide set. (http://www.cdc.gov)
85. Wasley A, Samandari T, Bell BP (2005) Incidence of hepatitis A in the United States in the era of vaccination. JAMA 294:194–201
86. Samoilovich EO (2005) Personal communication. March 2nd 2005
87. Anonymous (1992) Prospects for control of hepatitis A: panel discussion. In: Hollinger FB, André FE, Melnick J (eds). Proceedings of International Symposium on active immunization against hepatitis A. Vaccine 10(Suppl.1):S170–S174
88. Bell BP, Feinstone SM (2004) Hepatitis A vaccine. In: Vaccines, 4th ed. Plotkin SA, Orenstein WA (eds.) Elsevier Inc., pp 269–297
89. Scheifele DW (2005) Hepatitis A vaccines: the growing case for universal immunisation of children. Expert Opin Pharmacother 6:157–164

Mass Vaccination Against Hepatitis B: The French Example

F. Denis[1] (✉) · D. Levy-Bruhl[2]

[1]Department of Bacteriology-Virology-Hygiene,
2 Av. Martin Luther King, 87042 Limoges, France
francois.denis@unilim.fr

[2]Department of Infectious Diseases, Institut de Veille Sanitaire,
12 rue du Val d'Osne, 94415 Saint-Maurice Cedex, France

1	Introduction	116
2	Epidemiology and Carrier Rate of HBV in France	117
3	French Immunization Strategies	119
3.1	Availability of Hepatitis B Vaccines in France	119
3.2	Targeting At-Risk Groups	119
3.3	Universal Immunization	120
4	Hepatitis B Immunization Coverage	124
4.1	Global Coverage	124
4.2	Age-Specific Coverage	125
4.3	High-Risk Groups Coverage	125
4.4	Health Impact of Vaccination Programmes	127
5	Conclusion	127
	References	128

Abstract Mainland France is considered as a low endemicity area for hepatitis B, but the French Caribbean and Pacific territories are classified into areas of intermediate and high endemicity. In France vaccination programmes aimed at high-risk groups were started in 1982 (including health care workers and patients receiving blood products) and the immunization of babies born of hepatitis B virus surface antigen (HBsAg)-positive mothers was reinforced in 1992. Considering the drawbacks and limited effect of targeted vaccination policies, universal vaccination targeted particularly to the preadolescent and adolescent population was initiated in 1994. In 1995, hepatitis B virus (HBV) vaccination was included in the infant immunization schedule. However, the emotion generated by the claim that HBV vaccination could have led to the development of central nervous system demyelinating disorders resulted in a marked decline of HBV vaccine use, both in the pediatric (23.3% vaccination coverage in children less than 13 years old) and in the adult population. The current coverage rates are likely to be insufficient to bring about a significant reduction in the control of hepatitis B in France. The success of universal immunization is highly dependent on reinstating the confidence of the public and health care professionals in the safety and efficacy of hepatitis B vaccines.

1
Introduction

During the last two decades, considerable progress has been made in implementing a hepatitis B vaccination programme in France. As in all industrialized countries, as soon as the first generation vaccine was made available in the early 1980s vaccination was recommended for high-risk groups (health care workers in contact with high-risk patients, homosexuals, patients undergoing haemodialysis or receiving blood products, close family contacts of persons with chronic HBV infections, and travellers to high endemicity regions). In 1992, the screening of pregnant women for hepatitis B virus surface antigen (HBsAg) was made compulsory in order to prevent perinatal hepatitis B virus (HBV) transmission. In the early 1990s, the evaluation of the implementation of the targeted strategy, carried out in North America, lead to the conclusion that the spread of HBV could not be effectively controlled by vaccinating only high-risk groups [1, 2]. In 1992, the World Health Assembly recommended HBV vaccination in all countries for either newborns, infants or pre-adolescents, depending on the level of hepatitis B endemicity and the local epidemiology [3]. Accordingly, in 1994/1995, France included HBV vaccination in the infant immunization schedule, in addition to the high-risk groups vaccination strategy. To have a more rapid epidemiological impact, annual vaccination campaigns in schools targeting preadolescents in the first year of secondary school (10–12 years of age) were also launched. These campaigns were to be discontinued after 10 years, when the first cohort of children vaccinated as infants reached secondary-school age [4]. Unfortunately, the immediate success of the programme was shadowed after the safety of the vaccine had been questioned. This resulted in a decreased confidence in hepatitis B vaccination that resulted in a rapid fall in coverage. Therefore, the success of the recommendations for universal infant and adolescent immunization is highly dependent on reinstating confidence among the public and heath care professionals in the safety and efficacy of HBV vaccines. The analysis of the results showed the success but also the challenges encountered when a hepatitis B vaccination programme was implemented in France.

2
Epidemiology and Carrier Rate of HBV in France

The world can be separated into areas of low, intermediate and high endemicity of HBV carriage. In these areas, the HBsAg carrier rate in the population ranges from less than 2%, 2%–8% and more than 8%, respectively. Mainland France is considered as a low endemicity area, but the French Caribbean and Pacific territories are classified respectively into areas of intermediate and high endemicity (Table 1).

In countries of high and intermediate endemicity, as well as horizontal person-to-person spread, the perinatal transmission from a chronically infected mother to her infant at the time of birth is one of the most effective routes of transmission. In countries with low endemicity, most HBV infections result from sexual activity and exposure to infected blood and other body fluids and therefore occur at an older age. The outcome of HBV infection varies according to the age of infection. The large majority of infections acquired in infancy are asymptomatic but present a higher risk of developing chronic infection. As many as 90% of those infected in the first year of life become chronic carriers. In contrast, almost 50% of adult infections are asymptomatic, but only 5%–10% of those infected in adulthood become chronic carriers.

In the 1990s, the estimates of the carriage rate of HBV in the population of mainland France ranged from 0.2% to 0.5% (corresponding to more than 100,000 chronic carriers). Important regional variations were observed, due in part to differences in the importance of populations of various ethnic origins. For example, important geographical variations were observed among the carriage rate in pregnant women, ranging from 0.13% to 2.99%. The global HBsAg crude prevalence (0.72%) was significantly higher among women from countries with a high prevalence of hepatitis B (2.56%) than among women of French origin (0.15%). HBsAg prevalence increased from 1.75% in women from Mediterranean area, 2.83% in those from the Caribbean, 4.61% in those

Table 1 Distribution of HBV markers in France (mainland and overseas territories)

Prevalence	Endemicity		
	Low	Intermediate	High
HBsAg	<2%	2%–7%	8%–15%
All markers	<20%	20%–60%	>60%
Distribution	France	West Indies	French Polynesia
	Reunion	French Guiana	New Caledonia

from sub-Saharan Africa to 5.45% in those from South East Asia [8]. Recently, we observed that pregnant women from eastern European countries had an even higher HBsAg prevalence.

Before the introduction of systematic antenatal screening, it was estimated that as many as 1000 infants born each year in France from French infected mothers developed a persistent infection. This was the confirmation that even in low endemicity areas, the risk for newborns is substantial. This led to the implementation, in 1992, of the mandatory testing of pregnant mothers for HBsAg and immediate prophylaxis at birth in the case of positivity, based on the simultaneous administration of vaccination and specific immunoglobulins.

In the general population, a sentinel surveillance of acute hepatitis B has shown that the period of hepatitis B highest incidence was in young adulthood in the early 1990s (Fig. 1) reflecting–in particular–sexual exposure. Data from 1991 to 1996 revealed that sexual exposure (35%) and parenteral drug use (20%) were the main sources of contamination. Based on the data generated by this surveillance, the incidence rate in the early 1990s was estimated around 20,000–25,000 new HBV infections and around 1000 new chronic carriers per year.

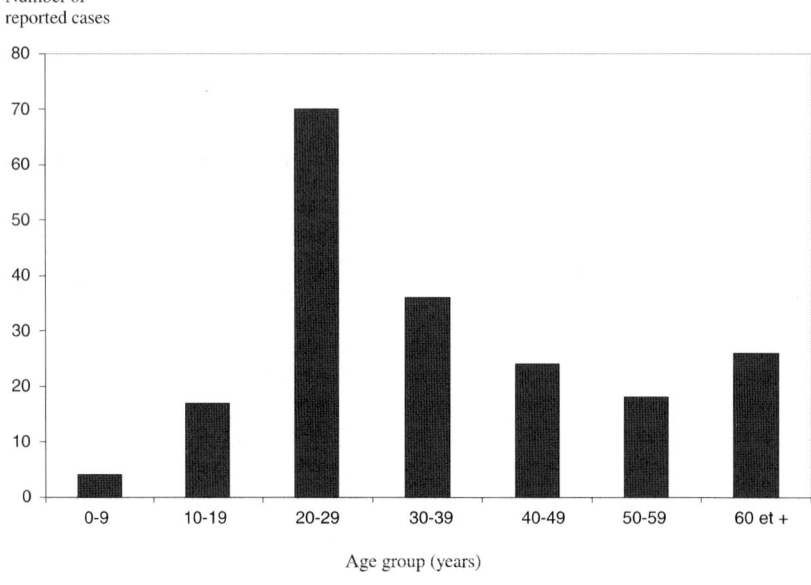

Fig. 1 Age distribution of reported acute hepatitis B cases, France, 1991–1996. (Source, Réseau "Sentinelles" INSERM U444)

The routes of transmission of HB in France has changed over the last few decades due to improved hygiene, prevention of risk behaviours regarding blood-borne infections and measures implemented to ensure the safety of blood related products, as well as high-risk group vaccination.

Recently, in 2005 the number of HBV chronic carriers was reevaluated to 300,000 in the population of mainland France.

3
French Immunization Strategies

3.1
Availability of Hepatitis B Vaccines in France

The first effective vaccine used the plasma of carriers as a source of viral antigen. The 22-nm particle-containing vaccines underwent multiple purification steps and treatment with formalin. It was associated with satisfactory immunogenicity and protective efficacy since introduction in 1976 in France [10] and later in the US [12].

In France, the HB plasma-derived vaccine was granted a license in 1981. A French group described vaccine immunogenicity among children and newborns that same year [1, 5].

Second generation vaccines containing recombinant HBsAg produced in eukaryotic (yeast or mammalian) cells have been available in France since 1986. Rapidly, as observed in other developed countries, the recombinant vaccine replaced the plasma-derived vaccine.

3.2
Targeting At-Risk Groups

Vaccination programmes aimed at high-risk groups (including health care workers and those receiving regular blood transfusions or blood products) were adopted when plasma-derived vaccines first became available in limited supply.

However, the drawbacks of this vaccination policy became apparent within 10 years of introduction. According to Bonanni, based on the US and Canadian experience [3], this can be explained by the fact that no risk factor is found in about one-third of cases of acute hepatitis B cases, and also because certain high-risk groups, such as intravenous drug users and those at risk because of their sexual behaviour, are difficult to access and are often already infected by the time they are targeted. Finally, transmission to babies from infected mothers was originally underestimated as poorly evaluated.

Table 2 Chronology of events in the implementation of the hepatitis B immunization programme in France

March 1981	Plasma derived Hepatitis B vaccine licensed (schedule with four doses: 0, 1, 2, 12 months)
June 1982	Vaccination recommended for healthcare workers and other high-risk groups
December 1984	Selective vaccine reimbursement by Social Security
January 1991	Mandatory vaccination to health care workers
February 1992	HBsAg screening for pregnant women Recombinant HBsAg vaccine licensed
January/February 1993	Immunization against Hepatitis B to students and teachers exposed through their school activities
December 1993	Vaccination recommended in the National Immunization Schedule to those travelling to areas of high prevalence
September 1994	General immunization campaign initiated by the French Health Minister for preadolescents and adolescents— General vaccine reimbursement by Social Security
October 1994	License for the vaccination schedule with three doses (0, 1, 6 months) granted
December 1994	Free school-based vaccination programs for adolescents
January 1995	Hepatitis B vaccination included in the infant and adolescent immunization schedule
October 1998	The French Minister of Health decided to stop hepatitis B vaccination in schools
2000	Hexavalent vaccines licensed in Europe
September 2003	Recommendations of the Consensus Conference on hepatitis B vaccination INSERM/ANAES

In France (Table 2), the vaccination of healthcare workers was initially recommended in 1982 and became mandatory in 1991. But the recommendation to vaccinate individuals who change sexual partners frequently, travellers to areas of high prevalence, close contacts of an acute case or carrier and other risk groups in the general population was, at least up to the mid 1990s, not satisfactorily implemented.

The immunization of babies born to HBsAg-positive mothers was reinforced by the mandatory screening of pregnant women in 1992.

3.3
Universal Immunization

The World Health Assembly in 1992 stated that low endemicity countries should be considering immunization of all adolescents as an alternative or addition to infant immunization. In 1994, the World Health Assembly also added a disease reduction target for hepatitis B, calling for an 80% decrease in the incidence of new HBV carriers in children by the year 2001.

Considering the drawbacks and limited effect of targeted vaccination policies, foreseeable by the Margolis model (Fig. 2), universal immunization was announced by the French government. A national campaign was initiated in September 1994 by the French Health Minister and targeted in particular the preadolescent and adolescent populations.

The uptake was very satisfactory among preadolescents and adolescents, especially when vaccinated at school. Older adolescents and young adults were vaccinated in other settings, such as paediatricians' or general practitioners' clinics or at university. A survey of school children in eight departments confirmed the success of the adolescent campaign and the high coverage rates achieved in the 11–13-years old population (Fig. 3) [9]. It also highlighted the positive effect of the campaign on other pupils who were not directly included in the school campaign, but who decided to be vaccinated.

In 1995, HBV vaccination was included in the infant immunization schedule. Acceptability for infants was however lower, as the risk of possible future contamination of their children–through sex or intravenous drug use–was felt too remote by parents to justify immediate vaccination. Moreover, immu-

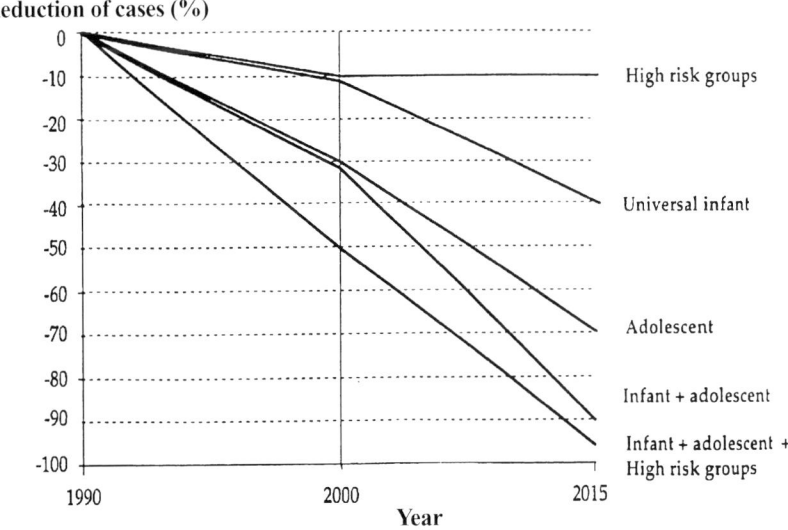

Fig. 2 Estimated proportion of cases of hepatitis B prevented, based on different vaccination strategies. (Source: H. Margolis, CDC, US, adapted)

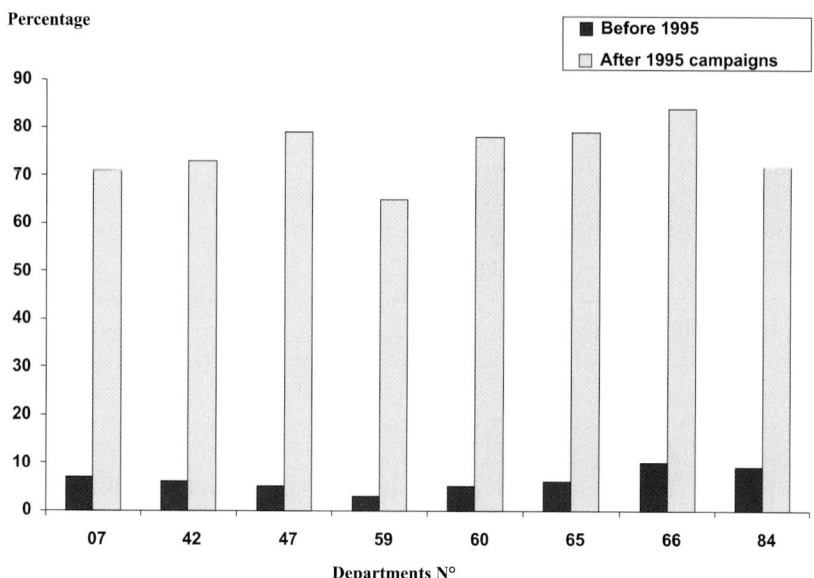

Fig. 3 Hepatitis B. Coverage in school children. (Source: National Institute for Public Health Surveillance, 8 Departments; France 1995)

nization of infants was required four extra injections plus, at least up to 1998, regular boosters.

After an initial phase of high demand for HBV vaccination in older children and adults, the confidence towards the vaccine decreased significantly. Several factors contributed to this negative evolution.

Insufficient information on vaccine characteristics (such as efficacy, side effects and duration of protection), on the reasons of the modifications of the vaccination protocol (four injections initially, modified to three injections, discontinuation of boosters), and on the disease (clinical symptoms and potential complications, risk of getting the disease according to age) contributes to latter difficulties. More generally, weaknesses in the planning, monitoring and evaluation process of the campaigns (for instance insufficient data on the epidemiology of hepatitis B, both before and after the promotion of HBV vaccination, and on the evolution of vaccination coverage according to age and risk group) have undermine confidence of both the professionals and the general public on the HBV vaccination policy.

In that context, reports in the media of hundreds, then thousands of "victims" of the HBV vaccination found an echo in the population. The emotion generated by the claim that hepatitis B vaccination could have led to the development of central nervous system demyelinating disorders (particularly multiple sclerosis) led, in October 1998, to the French government (French Health Minister) temporally suspending its school-based programme of adolescent vaccination (but not the universal vaccination of infants, nor the vaccination of adolescents or high-risk groups by family physicians). This decision was followed by a period of high-profile media attention to these allegations, went against expert consensus (reviewed elsewhere) that available scientific data did not justify a change in policy, and resulted in a marked decline in hepatitis B vaccine use, both in the paediatric and adult population.

The fall in coverage resulted from a loss of confidence not only from the public but also from physicians. Since 1998, in France, the number of hepatitis B vaccine doses administered has decreased dramatically (Fig. 4). Despite recommendations from national or international bodies (World Health Organization) and the publications of expert committees and consensus meeting conclusions (ANAES-INSERM) [13], confidence in vaccination was not restored.

Another more recent and potential threat to the perception on the safety of hepatitis B vaccines is a polemic that emerged in 1999 in the US about thimerosal, a mercury derivate, that has been used as a preservative in many other vaccines over the past 50 years. Also in France, another compound used in vaccine as an adjuvant, namely aluminium hydroxide has been suspected to lead to the development of a specific disease called macrophagic myofasciitis.

Considering, following Margolis, that the most important drawback to in-

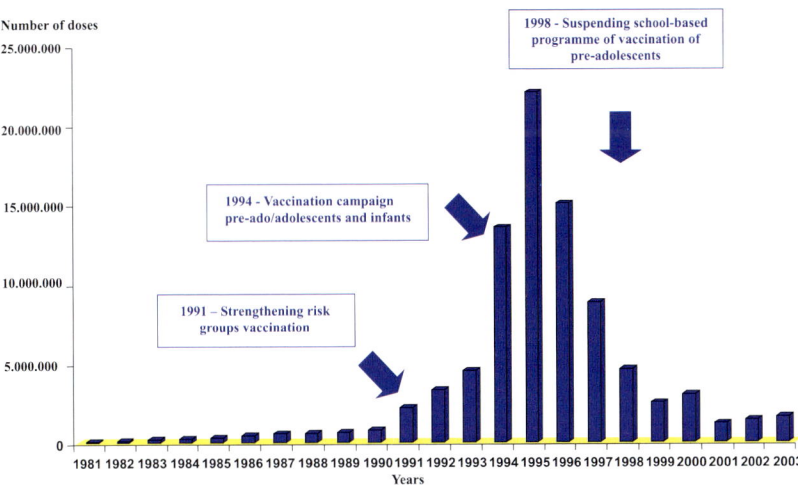

Fig. 4 Evolution of the hepatitis B vaccine market in France

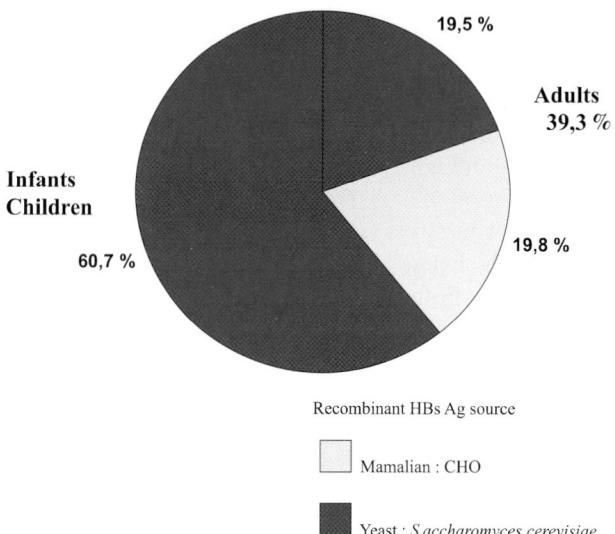

Fig. 5 Market of hepatitis B vaccines in France, 2003

fant immunization is that a major impact on the incidence of disease would not be seen for 15–20 years after the start of the immunization programme and the relative secondary failure of pre-adolescent immunization in France, promotion of immunization in childhood was favoured by consensus meetings during 2003 and published in the French immunization schedule that same year. It was confirmed in the recent international consensus meeting on 9 November 2004 [13].

In 2003, the market of hepatitis B vaccine remained stable (1,625,000 doses sold), with around 61% of the vaccinations given before adult age (Fig. 5).

It was hoped that the marketing of hexavalent combination vaccines would increase coverage in infants in France. However, these vaccines have not yet been admitted to the list of refundable drugs, thus limiting their acceptability.

4
Hepatitis B Immunization Coverage

4.1
Global Coverage

GlaxoSmithKline and Taylor Nelson Sofres Sante have conducted a survey on hepatitis B immunization coverage rate among 50,888 persons in 2002. The

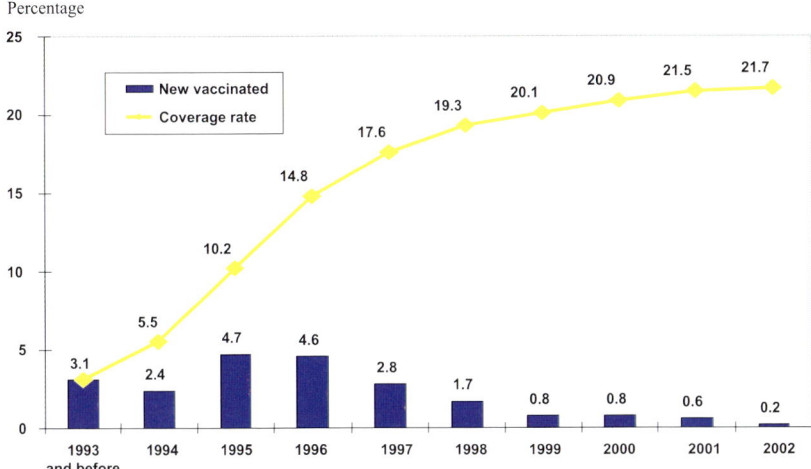

Fig. 6 Evolution of the immunization coverage rate in France (three doses)

cumulative coverage rate in the general population from 1993 to 2002 was around 21.7%. It has been increasing sharply since 1993, with a much slower progression since 1998 (Fig. 6) [6].

4.2
Age-Specific Coverage

In the same study, it was observed that vaccination coverage with three doses was low in children (23.3% in children less than 13 years old). The coverage was 19.8% in infants, and 46.2% in adolescents 14–18 years old, this age range including some births cohorts involved in the school based vaccination campaigns [6, 7]. Coverage rates by age group are shown in Figs. 7 and 8.

4.3
High-Risk Groups Coverage

A review of several national data on the coverage rates according to high-risk groups is summarized in Table 3.

Around 80%–90% of physicians and healthcare personnel in public or private hospitals were vaccinated against hepatitis B and the level of coverage was higher among those members of staff accidentally exposed to blood (90%–100%) [7]. Data also showed that between 25% and 45% of intravenous drug abusers, prisoners, or sexually transmitted disease patients were vaccinated [7].

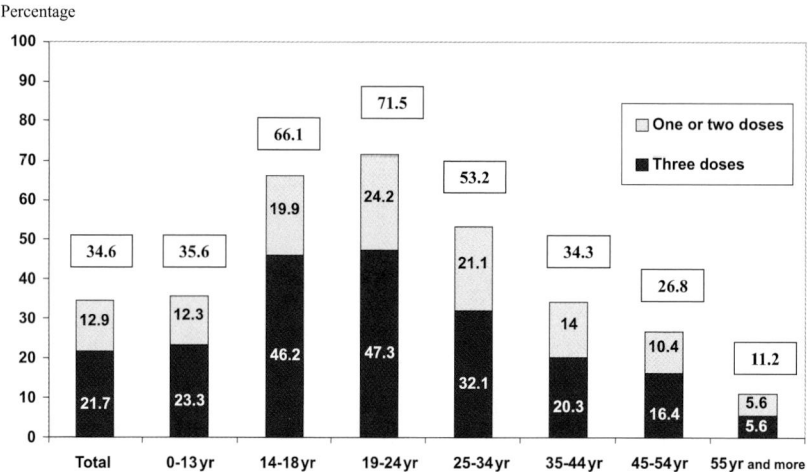

Fig. 7 Hepatitis B vaccination coverage rates in France, 2002 (Denis)

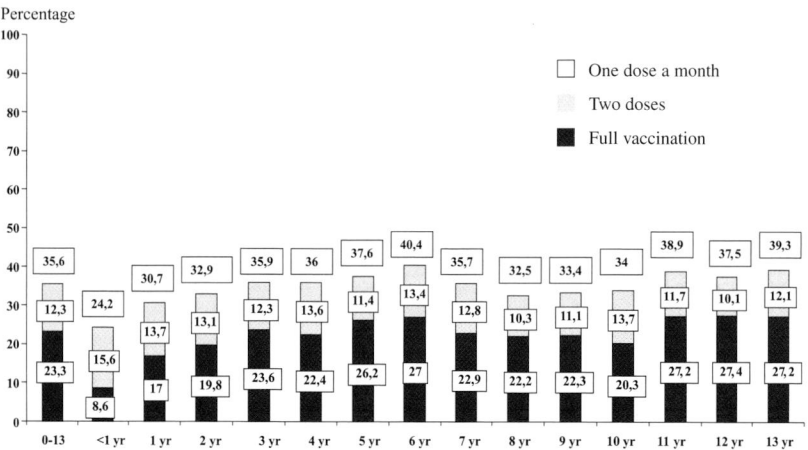

Fig. 8 Hepatitis B vaccination coverage rates in children, France 2002 (Denis)

Recently, we observed that the national specific prevention programme against mother-to-infant transmission was unevenly applied. A regional investigation revealed that among pregnant women, 20% were not screened for HBsAg. At national level, several cases of acute or fulminant hepatitis B were reported among babies born to infected mothers not screened for HBsAg.

Table 3 Hepatitis B vaccination among the health care workers submitted to blood exposures (BE) in Limoges hospital

Hospital workers	Limoges[a] (842 BE)	Southwest France[b] (6221 BE)
Nurses	98.3	90.8
AS/AH	97.7	90.5
Health students	96.2	95.3
Doctors	97.6	88.0
Surgeons	100	80.9
Others	91.6	84.4
Total	97.0 (+0.8)	89.9 (+1)

[a] 2000–2002 period [b] 2000–2001 period

4.4
Health Impact of Vaccination Programmes

The impact of vaccinating healthcare workers was rapidly observed with a dramatic fall in the number of occupational infections from 700 in 1981 to 76 in 1992. Since 1992, very few cases have been notified.

There are no data on the incidence of acute viral HBV hepatitis over a long period of time in France, as there are in other countries such as Italy or the US. Extrapolation at the national level from cases seen by general practitioners participating in the sentinel surveillance yielded an average estimated incidence of 8,000 new acute symptomatic infections each year during the first half of the 1990s. Data from the mandatory notification of hepatitis B acute infections, implemented in 2003, show an incidence of about 160 cases for the first year. Although, the level of under-notification is not known, these data are in favour of an epidemiological impact of the intense HBV vaccination activities in the second half of the 1990s. This conclusion is further reinforced by the observed shift in age towards older age groups (the age range of maximum incidence being 30–39 years old as compared to 20–29 years old in the early 1990s), which is probably a result of the high coverage reached in adolescents during 1994–1998. A decrease in the incidence of acute fulminating hepatitis B has also been observed in the recent years.

5
Conclusion

Significant progress has been made in implementing a comprehensive strategy to eliminate HBV transmission in France. The impact of this programme can be measured through the high vaccine coverage reached in some age groups and declining rates of acute hepatitis B. Future efforts will need to focus on improving the management of babies born to HBsAg positive mothers, on increasing coverage in infants, in 11–12-year old children and in high-risk adolescents and adults [13].

These objectives, however, will be achieved only if an appropriate response to the current confidence crisis is provided to the public through the media and the professionals to counteract the unjustified allegations about hepatitis B vaccination that have negatively affected coverage. Similarly, high-quality scientific information should be provided to professionals in order to restore their confidence in the safety and efficacy of HBV vaccination.

The current coverage rates are likely to be insufficient to observe, in the long run, a significant reduction and a control of hepatitis B infections in France.

Lessons learned from the French experience show the paramount importance of monitoring tools, when large scale vaccination activities are undertaken. Sound epidemiological data, such as age specific incidence rates, are needed to justify the strategy and to able to show its impact. Age and population specific vaccination coverage data allow the assessment of progress and identification of un-immunized pockets which could require specific action [2]. It also allows the identification of deviation from the initial target populations of the vaccination strategies decided upon by the health authorities. The very large HBV vaccination of the adult population in France in the 1994–1998 period, well beyond the targeted high-risk groups, appears retrospectively to have been counterproductive. The large number of adverse events notified in adults to the French Drug Safety Agency, probably in reality only temporally linked with vaccination, has led to a crisis that negatively affected the coverage in the priority populations.

References

1. Barin F, Goudeau A, Denis F, Yvonnet B, Chiron JP, Coursaget P, Diopmar I (1981) Immune response in neonates to hepatitis B vaccine. Lancet, i: 251–253
2. Bartlett S, Van Damme P on behalf of the viral Hepatitis Prevention Board (2000) Behavioural issues in hepatitis B vaccination. Report of a meeting organized by the viral Hepatitis Prevention Board, University of Antwerp
3. Bonanni P (1998) Universal hepatitis B immunization: infant and infant plus adolescent immunization. Vaccine 16:S17–S22
4. Calendrier vaccinal 2004. Avis du Conseil Supérieur d'Hygiène Publique de France (2004) Bull Epidemiol Hebd 28–29:121–125
5. Coursaget P, Chiron JP, Barin F, Goudeau A, Yvonnet B, Denis F (1981) Hepatitis B vaccine: immunization of children and newborns in an endemic area. Develop Biol Standard 54:245–257

6. Denis F (2004) Hepatitis B vaccination in France: vaccination coverage in 2002. Bull Acad Natle Med 188:115–123
7. Denis F, Abitbol V, Aufrere A (2004) Evolution of strategy and coverage rates for hepatitis B vaccination in France country with low endemicity. Med Mal Inf 34:149–158
8. Denis F, Tabaste JL, Ranger-Rogez S and multicentric group (1994) Prevalence of HBsAg in about 21500 pregnant women: a study of 12 French university hospitals. Path Biol 42, (5):533–538
9. Guerin N (1998) Assessing immunization coverage: how and why? Vaccine 16: S81–S83
10. Maupas P, Goudeau A, Coursaget P, Drucker J (1976) Immunization against hepatitis B in mass. Lancet i:1367–1370
11. RNSP. Cellules interrégionales d'épidémiologie. SPSFE (1997) Evaluation de la couverture du programme de vaccination hépatite B dans les collèges (1ère campagne 1994–1995). Bull Epidemiol Hebd 51:225–227
12. Szmuness W, Stevens CE, Harley EJ, et al. (1980) Hepatitis B vaccine demonstrating of efficacy in a controlled clinic trial in a high-risk population in the United States. N Engl J Med 303:833–841
13. Vaccination contre le virus de l'hépatite B et sclérose en plaque : état des lieux (2004). Rapport d'orientation de la commission d'audition. INSERM/ANAES. Paris www.inserm.fr

Mass Vaccination for Annual and Pandemic Influenza

B. Schwartz (✉) · P. Wortley

Immunization Services Division, National Immunization Program, Centers for Disease Control and Prevention, 1600 Clifton Road NE, Atlanta, GA 30333, USA
bxs1@cdc.gov

1	Influenza Disease and Vaccine	132
2	Mass Vaccination for Annual Influenza Epidemics	134
3	Mass Vaccination for Pandemic Influenza	139
3.1	Coordination	143
3.2	Staffing	144
3.3	Location of Clinics	145
3.4	Clinic Lay-Out	145
3.5	Security and Crowd Control	146
3.6	Communication and Public Education	146
3.7	Exercises	146
4	The Future of Mass Vaccination for Annual and Pandemic Influenza	148
	References	150

Abstract Influenza virus causes annual epidemics and occasional pandemics. Frequent mutations in circulating influenza strains ("antigenic drift") result in the need for annual vaccination. More than two-thirds of persons in the U.S. are recommended for annual vaccination. Because influenza vaccine is available seasonally, mass vaccination strategies are well suited to its delivery. Although doctors offices are the most frequent setting for influenza vaccination overall, workplaces, clinics, and community sites (retail stores and pharmacies) also are common vaccination settings. Influenza vaccination also is delivered in mass vaccination clinics to health care workers and military personnel. Universal influenza vaccination, which has been recommended as a strategy to improve prevention by increasing vaccination coverage and providing indirect protection of adults by decreasing infection and transmission among children, would require expanded use of mass vaccination, for example in schools, as well as in the community. Influenza pandemics occur when a new influenza A subtype is introduced into the population ("antigenic shift"). Most or all of the population is susceptible to the pandemic virus and two doses of vaccine may be needed for protection. U.S. pandemic preparedness and response plans indicate that the entire population should be vaccinated beginning with defined priority groups including those who provide essential services including healthcare and those at highest risk of severe illness and death. Pandemic influenza vaccination will occur primarily through the public sector in mass clinic settings. Vaccination program planning must consider issues including coordination, staffing, clinic location and lay-out, security, record keeping, and communications. Exercising vaccination clinics is important for preparedness and can be done in the context of annual influenza vaccination.

1
Influenza Disease and Vaccine

Influenza is an acute viral infection characterized by fever, cough, myalgia, and malaise. Complications include pneumonia – either from the viral infection or a secondary bacterial pathogen – otitis media, myositis, myocarditis, and encephalitis. Illness generally is mild and self-limiting but occasionally, severe or complicated disease results in hospitalization and death. In temperate climates, influenza causes annual epidemics, typically during winter months. Attack rates of infection are highest in children who often are the source of transmission within families and communities. In community outbreaks, as many as 40% of children may become infected compared with 10%–20% of adults. By contrast, the burden of severe influenza is concentrated among the elderly; in the US, about 90% of deaths and half of influenza hospitalizations occur among those aged 65 years or more. High high-risk groups also include persons with chronic underlying illnesses, children less than 2 years old, and pregnant women. Recent US estimates suggest that about 36,000 persons die each year from influenza (Thompson et al. 2003), more than for all other vaccine preventable diseases combined, and about 200,000 are hospitalized (Thompson et al. 2004).

Protection against influenza following infection or vaccination is mediated by antibody to hemagglutinin and neuraminidase antigens. These glycoproteins change antigenically through mutation ('antigenic drift') resulting in the continual formation of new viruses. Antibodies induced by prior infection or vaccination may partially protect against infection with a drifted strain. Rarely, reassortment of genetic material between two influenza viruses occurs, resulting in a strain with markedly different HA and/or NA antigens ('antigenic shift'). Antigenic shift among influenza A viruses can result in global epidemics, or pandemics, with circulation of a new virus subtype to which there is little or no prior immunity. The 1918 influenza pandemic, in which an H1N1 strain was introduced into a largely immunologically naive population caused over 500,000 US deaths and, according to some estimates more than 50 million deaths globally. Other twentieth century pandemics, occurring in 1957 (H2N2) and 1968 (H3N2), caused about one-tenth of the number of deaths. Although the timing and severity of influenza pandemics are unpredictable, most experts agree that they are inevitable. Recent transmission of H5N1 influenza viruses from domestic poultry to humans in the context of widespread avian infection in Asia, and other recent instances of animal to human transmission of novel influenza strains, highlight the ongoing pandemic threat (World Health Organization 2005).

Influenza vaccine protects against disease by inducing antibody primarily to the HA protein. Current influenza vaccines are trivalent, targeting two influenza A (H1N1 and H3N2) and one influenza B strain. Because circulating influenza strains may change with each influenza season, vaccination is needed annually. About 50 countries worldwide have influenza vaccination recommendations. In the US vaccination is recommended by the Advisory Committee on Immunization Practices (ACIP) for those who are at high risk for severe illness and their contacts (Table 1), which includes almost two-thirds of the entire population (CDC 2004a). Annual vaccination coverage, however, falls far short of that recommended; only about 83 million doses of influenza vaccine were distributed during the 2003–2004 season for the 186 million persons in the target population. The substantial ongoing mor-

Table 1 Groups targeted for annual influenza vaccination in the US. Recommendations are from the Advisory Committee on Immunization Practices, 2004

Persons at increased risk for influenza complications
- Children 6–23 months old
- Adults 65 years old or older
- Adults and children who have chronic disorders of the cardiovascular or pulmonary systems, including asthma, or who required regular medical follow-up or were hospitalized during the preceding year because of chronic metabolic disease, including diabetes mellitus, renal dysfunction, hemoglobinopathy, or immunosuppression, including that caused by medication or human immunodeficiency virus (HIV) infection
- Women who will be pregnant during the influenza season
- Residents of nursing homes and other chronic-care facilities that house persons of any age who have chronic medical conditions
- Children and adolescents who are receiving long-term aspirin therapy and may be at risk for Reye syndrome after influenza infection

Other recommended groups
- Persons aged 50–64 years
- Health care workers
- Care givers and household contacts of persons in high-risk groups for whom vaccination is recommended, and for infants aged 0–5 months for whom influenza vaccines have not been licensed

bidity and mortality from influenza and the difficulty achieving high rates of vaccination coverage in the elderly and high-risk groups has led to consideration of expanded vaccination recommendations. Universal influenza vaccination may enhance prevention by stimulating increased vaccine uptake by groups currently recommended to be vaccinated, and by decreasing transmission of infection and indirectly protecting vulnerable populations through vaccination of children. Ontario, Canada, adopted a universal vaccination recommendation in 2000, resulting in a significant increase in coverage; disease impacts have not yet been assessed.

2
Mass Vaccination for Annual Influenza Epidemics

Influenza vaccine is particularly well suited for delivery by mass vaccination strategies. Annual vaccine for the Northern Hemisphere becomes available in late-summer or early-fall and must be administered before disease becomes widespread. By contrast with routine vaccination of infants where age-defined medical care visits provide an opportunity for immunization, influenza vaccine is delivered seasonally and most vaccine is administered to adults who seldom make routine medical care visits. Even among children, influenza vaccination visits at medical practices may create a substantial burden. Researchers analyzed a large administrative database to assess the number of additional provider visits that would be required to fully implement a recommendation for vaccination of 6–23-month-old children. If vaccination occurred during a 3-month window and only well child care visits were used for vaccination, 39% of children would require one additional visit and 35% would require two additional visits to be fully immunized (Szilagyi et al. 2003a). The same investigators also assessed the time required for influenza vaccination visits among children at four urban and three suburban practices. The median visit length was 14 min (urban, 22 min; suburban, 9 min) with the majority of that time spent waiting in an examination room (Szilagyi et al. 2003b). The investigators concluded that influenza vaccination of young children at provider's offices would place a substantial burden on busy pediatric practices and that office-based mass vaccination strategies such as vaccination clinics would increase efficiency. Vaccination clinics also may decrease costs which, in a setting of individual, provider-based influenza vaccination, may exceed reimbursement rates when all staff time costs and office overhead are considered. Both facility-based and 'drive-through' vaccination clinics have been implemented as part of a strategy to efficiently increase vaccination rates in children and adults. Other components required for an effective approach include standing orders for vaccination, use of reminder systems, and careful planning of logistics (National Foundation for Infectious Diseases 2003).

Mass influenza vaccination among adults also has been implemented in a variety of settings. Data on where persons were vaccinated against influenza during the previous year were collected in the Center for Disease Control and Prevention's 1999 Behavioral Risk Factor Surveillance System (Table 2) (CDC, unpublished data). Workplaces were the second most common site for influenza vaccination (17.8% of vaccinations), and were the most common site among persons 18–49 years old. Other community vaccination sites in nonhealth care settings contributed an additional 12.4% of influenza vaccinations. Receipt of influenza vaccination in community settings was more common among persons who were younger, healthy, employed, white, college-educated, and who had not had a recent routine check-up. While Black and Hispanic adults were less likely to receive their influenza vaccine at workplaces or other community sites, it is unclear whether this was related to the acceptability of community-based vaccination or access to the locations where vaccine was offered. Influenza vaccination at sites other than provider offices, in addition to decreasing the burden on office-based providers, may offer greater convenience and decreased costs both to the vaccinee and the health care system. Given the importance of influenza vaccination in settings other than physicians' offices, guidelines have been established defining quality standards for immunization in nontraditional settings to assure that the immunizations delivered are safe and effective (Table 3) (CDC 2000).

Table 2 Sites where adults received influenza vaccine, 1998–1999. Data are from the US Behavioral Risk Factor Surveillance System, 1999

Setting	Percent of age group			Total
	18–49 years	50–64 years	≥65 years	
Doctors office. HMO	32.5%	44.6%	62.8%	47.0%
Hospital/emergency department	8.1%	6.7%	5.9%	6.9%
Health department	6.4%	6.8%	6.4%	6.5%
Other clinic/health center	9.0%	9.2%	9.0%	9.1%
Workplace	33.2%	20.1%	1.4%	17.8%
Store	4.5%	6.5%	4.8%	5.1%
Senior/recreational/community center	1.4%	2.7%	6.8%	3.8%
Other nontraditional setting sure	4.7%	3.3%	2.5%	3.5%
Not sure	0.3%	0.2%	0.4%	0.3%

Table 3 Quality standards for adult immunization programs in nontraditional settings based on a report of the US National Vaccine Advisory Committee (MMWR, 2000)

---

1. Information and education for vaccinees

    Provide information on benefits and risks of vaccination and on the importance of having a medical home and receiving other preventive services

2. Vaccine storage and handling

    Adhere to recommendations in package inserts, especially regarding storage temperature, and maintain records for documentation

3. Immunization history

    Screen before vaccination for immunizations received, health history, allergies, and adverse events following previous vaccinations

4. Contraindications

    As part of the history, assess whether any contraindication exists to vaccination

5. Record-keeping

    Record vaccination information (vaccinees name and age, pre-existing health conditions, vaccination date, vaccine type, dose, site and route of administration, name of the vaccine provider, manufacturer, lot number, and the date the next dose is due). Copies should be given to the vaccinee and their primary-care provider or local health department if no provider is identified

6. Vaccine administration

    Providers who administer vaccine must have the legal authority to do so and must administer vaccine according to information in the package insert

7. Adverse events

    Vaccinators must be trained to recognize and manage adverse reactions. If adverse events occur, they should be reported to the Vaccine Adverse Event Reporting System

---

Influenza vaccination of residents and staff of nursing homes and other long-term care facilities has been documented to decrease influenza disease and mortality. In a 1991 Canadian survey of nursing homes, the reported mean vaccination coverage at 1,270 responding facilities was 78.5%. Factors associated with higher vaccination coverage among residents included vaccine being offered to all residents, obtaining consent for vaccination at admission rather than annually, automatically vaccinating incompetent residents whose guardians could not be contacted, having a single nonphysician staff member organize the program, and having more program components covered by written policies. Higher coverage among staff was associated with promoting vaccination and holding vaccination clinics in the facility (McArthur et al. 1999).

Occupation-based strategies are an effective approach to vaccinate health care workers, who are recommended for annual vaccination to decrease transmission of infection to patients. Surveillance at one academic medical center found that nosocomial cases accounted for 32% of all influenza among hospitalized patients during the 1987–1988 influenza season when only 4% of health care workers were vaccinated. Following implementation of a program to vaccinate hospital staff, coverage among health care workers increased to 67% for the 1999–2000 season; that year no nosocomial influenza cases were identified. Logistic regression analysis showed a statistically significant inverse association between the rate of health care worker vaccination and the rate of nosocomial influenza among patients (Salgado et al. 2004). Hospital vaccination clinics have succeeded in increasing coverage rates among health care providers by reducing financial barriers and facilitating access (D'Heilly and Nichol 2004). Mobile cart programs, bringing vaccination directly to patient care units (Sartor et al. 2004), represents one innovative and successful strategy.

Vaccination clinics at workplaces outside the health care system also have been implemented to prevent influenza disease-associated absenteeism among employees. A placebo-controlled trial in Minnesota in 1994–1995 showed that vaccination of healthy working adults 18–64 years old resulted in 25% fewer episodes of upper respiratory illness (URI), 43% fewer days of URI-associated sick leave, 44% fewer physician office visits for URI, and a cost savings estimated at almost $47 per person vaccinated (Nichol et al. 1995). However, a similar controlled trial over two influenza seasons (1997–1998 and 1998–1999) at a US manufacturing company found substantially less impact on health outcomes and worker absenteeism, and calculated net societal costs that exceeded benefits (Bridges et al. 2000). Differences between the two studies may relate to rates of influenza disease and vaccine efficacy in the different influenza seasons or differences in leave-taking behaviors; workplace vaccination may be cost-effective in some years or some industrial settings and not in others.

Mass vaccination of military personnel also has been implemented to decrease health impacts and time lost to influenza illness. Crowded living conditions and increased exposure from deployment to areas where outbreaks may be occurring contribute to high rates of respiratory infections in military settings (Gray et al. 1999). Annual influenza vaccination of US military personnel was implemented in the 1950s. This program has been successful in decreasing infections and preventing epidemics. Disease outbreaks, however, may occur when the strains in the vaccine do not match those that are circulating. In 1996, 42% of crew members on a US navy ship developed influenza despite 95% having been appropriately immunized; the H3N2 virus isolated from patients was antigenically distinct from the strain included in the vaccine (Earhart et al. 2001). Military personnel also have been at high risk when antigenic shifts occur. Service personnel experienced substantial mortality and morbidity in the 1918 pandemic; a military unit that traveled to Asia experienced the initial outbreak among Americans in the 1968 pandemic; and a large cluster of cases in 1976 at Fort Dix, New Jersey, led to the swine influenza vaccination program.

Retail stores provide another venue for annual mass vaccination. In many states, pharmacists are allowed to provide immunizations. By dispensing prescription medications, pharmacists are able to identify persons with high-risk conditions and can offer influenza vaccination to this target population. A survey of persons vaccinated by pharmacists in 17 cities found that 84% visited the pharmacy intending to be vaccinated, while 10% went to the pharmacy to receive a prescription medication and 7% to purchase other merchandise. A majority of vaccinees cited convenience as the primary reason for seeking vaccination at a pharmacy compared with other locations (Grabenstein et al. 2001). By contrast with pharmacies where vaccinations are administered throughout the influenza vaccination season, immunization at grocery stores usually is provided by contracted nurses in campaigns lasting 1 or 2 days.

Although mass influenza vaccination clinics in health care and community settings and in institutions increase access to vaccination, access alone is not sufficient to achieve high vaccination coverage. The most important factor associated with receipt of any vaccination is the recommendation of a health care provider, which can easily be made in the context of office visits but not at the time of mass vaccination in a community or workplace setting. Therefore, other mechanisms must be used to motivate and educate potential vaccine recipients, and to overcome barriers to influenza vaccination such as fear of side effects, perception that influenza is a mild disease and that immunization is not important, and cost. Factors associated with a successful occupational program were assessed in a survey of occupational health nurses employed by health care and nonhealth care companies. Successful workplace vaccination programs (those vaccinating more than 50% of employees) were significantly more likely to be implemented by a health care company, to have the costs of vaccination covered by the employer, to have management encouragement of vaccination, and to be implemented by a company having more experience with workplace vaccination (D'Heilly and Nichol 2004).

The features that contribute to a successful community-wide vaccination program are illustrated by a program implemented collaboratively between a hospital system and the health department in a mid-sized US city (Parry et al. 2004). Public awareness was fostered through a variety of media events. A consent form and vaccination cards were developed and an electronic database created to track vaccinations, facilitate roster billing to Medicare for elderly vaccinees, and generate patient recall reminders. Several clinic sites were established, contracts were established with area corporations, and health department staff visited long-term care facilities for the elderly to provide on-site vaccinations. Cost of vaccination was low and health department and hospital employees received free vaccine. The first year following implementation, this program increased the number of influenza vaccinations administered by 70% and at the end of the third program year, by 150%. Emergency department visits for all respiratory diagnoses decreased by 34% and for chronic obstructive lung disease by 46% compared with other areas of the county without this program (Parry et al. 2004).

3
Mass Vaccination for Pandemic Influenza

Several critical factors distinguish vaccination for annual influenza epidemics and for an influenza pandemic. The entire population may be susceptible to a pandemic strain, leading to universal vaccination recommendations. Two vaccine doses may be required to induce an acceptable antibody response to a subtype that has not circulated previously among people. And groups at high risk for severe illness may differ from annual risk groups. During the 1918 pandemic, the age-specific mortality curve was 'W' shaped, with a high risk of death in young adults along with those at the extremes of age.

In the face of increased pandemic vaccine needs, it is likely that vaccine initially will be unavailable as at least 4 months are needed to develop and obtain regulatory approval for the new product. Once production begins, supply in countries with domestic producers will be limited based on manufacturing capacity; in countries without domestic production, vaccine likely will be unavailable as countries will retain what they produce for their own population. Six manufacturers produced influenza vaccine in the US at the time of the 1957 Asian influenza pandemic, this number decreased to four by the 1976 swine influenza program, and currently a single manufacturer produces influenza vaccine from a completely US-based supply chain. Based on current estimates of production capacity from that manufacturer and assuming that 15 µg of antigen will be required per dose and a two-dose vaccination schedule, it is likely that less than half of the US population could be fully vaccinated during the first year of pandemic vaccine production.

Delayed vaccine availability and limited supply will require that pandemic vaccine be targeted to defined priority groups, which would differ from those for annual vaccination. Priority groups likely will include health care workers, persons critical to the pandemic response, public safety workers such as police and fire fighters, and other essential community service providers, in addition to those at high risk for severe disease. The need to effectively target vaccine to priority groups, many of which will be defined by occupation, and to eventually vaccinate the entire population make mass vaccination strategies critical during a pandemic.

Influenza vaccine was used during the 1957 and 1968 pandemics as well as during the swine influenza scare in 1976. In 1957, disease caused by the pandemic strain first occurred in China in February. A vaccine reference strain was delivered to manufacturers in May and the first doses of monovalent vaccine were available in September, over a month after the initial US outbreak in Louisiana. At the peak of the US pandemic in mid-October, fewer than half of the approximately 60 million doses eventually produced had been delivered. Health care workers, essential public servants, and persons at high risk were recommended as priority groups. While manufacturers, at the urging of the Public Health Service, voluntarily distributed vaccine equitably between states, no attempt was made by the public health care sector to control vaccine distribution or enforce vaccination priorities. Consequently, virtually all vaccine doses were delivered by the private sector without regard to the recommendations (US Public Health Service, unpublished data).

The emergence of a new influenza strain in 1968, resulting in the Hong Kong influenza pandemic, occurred relatively late in the year. The ACIP issued influenza vaccination recommendations in late-June for a polyvalent vaccine incorporating older influenza A and B strains (CDC 1968a). In July, an influenza outbreak caused by the new strain was recognized in Hong Kong and in August, US military personnel were infected following a trip to Asia. A new monovalent vaccine, containing the Hong Kong strain was prepared but supply was limited. Therefore, ACIP limited recommendations to adults and children with 'chronic debilitating diseases' and those in older age groups (CDC 1968a). Limited supply of monovalent vaccine before the occurrence of disease outbreaks decreased implementation of a mass vaccination response to the pandemic. However, a landmark study was done to evaluate the impact of mass vaccination of school children on the course of the influenza outbreak in a Michigan community (Monto et al. 1969). In the intervention community, school-based vaccination was implemented with coverage of almost 92% among elementary school children and 75% among high-school students. School absenteeism and rates of respiratory illness were compared for this community and a nearby control community. School absenteeism peaked at about 14% in the control community but never exceeded 8% in the community with the school-based program. Compared with the control community, rates of respiratory illness were substantially lower among the children who had been immunized and also among unvaccinated children attending the same schools. Rates of respiratory illness also were less among young adults in the intervention community, documenting indirect protection (herd immunity) associated with vaccination of children (Monto et al. 1969).

The swine influenza episode in 1976 generally is remembered as a debacle because of vaccine-associated cases of Guillain–Barré syndrome (GBS) and the absence of swine influenza disease. The swine influenza vaccination program also was the first public sector mass vaccination campaign for a pandemic influenza threat. Following identification of H1N1 'swine influenza' disease and person-to-person spread of infection among military personnel at Fort Dix, New Jersey, it was decided to mount a campaign with the goal of vaccinating all Americans. Federal funding was appropriated for vaccine purchase and manufacturers made about 150 million monovalent vaccine doses. State-based mass vaccinations began in October, about 8 months after manufacturing activities began. Within the first 10 days of the program, over one million people had been vaccinated, almost exclusively by mass public sector campaigns. Program intensiveness and vaccination coverage varied greatly between and within states. By the time the program was halted in mid-December following detection of the link with GBS, over 40 million persons had been immunized (Neustadt and Feinberg 1978).

Lessons learned from these pandemic vaccination experiences, along with those from vaccination for annual influenza, have laid the foundation for vaccination strategies for the next pandemic. In 2004, the US released a national pandemic influenza preparedness and response plan to provide guidance to all levels of government and to the health care system regarding critical activities to undertake before and during a pandemic (US Department of Health and Human Services 2005). As in 1957, the plan recommends focusing initially available pandemic vaccine supply to designated priority groups, while similar to 1976 is the recommendation that the entire US population be vaccinated as supply becomes available. Recognizing the difficulty targeting vaccine in 1957 given a private sector program, greater public sector involvement, as in 1976, is proposed.

The goals of a pandemic response include reducing influenza-associated morbidity and mortality, and decreasing societal disruption and economic loss. Vaccination is likely to be the most important intervention to achieve these goals. Global influenza surveillance systems have been strengthened to provide earlier warning of the spread of a new influenza subtype among people, increasing the window for vaccine development, production, and administration before pandemic disease is widespread. Nevertheless, with limited influenza vaccine production capacity and the potential rapid spread of disease globally, vaccine shortages appear inevitable. Optimally achieving pandemic response goals, therefore, requires that available vaccine be effectively targeted to defined priority groups.

A critical strategy to reduce pandemic health impacts – among persons with influenza as well as those with other life-threatening diseases that require care during a pandemic – is to preserve the quality of medical care, particularly in hospitals. Vaccinating hospital personnel would reduce absenteeism due to illness or fear of acquiring disease in the workplace. Because of limited vaccine availability and the need to vaccinate multiple priority groups, targeting vaccination to those hospital personnel who are most essential to quality patient care during a 6–8-week community pandemic outbreak would improve efficiency. Protecting outpatient primary care providers also would be important as delivery of health care in the community will be needed to keep hospitals from becoming overwhelmed.

Maintaining public safety and other essential community services also is important to achieving pandemic response goals. The specific occupational groups to include in this category are not clear and may differ between regions or communities. Limited vaccine supply may dictate a more restricted definition than would be optimal. A critical benchmark to guide decision-making on priority groups may be the question: could the service be adequately maintained despite the loss of one-third of employees who would likely become ill during the outbreak period?

Protecting persons at high-risk for severe or fatal influenza is the focus of annual influenza recommendations and also will be a priority during a pandemic. Based on current ACIP recommendations, almost 30% of the US population is included in this category. Risk groups in a pandemic, however, could differ from those for annual disease. For example, if an H2 strain were to cause the next pandemic, some elderly persons may have partial immunity because of prior exposure to this subtype. Most 2004 human cases and deaths from H5N1 avian influenza in Asia have occurred in children and young adults although it is unclear whether this reflects increased risk of severe illness or more frequent exposure to the poultry vector. An assumption that risk groups will be similar to those for annual disease can be used for pandemic planning but actual vaccination recommendations and programs will need to be based on the epidemiology of the pandemic. A strategy of indirectly protecting persons at high risk by vaccinating children, who are most likely to transmit infection, could be considered (Monto et al. 1969). However, this approach would be a radical departure from past and current practices and would not likely be adopted in the absence of strong supportive data from mathematical models and community trials.

Mass vaccination campaigns coordinated by public health personnel would be most efficient and effective in delivering vaccine to priority groups in a pandemic. Evaluations of adherence by office-based clinicians to special recommendations during shortages of influenza and other vaccines have shown doses frequently being administered to persons not in recommended groups (Broder et al 2005; CDC 2004b). The risks and consequences of misallocation would be exacerbated in a pandemic when risk of severe disease is high and vaccine supply limited. Public sector control of vaccine supply and administration in occupational and community clinic settings would optimize targeting and enhance meeting response goals early in a pandemic. As vaccine supply increases and key priority groups are protected, strategies for vaccine delivery may evolve toward the primarily private sector program used in annual influenza outbreaks, possibly with a greater public sector role to ensure equity in access to vaccine among all racial and ethnic groups.

The national pandemic influenza preparedness and response plan outlines goals for pandemic vaccination and offers guidance regarding priority groups, but planning and implementing specific public sector vaccination activities will be a responsibility of the state and local health departments. State pandemic plans define preparedness activities that will be undertaken during the interpandemic period and response activities that will be implemented during the pandemic (Table 4). State functions include receiving vaccine and storing it securely, distributing vaccine to local health departments, administering it to state level personnel in priority groups, monitoring vaccine coverage and adverse events, and coordinating communications and education. Local leadership will be needed as plans must be tailored to the specific needs of communities, partnerships must be developed with local health agencies and others, and vaccination programs must be implemented.

Mass vaccination for a pandemic will be similar to programs for other public health emergencies. The major components of a mass vaccination plan are summarized with specific reference to issues relevant to an influenza pandemic.

3.1
Coordination

Mass vaccination programs require coordinating large numbers of people and multiple agencies. Incident command provides a standardized structure that is appropriate for a range of public health emergency response programs and can be included in an all-hazards plan. Characteristics of an incident command structure include pre-defied roles and responsibilities for all staff, a clear and uniform chain of command, scalability to meet different levels of program needs, and integration into a community's emergency operations system. Because all communities will be affected by a pandemic, defining the command structure at national, state, and local levels and the interactions between these will be important.

Table 4 Pandemic influenza vaccination preparedness activities to be implemented by State Health Departments

- Improve vaccine delivery during the interpandemic period for recommended groups
- Define vaccination priority groups specifically within the guidance provided from the national level
- Develop and translate educational materials for the public, including CDC's Vaccine Information Statement, which is required by law to be given to all vaccinees
- Develop standing orders allowing influenza vaccination without an individual order by a physician
- Identify health care workers who can assist in a mass vaccination program during a pandemic
- Define the legal basis for licensed and nonlicensed health care personnel providing vaccinations
- Identify whether state statutes provide for mandatory vaccination in specific settings during a pandemic
- Develop a mass vaccination plan and clinic flow-charts
- Develop a mechanism for local health departments (LHDs) to order vaccine from the State
- Develop plans for secure vaccine storage and secure delivery to LHDs
- Develop a registry to track vaccination and provide reminders if a two-dose schedule is needed
- Develop a system to monitor vaccine adverse events in collaboration with CDC and national adverse event surveillance systems
- Review vaccination plans developed by LHDs and assure their adequacy
- Conduct tabletop and field exercises of vaccine preparedness and vaccination

3.2
Staffing

The first step in determining staffing is to define the size of the population to be vaccinated and the strategies needed to reach those populations. Uncertainties regarding priority groups and vaccine supply complicate the planning process. Neighboring jurisdictions would benefit from joint planning activities as persons who live in one state may be vaccinated in a neighboring state where they are employed. Because many vaccinations are likely to be provided in health care and other occupational settings, staff and other human resources already may be on-site. After determining the number of persons to be served, rough calculations can be made to determine the number of staff needed to vaccinate a given population in a given time period. At least two software programs exist to help determine staffing needs (Hupert and Cuomo 2003; CDC 2004c). Although increasing the number of clinics enhances convenience to the public, the number of clinics must be balanced against available staffing as economies of scale are greatest for large clinics.

Identifying sufficient staffing is one of the greatest challenges of mass vaccination. While vaccination early in a pandemic likely will be coordinated by the public sector, staffing needs far exceed what health departments alone can provide, particularly since public health staff likely will have additional pandemic response tasks and may be impacted by pandemic disease. Thus, public health must partner with the private sector to staff mass vaccination clinics. Establishing agreements during the interpandemic period with health care agencies that provide mass vaccination annually in workplaces and other community sites is one potential strategy. Volunteers also may be used in some mass vaccination clinic roles. It may be necessary to relax scopes of work so that persons not normally licensed to vaccinate can legally perform this function in emergency circumstances. Issues of liability protection for vaccinators and other clinic staff may need to be addressed.

Given the uncertainty of when a pandemic will occur and who specifically would staff a vaccination program, training is likely not possible before the event except for persons who will be responsible for training others. Training plans need to be developed in such a way that a relatively small number of persons can train others on a 'just in time' basis.

3.3
Location of Clinics

Clinic location will depend on the target groups for vaccination, characteristics of the community, and human and physical resources available. In an exercise conducted in San Francisco, many neighborhood clinics were held, an ideal approach for a densely populated area where people could walk to clinics and important given limited parking space. In other settings, where the population is more dispersed, availability of adequate parking may be crucial. The need to assure equity in access between racial, ethnic, and socioeconomic groups requires an understanding of issues and needs specific to different subgroups within a community. Clinics located in occupational settings may be optimal for vaccination of some priority groups. Potential locations for community clinics include schools, churches, or auditoriums.

3.4
Clinic Lay-Out

The clinic must be laid out with a number of sequential stations, including for example eligibility screening, registration, medical screening, and vaccination areas. Clinics should have a separate area for special needs patients (e.g., advanced age, infirm) who may not be able to walk through the clinic stations. Ideally, all vaccination clinics in a jurisdiction will share the same floor plan making it easier for staff to move between clinics. Translation services will be important in some communities. Buildings where clinics are to be held need to have separate entry and exit doors to allow for unidirectional flow, functional and accessible restrooms, adequate space for all clinic functions, and separate areas for vaccine preparation and staff breaks.

3.5
Security and Crowd Control

The importance of security for mass vaccination clinics and the number of persons needed for this purpose should not be underestimated. Security staff will be needed for crowd control, traffic movement and personnel safety. In a setting where vaccination priorities are strictly enforced, security personnel may need to help turn away those not in the designated groups. Limiting the number of controlled entry and exit portals will facilitate clinic security.

3.6
Communication and Public Education

The scale of a mass vaccination campaign in a pandemic and the anxiety inherent to a health emergency when a key preventive intervention must be rationed call for clear and consistent communication with the public. The public must be informed of the need to target vaccine supplies, the rationale and the approach to defining priority groups, and the eventual availability of vaccine for everyone. In addition, people must be informed of the procedures to be used in the vaccination campaign before it begins. This includes informing them where and when they need to present for vaccination, the expected processes, and the importance of follow-up if a two-dose vaccination schedule is required. Information must be disseminated through the appropriate channels to reach all the target populations and must be disseminated in multiple languages as needed.

3.7
Exercises

Clinic drills offer an opportunity to test a clinic lay-out, identify and remedy bottleneck areas, and optimize staffing. Exercises are important not only to determine how well the plan will function, but also to help develop partnerships with other agencies and between the public and private sectors. By contrast with other emergency preparedness vaccination programs where opportunities to realistically test vaccination plans are not available, with influenza such opportunities occur annually. Thus, exercises to vaccinate hospital-based heath care workers can help achieve annual influenza prevention goals while also enhancing pandemic preparedness.

Monitoring and evaluation of pandemic influenza vaccination programs are an important shared responsibility of national, state, and local public health personnel. Systems must be developed or existing immunization registries adapted to capture pandemic vaccination data. The ability to use such systems to automatically generate reminders for a second dose, if needed, would be of benefit. Analysis of coverage data at community level should be done periodically during the pandemic to determine whether persons are completing their vaccination schedule, to assess whether vaccine is being effectively targeted to priority groups, and to determine whether disparities in coverage exist between segments of the population among the target populations.

Careful monitoring for adverse events is important for any vaccination program but particularly for pandemic influenza vaccination given the occurrence of GBS associated with swine influenza vaccination in 1976. During a pandemic, national adverse event surveillance may be augmented by state-based systems to stimulate reporting and analyze and investigate signals of potentially vaccine-linked adverse events. The ability to distinguish between coincidental and vaccine-associated events is a particular challenge. Within the first 2 weeks after implementing the swine influenza vaccination program in October 1976, three elderly persons in Pittsburgh died of cardiac disease within a day after vaccination. The local coroner would not rule out vaccination as a contributing factor, the media disseminated the story widely, and several states suspended their vaccination programs. Subsequent analysis of data on cardiac mortality showed that in the context of a mass vaccination campaign, three deaths shortly after vaccination could be expected to occur. The furor subsided, the President demonstrated confidence in the program by being vaccinated, and vaccinations resumed (Neustadt and Feinberg 1978). This episode illustrates, however, the potential for mass vaccination activities to be derailed by vaccine safety concerns and the importance of communication and education before the campaign about the occurrence of coincidental health events, and the value of having calculated, in advance, the expected frequencies of common health events.

4
The Future of Mass Vaccination for Annual and Pandemic Influenza

The significant annual health impacts of influenza, the difficulty achieving high coverage rates among older adults and those at high-risk for severe disease, and lower vaccine efficacy in these populations, have led to consideration of expanded vaccination recommendations. Children experience the highest rates of influenza and transmit infection to household contacts (Neuzil et al. 2002; Principi et al. 2004). Community-based studies have shown that vaccinating children against influenza also decreases influenza disease among adults (Monto et al. 1969; Glezen 2004). A longitudinal study of excess pneumonia and influenza mortality in Japan suggests that rates dropped between 1962 and 1987 when the influenza vaccination program was targeted at school children but increased once the program was discontinued in favor of vaccinating the elderly and those at high risk (Richert et al. 2001). Results from mathematical models also predict greater vaccination program impacts when vaccine is targeted to children (Weycker et al. 2005), with adults indirectly protected because of decreased exposure to influenza as transmission within the community is decreased.

Major challenges exist to implementing a childhood influenza vaccination strategy, potentially under a universal vaccination recommendation. Influenza vaccine supply delays and shortages have occurred in the US during recent years and influenza vaccine manufacturing capacity falls short of that needed to support implementation of expanded recommendations. Developing feasible strategies to reach children and achieve high vaccination coverage, and acceptability of annual vaccination to children, their parents, and medical care providers are additional challenges. Vaccination campaigns in schools would be an ideal approach to achieve access to the large majority of children. In the Michigan community-based study, 86% of all school children were vaccinated: 92% of those in elementary school and 75% of high-school students. Under Ontario, Canada's universal vaccination recommendation, coverage among children tended to be greater in health districts that held school-based clinics compared with those that did not (S. Tamblyn, personal communication). Mass vaccination in schools would be facilitated by use of more acceptable vaccine delivery methods than injection. Intranasal administration of live-attenuated influenza vaccine, licensed in the US for use in healthy persons 5–49 years old, offers an alternate approach. This vaccine also may offer greater cross-protection against drifted influenza variants leading to better effectiveness than inactivated vaccine when the match between the circulating and vaccine strain is less close or in a second year after vaccination the previous season (Gaglani et al. 2004).

If a universal influenza vaccination recommendation were made, in addition to school-based vaccination, implementation would require additional community-based strategies, including expansion of clinics at health departments, workplaces, retail locations, and community centers. Easier vaccine delivery methods also would be of value for adult vaccination; self-administration of the intranasal vaccine has been proposed but would require licensure. Achieving success in vaccinating adults also requires strengthening the public-sector adult immunization infrastructure, which has been a critical factor in the pediatric vaccination program. Key elements of proposals to strengthen adult immunization are enhancing capabilities at state health departments and increasing the public sector role in vaccination financing for adults, possibly through federal financing of vaccines for low income and uninsured adults who do not qualify for current entitlement programs. Some state health departments have conducted mass vaccination exercises for pandemic preparedness which may mimic their role if universal influenza vaccination were recommended annually.

Vaccination for pandemic influenza is constrained primarily by the limited vaccine supply that would be available. If manufacturing capacity were expanded or if innovations in vaccine formulation or delivery were studied and licensed before the next pandemic, approaches to pandemic vaccination also may change. Major expansions in production capacity are unlikely because manufacturers calibrate capacity to annual vaccine demand; in addition, building new facilities requires several years. A more promising solution is licensure of 'antigen-sparing' approaches which would expand the number of doses produced by decreasing the amount of vaccine antigen required in each dose. Adding an aluminum adjuvant to influenza vaccine (Hehme et al. 2002) and administering vaccine intradermally (Belshe et al. 2004; Kenney et al. 2004) have been shown to enhance immune response to vaccination for some circulating as well as novel influenza strains and may make possible lower antigen dose formulations; further investigation of these strategies is needed. An intervention that substantially expands pandemic vaccine availability may decrease the need for strict adherence to vaccination only of priority groups. Efficient mass vaccination programs would be more critical if more doses were available to be administered. Intradermal vaccination would pose special challenges due to the difficulty administering intradermal vaccination with needle and syringe. New intradermal or transcutaneous vaccine delivery methods are being developed to overcome this obstacle (Glenn et al. 2003).

The optimal long-term solution to pandemic and annual vaccination is the development of a new influenza vaccine that induces an immune response to an antigen that is present in all influenza subtypes and does not change. This will prove challenging as natural influenza infection one year does not protect against infection with another strain the following year. However, the availability of various strategies to enhance immune responses beyond what occurs in nature may make this goal possible. A common-epitope influenza vaccine would likely obviate the need for annual vaccination and would mean that persons vaccinated previously would be immune or partially immune to the pandemic strain, depending on the level and duration of protection afforded by vaccination. It also would mean that vaccine could be stockpiled and the risk of shortages eliminated. Although this is a long-term goal that may not be achieved by the time of the next pandemic, the nature of the influenza virus and inevitability of annual epidemics and periodic pandemics, makes it a goal worth pursuing vigorously.

References

Belshe RB, Newman FK, Cannon J, et al. (2004) Serum antibody responses after intradermal vaccination against influenza. N Engl J Med 351:2286–2294

Bridges CB, Thompson WW, Meltzer MI, et al. (2000) Effectiveness and cost-benefit of influenza vaccination of healthy working adults: a randomized controlled trial. JAMA 2000 284:1655–1663

Broder KR, MacNeil A, Malone S (2005) Who's calling the shots? Pediatricians' adherence to the 2001–2003 Pneumococcal Conjugate Vaccine Shortage Recommendations. Pediatrics (in press)

CDC (1968) Recommendations of the Public Health Service Advisory Committee on Immunization Practices: A2 influenza virus vaccine, monovalent, 1968–69. MMWR 17:368

CDC (1968a) Recommendations of the Public Health Service Advisory Committee on Immunization Practices: influenza vaccines – 1968–69. MMWR 17:246–247

CDC (2000) Adult immunization programs in nontraditional settings: quality standards and guidance for program evaluation: a report of the National Vaccine Advisory Committee. MMWR 49(RR-01)1–13

CDC (2004a) Prevention and control of influenza: Recommendations of the Advisory Committee on Immunization Practices. MMWR 53(RR-06):1–40

CDC (2004b) Estimated influenza vaccination coverage among adults and children – United States, September 1–November 30, 2004

CDC (2004c) Maxi-Vac 1.0 http://www.bt.cdc.gov/agent/smallpox/vaccination/maxi-vac/index.asp (accessed 12/17/2004)

D'Heilly SJ, Nichol KL (2004) Work site-based influenza vaccination in healthcare and non-healthcare settings. Infect Control Hosp Epidemiol 25:941–945

Earhart KC, Beadle C, Miller LK, et al. (2001) Outbreak of influenza in a highly vaccinated crew of U.S. navy ship. Emerg Infect Dis 7:463–465

Gaglani MJ, Piedra PA, Herschler GB, et al. (2004) Direct and total effectiveness of the intranasal, live-attenuated, trivalent cold-adapted influenza virus vaccine against the 2000–2001 influenza A (H1N1) and B epidemic in healthy children. Arch Pediatr Adolesc Med 158:65–73

Glenn GM, Kenney RT, Hammond SA, Ellingsworth LR (2003) Transcutaneous immunization and immunostimulant strategies. ImmunolAllergy Clin N Am 23:787–813

Glezen PW (2004) Control of influenza. Tex Heart Inst J 31:39–41

Grabenstein JD, Guess HA, Hartzema AG (2001) People vaccinated by pharmacists: descriptive epidemiology. J Am Pharm Assoc 41:46–52

Gray GC, Callahan JD, Hawksworth AW, Fisher CA, Gaydos JC (1999) Respiratory diseases among U.S. military personnel: countering emerging threats. Emerg Infect Dis 5:379–385

Hehme N. Engelmann H. Kunzel W. Neumeier E. Sanger R (2002) Pandemic preparedness: lessons learnt from H2N2 and H9N2 candidate vaccines. Med Microbiol Immunol 191:203–208

Hupert N, Cuomo J (2003) Bioterrorism and Epidemic Outbreak Response Model (BERM). DHHS Agency for Healthcare Research and Quality (AHRQ). Available at http://www.ahrq.gov/news/press/pr2003/btmodpr.htm (accessed 12/17/2004)

Kenney RT, Frech SA, Muenz LR, Villar CP, Glenn GM (2004) Dose sparing with intradermal injection of influenza vaccine. N Engl J Med 351:2295–2301

McArthur MA, Simor AE, Campbell B, McGeer A (1999) Influenza vaccination in long-term-care facilities: structuring programs for success. Infect Control Hosp Epidemiol 20:499–503

Monto AS, Davenport FM, Napier JA, Francis T Jr. (1969) Effect of vaccination of a school-age population upon the course of an A2/Hong Kong influenza epidemic. Bull World Health Org 41:537–542

National Foundation for Infectious Diseases (2003) Increasing influenza immunization rates in infants and children: putting recommendations into practice. http://www.nfid.org/publications/pediatricflu.pdf (accessed 2/7/05)

Neustadt RE, Feinberg HV (1978) The Swine Flu Affair: Decision-Making on a Slippery Slope. Government Printing Office, Washington DC pp 1–189

Neuzil KM, Hohlbein C, Zhu Y (2002) Illness among schoolchildren during influenza season: effect on school absenteeism, parental absenteeism, and secondary illness in families. Arch Pediatr Adolesc Med 156:986–991

Nichol KL, Lind A, Margolis KL, et al. (1995) The effectiveness of vaccination against influenza in healthy, working adults. N Engl J Med 333:889–893

Parry MF, Grant B, Iton A, Parry PD, Baranowsky D (2004) Influenza vaccination: a collaborative effort to improve the health of the community. Infect Control Hosp Epidemiol 25:929–932

Principi N, Esposito S, Gasparini R, Marchisio P, Crovari P (2004) Burden of influenza in healthy children and their households. Arch Dis Child 89:1002–1007

Richert TA, Sugaya N, Fesdon DS, Glezen PW, Simonsen L, Tashiro M (2001) The Japanese experience with vaccinating schoolchildren against influenza. N Engl J Med 344:889–896

Salgado CD, Giannetta ET, Hayden FG, Farr BM (2004) Preventing nosocomial influenza by improving the vaccine acceptance rate of clinicians. Infect Control Hosp Epidemiol 25:923–928

Sartor C, Tissot-Dupont H, Zandotti C, Martin F, Roques P, Drancourt M (2004) Use of a mobile cart influenza program for vaccination of hospital employees. Infect Control Hosp Epidemiol 25:918–922

Szilagyi PG, Iwane MK, Humiston, et al. (2003b) Time spent by primary care practices on pediatric influenza vaccination visits: implications for universal influenza vaccination. Arch Pediatr Adolesc Med 157:191–195

Szilagyi PG, Iwane MK, Schaffer S, et al. (2003a) Potential burden of universal influenza vaccination of young children on visits to primary care practices. Pediatrics 112:821–828

Thompson WW, Shay DK, Weintraub E, Brammer L, Bridges CB, Cox NJ, Fukuda K (2004) Influenza-associated hospitalizations in the United States. JAMA 292:1333–1340

Thompson WW, Shay DK, Weintraub L, Cox N, Alderson LJ, Fukuda K (2003) Mortality associated with influenza and respiratory syncytial virus in the United States. JAMA 289:179–186

US Department of Health and Human Services (2005) http://www.hhs.gov/nvpo/pandemicplan/ (accessed 2/7/05)

Weycker D, Edelsberg J, Halloran ME, et al. (2005) Population-wide benefits of routine vaccination of children against influenza. Vaccine (in press)

World Health Organization (2005) http://www.who.int/csr/disease/avian_influenza/en/ (accessed 2/7/05)

Is Global Measles Eradication Feasible?

C. A. de Quadros (✉)

Sabin Vaccine Institute and Pan American Health Organization,
Washington, DC, USA
ciro.dequadros@sabin.org

1	Background	154
2	Measles Eradication in the Western Hemisphere	154
3	Strategies	156
4	Results	160
5	Lessons Learned	161
6	Conclusion	162
	References	163

Abstract Measles is one of most infectious diseases. Before the introduction of the measles vaccine, practically all children in the long run contracted measles. By the end of the 1980s most countries of the world had incorporated measles vaccine into their routine vaccination programs. Globally, some 800,000 deaths due to measles still occur every year, half of them in Africa. Eradication of measles would play an important role in improving child survival. The goal to eradicate measles from the Americas was set by the Pan American Sanitary Conference in 1994. Progress to date has been remarkable. Measles is no longer an endemic disease in the Americas and interruption of transmission has been documented in most countries. As of August 2005, 3 years have elapsed since the detection of the last indigenous case in Venezuela in September 2002. This experience shows that interruption of measles transmission can be achieved and sustained over a long period of time and that global eradication is feasible if appropriate strategy is implemented. Even in a new paradigm in which eradication is not followed by the discontinuation of vaccination, eradication of measles will be a good investment to avoid expensive epidemics and save the almost one million children that die every year to infection with the measles virus. It is not a dream to think that we will se a world free of measles by the year 2015.

Reproduced with permission of the Pan American Health Organization (PAHO). This article was originally published in PAHO´s book: "Vaccines. Preventing Disease and Promoting Health". To obtain information about PAHO publications visit their website at: http://publications.paho.org

1
Background

Measles is one of the most infectious diseases. Before the introduction of the measles vaccine, practically all children contracted measles in the long run. Human beings are the only reservoir of measles, although other primates, such as monkeys, also can have the infection. The most infectious phase is the prodromic one, before other symptoms, such as fever and exanthema, appear. The communicability diminishes rapidly after the appearance of exanthema [1].

At the end of the 1970s an attenuated live measles virus vaccine, which was authorized for use in the US in 1963, had already been widely disseminated in several parts of the world. It is documented that this vaccine protects for more than 20 years, but it is believed that the immunity conferred by the vaccine lasts for the entire life [2]. Its effectiveness is around 90% to 95%. Due to the interference of maternal antibodies, the effectiveness of the vaccine increases after the first 6 months of life, reaching the maximum level of 95%–98% at 12–15 months of age [3]. By the end of the 1980s, most countries of the world had incorporated measles vaccines into their routine vaccination programs, and immunization coverage with this vaccine has increased considerably. By 1990, the world reported coverage of children aged 2 years was approximately 70%.

Data from the World Health Organization (WHO) indicate that measles is responsible for 10% of deaths worldwide in children under 5 years of age. Worldwide, some 40 million cases and 800,000 deaths due to measles still occur every year; more than half of the deaths occur in Africa. The eradication of measles would, therefore, play an important role in improving child survival.

To answer the question posed in this chapter's title it is necessary to review the experiences with measles eradication in the Region of the Americas. To that end, what is briefly described here are the strategies being implemented in the Americas to interrupt indigenous measles transmission, as well as the results achieved so far.

2
Measles Eradication in the Western Hemisphere

The goal to eradicate measles from the Western Hemisphere was set by the Pan American Sanitary Conference in 1994, at the same time that that the International Commission for Certification of Poliomyelitis declared the Region polio free [4]. The rationale for the strategy used to achieve this goal was based in the epidemiology of measles before and after the vaccine was

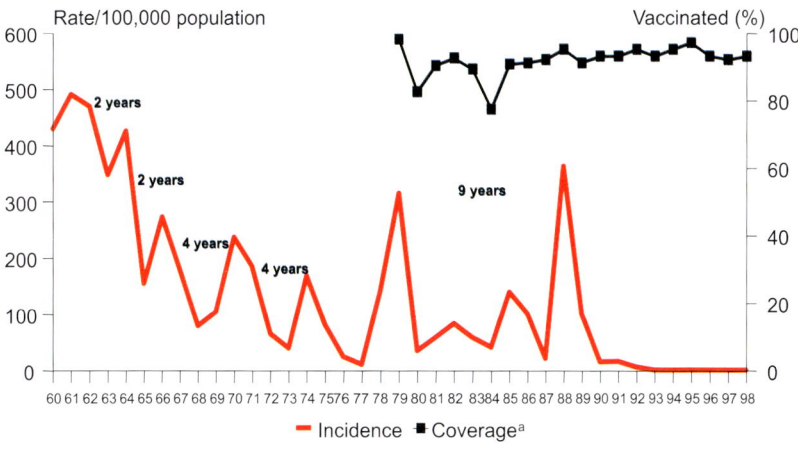

Fig. 1 Measles interepidemic periods, post-vaccine era, Chile, 1960–1998. Vaccination coverage in children <1 year of age. (Source: Immunizations Unit, PAHO)

introduced. Before the vaccine was introduced, measles epidemics occurred every couple of years, emerging as soon as a pool of susceptibles provided by every birth cohort was available to fuel transmission when the virus was introduced in a given population. After the introduction of the vaccine and with subsequent increases in vaccination coverage, the interepidemic periods lengthened, sometimes stretching for several years between one epidemic and the next. For example, the interepidemic period spanned 9 years in Chile (Fig. 1) and 12 years in the US.

Furthermore, in the pre-vaccine era, measles cases occurred in very young children and by the age of 5 years almost all had already suffered the diseases. With the introduction of the vaccine, and with increased coverage, the age specific rate increased in older children and even young adults and adults suffered measles [5].

Another important factor to consider is that a considerable number of children remain susceptible because they never received the vaccine. In addition, because vaccine effectiveness is not 100%, a small proportion of those vaccinated who were primary failures also remain susceptible. The result is that over a few years, even with a very good immunization program in place, accumulation of susceptible children will occur (Fig. 2). In other words, vaccine coverage does not equal population immunity.

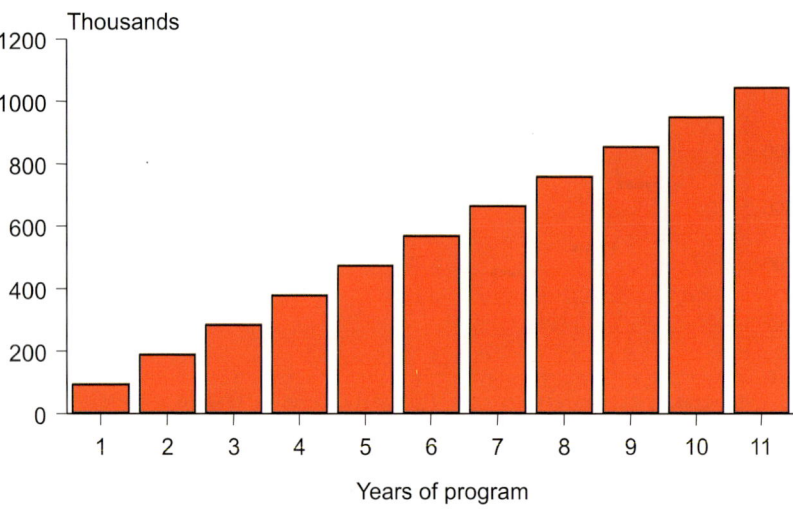

Note: 500,000 newborns: vaccine coverage, 90%; vaccine efficacy, 90%
Source: de Quadros, C.A., et al. (JAMA-January 17, 1996)

Fig. 2 Accumulation of susceptibles while an immunization program is in place. Note: 500,000 newborns, vaccine coverage, 90%; vaccine efficacy, 90%. (Source: de Quadros et al. [6])

3
Strategies

Given this background, the strategy recommended by the Pan American Health Organization called for high vaccination coverage of the susceptible population at all times and effective surveillance to detect measles transmission and respond accordingly. The vaccination strategy [6] is three-pronged. First, a one-time-only "catch-up" campaign, implemented during the low season targets all children 1–14 years of age, to attempt interruption of all chains of measles transmission. This age group was chosen because it was among them where more than 90% of the cases were occurring by the time this program started in the Americas. The strategy's second component is to "keep up" with vaccination in routine services to achieve the highest level possible of coverage in the new birth cohorts in every district of every country in order to delay the accumulation of susceptibles.

However, even with high coverage in every district, susceptibles will accumulate because some children will be missed and a few that received the vaccine are primary failures as indicated above. With average vaccination coverage of 80%, it is estimated that it takes about 5 years for the accumulation of susceptible children to be equivalent to one birth cohort. When this number is reached, it is suggested that a "follow-up" campaign be undertaken in all children aged 1–4 years, regardless of previous vaccination status. This, then, is the third component of the vaccination strategy—"follow-up" campaigns designed to address the accumulation of susceptibles. These campaigns are conducted every 4 years and target all children 1–4 years of age, regardless of previous vaccination status. The campaigns' main objective is to reach those children who never received a single dose of measles vaccine, but those children that did receive a previous dose will benefit from a second dose. This strategy offers children a "second opportunity" to receive their first measles vaccine dose. The first country to utilize this strategy in the Americas was Cuba, which successfully interrupted measles transmission in the late 1980s (Fig. 3).

The surveillance component was designed to be very simple and timely, as well as sensible to detect outbreaks and to be understood by every health worker, allowing for a prompt and adequate response (Fig. 4). Basically it works this way: if a health worker suspects measles, the suspected case should be visited by a trained epidemiologist who decides whether the case should be classified as a suspected measles case requiring further investigation and collection of a blood specimen for confirmation through an IgM capture test. If no adequate specimen was taken but there was an epidemiological link with

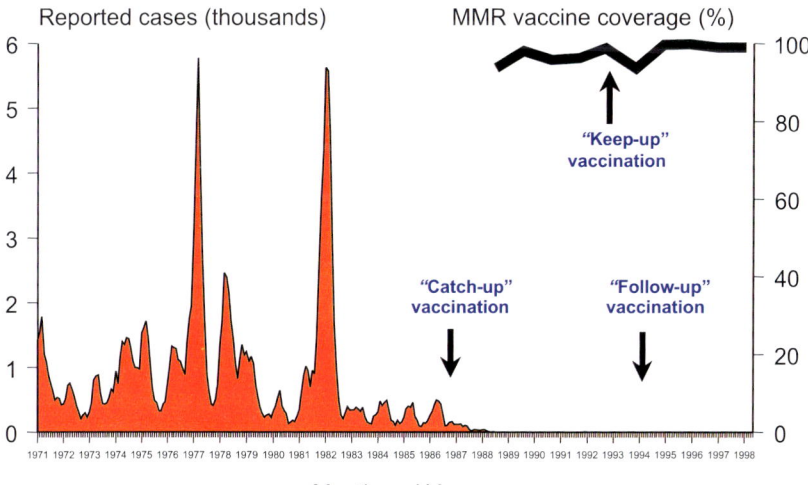

Fig. 3 Reported measles cases, by month, Cuba, 1971–1998. (Source: Ministry of Health, Cuba)

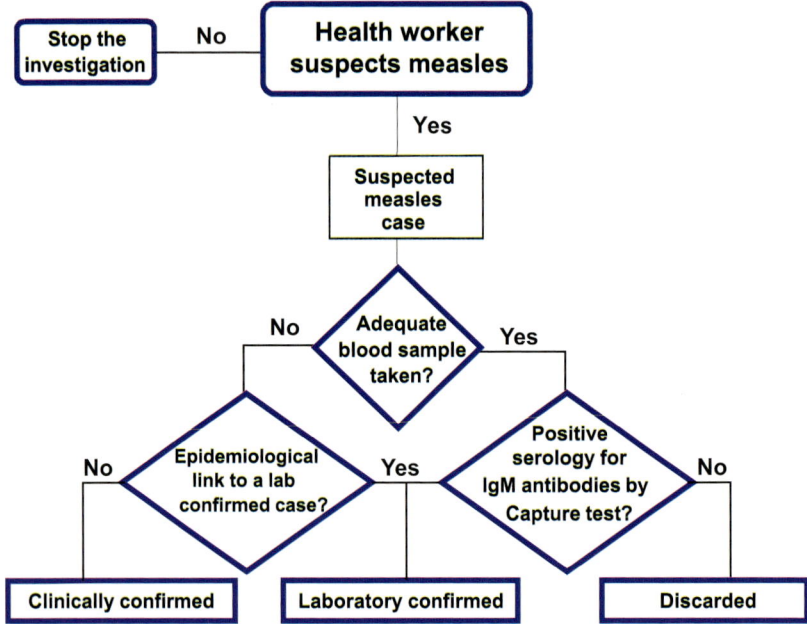

Fig. 4 Surveillance strategy for measles cases

a laboratory-confirmed case, the case also would be laboratory confirmed, otherwise it would be clinically confirmed. This last category of cases was the result of deficiencies in the surveillance system.

At the beginning of the program, a major proportion of cases were clinically confirmed, while at present nearly 100% of cases are discarded because they have adequate specimens and negative laboratory results. Surveillance was integrated with rubella surveillance to maximize the activities related to rubella control. If a suspected measles case is laboratory-negative, tests are performed to investigate for rubella, and vice versa. Management indicators have been introduced, such as the proportion of suspected cases investigated within 48 h of reporting; the proportion of those that have adequate specimens collected and sent to the lab; and for each outbreak, urine samples are taken for virus isolation. The proportion of laboratory results that is available within 5 days of receipt at the laboratory serve to measure the network performance. Active search for cases also is conducted periodically in areas that have suffered recent outbreaks or have low coverage, have reported suspected cases for some time, or where the population has low access to health services.

Is Global Measles Eradication Feasible?

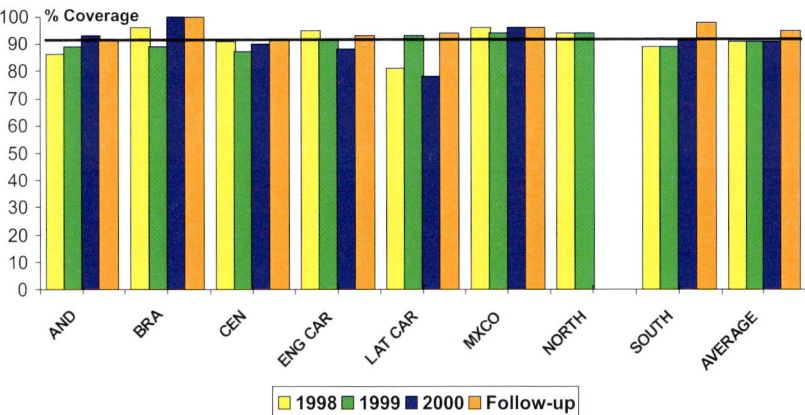

Source: Country reports. US data are from national survey for children ages 19-35 months

Fig. 5 Measles vaccination coverage, by subregion, 1998–2000, and last "follow-up" campaign. (Source: Country reports. US data are from national survey for children ages 19–35 months)

Progress to date has been remarkable. Most of the countries have conducted "catch-up" campaigns with very high coverage levels, and now most of them are in the phase of implementing "follow-up" campaigns. These campaigns usually have achieved very high coverage, more than 90% at the national level (Fig. 5).

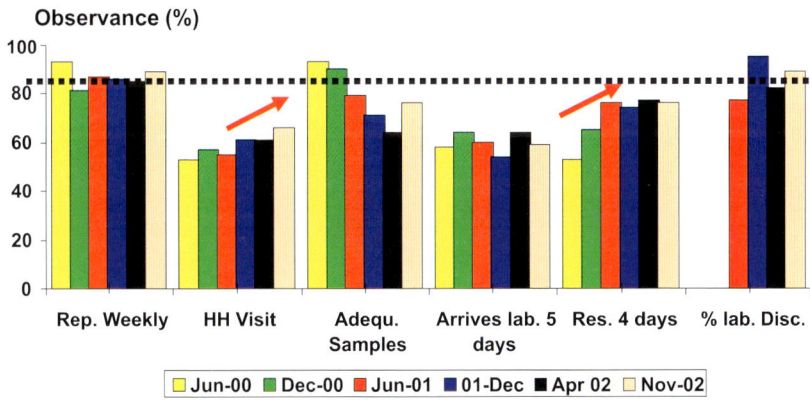

Source: Country reports, data as of November 15, 2002.

Fig. 6 Average observance, measles surveillance indicators (%), Region of the Americas, July 2000–November 2002. (Source: Country reports, data as of 15 November 2002)

Districts that are below the national average are identified, and additional "mopping-up" campaigns are then implemented in districts at risk.

Surveillance indicators have been kept at acceptable levels (Fig. 6). Laboratory response within 5 days has improved, and the laboratory-discarded cases now reach over 80% [7].

4
Results

In 1990, there were more than 240,000 cases reported in the region. In 1996, only 2,106 cases of measles were reported in the Western Hemisphere. Of these, some 50% were laboratory confirmed. By the end of 1996, the number of measles cases in the Americas had been reduced by 99%, compared with 1990. In 1997 there was a resurgence of measles in São Paulo, Brazil, that country's only state that did no implement a follow-up campaign due in the country for 1996. An outbreak that started in early 1997, originating from a probable importation from Europe, spread to other states and to several other countries in the region. By the end of 1997, more than 50,000 cases were reported in the Americas, with more than 90% originating in Brazil [8].

In 1998, the number of cases declined to 14,000 cases, following the epidemic generated in Brazil in 1997, with subsequent spread to Argentina, Bolivia, and eventually to the Dominican Republic and Haiti. During 2001

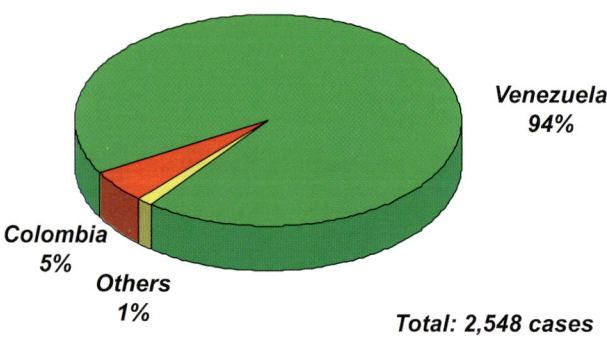

Fig. 7 Distribution of confirmed measles cases, Colombia, Venezuela, and all other countries, Region of the Americas, 2002. Data as of 16 November 2002. (Source: Pan American Health Organization, Immunizations Unit)

only 545 cases were reported in the entire region, with epidemic transmission at the end of 2001 only in Venezuela and a few importations into the northern border areas of Colombia.

Transmission in the Dominican Republic and Haiti was interrupted in mid-2001. The majority of cases reported in 2002 were from Venezuela, with other countries reporting a few cases related to importations from other Regions of the world (Fig. 7).

The last indigenous cases in the region were in Colombia in week 36 and in Venezuela in week 38. As of today, 4 months have elapsed without indigenous transmission being detected anywhere in the Western Hemisphere.

5
Lessons Learned

In summary, the "catch-up" campaigns, the "keep-up" activities, and the "follow-up" campaigns have been successful in interrupting measles transmission in the Americas.

Measles is no longer an endemic disease in the Americas, and interruption of transmission has been documented in most countries. Thirty-eight of 47 countries and territories have been free of indigenous measles transmission for more than 2 years. The Americas suffered a re-emergence of measles in 2001/2002 because of failure to fully implement the recommended strategy. In that instance, most cases were seen in vaccinated pre-school aged children and in unvaccinated young adults, with health professionals playing a very important role in the chain of transmission. A similar reemergence of measles occurred in 1997 and 1998 in Brazil for the same reason, failure to fully implement the strategy.

Importations of measles into countries that have followed the PAHO recommended strategies did not generate epidemics, and only occasionally generated a few secondary cases. This happened in El Salvador, for instance, which had the last case in 1996. In May 2001 two young adults who had been traveling in Europe, returned infected with measles, probably acquired in Switzerland. There was no secondary transmission in spite of an active search conducted throughout the country in which basically every household in was visited. Peru suffered several importations from neighboring Bolivia during the outbreak during 2000. Only in a few instances were there secondary cases within the household were the importation had occurred. Cases in Canada and the US also have been linked to importations from Europe. In Mexico, two cases were imported from Japan, into Cancún, a very busy tourist resort, but with no spread into the overall community.

Surveillance has improved considerably throughout the region, and active search has not detected transmission in any country. In the Dominican Republic and Haiti there were house-to-house vaccinations to control a vaccine-derived polio outbreak that occurred in 2000/2201. This polio outbreak was concomitant with the importation of measles into both countries, therefore the vaccination campaigns used polio and measles vaccines. Furthermore health workers were offered a US$ 100 reward dollars if they found a case of polio or measles during the house-to-house visits. No case of either disease was found.

Although the resurgence of measles in the Americas during 1997 represented an important increase compared with the number of cases reported in 1996, the total of 53,000 cases represents only about 10% of the cases reported in 1990. Nevertheless, important lessons can be extracted from this experience.

First, the lack of a timely "follow-up" vaccination campaign in 1996 in São Paolo for children 1–4 years old, combined with low coverage of routine vaccination ("keep-up") of infants with at least one dose of measles vaccine, allowed for a fast and dangerous accumulation of susceptible children. Second, the presence of a great many young adults who were not exposed to the natural infection and had never been vaccinated exacerbated the risk of an outbreak. Third, the measles virus was most likely introduced from Europe into São Paulo. Finally, the city's great population density facilitated contact between infected persons and the susceptible population.

Surveillance data for measles, combined with the results of molecular epidemiology studies, indicate that the countries of the Americas are continually exposed to measles virus from other regions of the world where measles continues to be endemic.

As of today, 4 months have elapsed since the detection of the last case in Venezuela. The eradication of the clade 9 of measles virus that was imported into Venezuela has been documented [9].

6
Conclusion

The experience of the last 5 years with the measles eradication program in the Americas shows that measles transmission can be interrupted and interruption can be sustained over a long period if countries fully apply the strategy of vaccination recommended by PAHO for all the countries of the region.

The experience described indicates that the PAHO strategy can effectively achieve and sustain the interruption of epidemic transmission in a very large geographical area, such as the Western Hemisphere. From this experience we believe that global eradication is feasible if an appropriate strategy is implemented. We also believe–and the experience in the America's proves this, that the current measles vaccine–although not perfect, has been adequate to stop measles transmission. The eradication of measles will have a major impact in childhood morbidity and mortality. Even in a new paradigm in which eradication is not followed by the discontinuation of vaccination, eradication of measles will be a good investment to avoid expensive epidemics of measles, but most importantly, to save the almost one million children that die every year due to infection with the measles virus.

However, before a global initiative on measles eradication is launched, it is necessary to demonstrate that poliomyelitis has been eradicated. There also will be programmatic, political and financial obstacles that will need to be overcome before global measles eradication is launched. Partnerships will be essential to support governments embarking on it.

It is not a dream to imagine a world free of measles by the year 2015.

References

1. Krugman S, Katz SL, Gershon AA, Wilfert C (1985) Infectious diseases of children. 8th ed. Mosby, St. Louis
2. Krugman, S, Giles, JP, Jacobs AM, Friedman H (1963) Studies with a further attenuated live measles-virus vaccine. Pediatrics 31:919–928
3. Markowitz LE, Preblud SR, Fine PE, Orenstein WA (1990) Duration of live measles vaccine-induced immunity. Pediatr Infect Dis J 9(2):101–110
4. Pan American Health Organization (1994) Measles elimination by the year 2000. EPI Newsletter 16(5):1–2
5. Clements CJ, Strassburg M, Cutts FT, Torel C (1992) The epidemiology of measles. World Health Stat Q 45(2–3):285–291
6. de Quadros CA, Olivé JM, Hersh BS, Strassburg MA, Henderson DA, Brandling-Bennett D, et al. (1996) Measles elimination in the Americas. Evolving strategies. JAMA 275(3):224–229
7. Hersh BS, Tambini G, Nogueira AC, Carrasco P, de Quadros CA (2000) Review of regional measles surveillance data in the Americas, 1996–99. Lancet 355(9219):1943–1948
8. Pan American Health Organization (1997) Measles in the Americas, 1997. EPI Newsletter 19(6):1–3
9. United States of America, Department of Health and Human Services, Centers for Disease Control and Prevention (2003) Absence of transmission of the d9 measles virus–Region of the Americas, November 2002-March 2003. MMWR Morb Mortal Wkly Rep 52(11):228–229

Measles Aerosol Vaccination

J. L. Valdespino-Gómez[1] (✉) · M. de Lourdes Garcia-Garcia[2] ·
J. Fernandez-de-Castro[2] · A. M. Henao-Restrepo[3] · J. Bennett[4] ·
J. Sepulveda-Amor[1]

[1]Coordination of the National Institutes of Health, Periférico Sur, No. 4118–1er. piso,
Col. Jardines del Pedregal, Del. Alvaro Obregón, C.P. 01900 Mexico
jvaldesp@insp.mx

[2]Instituto Nacional de Salud Pública/Escuela de Salud Pública de México,
Ave. Universidad 655, Mor. CP 62508 Cuernavaca, Mexico

[3]Initiative for Vaccine Research, Department of Immunization,
Vaccines and Biologicals, World Health Organization, 20 Avenue Appia,
1211 Geneva 27, Switzerland

[4]Department of Epidemiology, Rollins School of Public Health,
Grace Crum Rollins Building, 1518 Clifton Road, Atlanta, GA 30322, USA

1	Measles Disease Burden	166
2	New Approaches to Measles Control	166
3	Benefits of Measles Vaccination via the Respiratory Route	168
4	The Aerosol Method Using the Classic Mexican Device	168
4.1	The Classic Mexican Device	168
4.2	Aerosolization of Vaccine	168
4.3	Dose Administered by the Aerosol Method	169
4.4	Dose Reaching the Lung Parenchyma	171
4.5	Considerations on Vaccine Strain, Presentation and Manufacturer	171
5	Experience in Administration of Measles Vaccine via the Respiratory Route	172
5.1	In Vitro Studies	172
5.2	Animal Studies	172
5.3	Clinical Studies	173
5.3.1	Initial Studies	173
5.3.2	Mass Campaign	173
5.3.3	South African Studies	185
5.3.4	Recent Mexican Studies	185
6	Future Challenges	188
7	The Measles Aerosol Project	189

8   Conclusions 189

References 190

Abstract Measles ranks fifth among the five major childhood conditions which are responsible for 21% of all deaths in low and middle-income countries. Measles immunization is considered the most cost-effective public health intervention in the world. In recent years, there has been a critical need to identify alternative routes of measles immunization, which are rapid, reliable, cost-effective, needle-free, and suitable for use in mass campaigns. Aerosol administration of measles vaccines in mass campaigns was first proposed by Dr. Albert Sabin. We review the different clinical trials that have been conducted using the classic Mexican device as well as issues regarding vaccine strain, presentation, and manufacturer. Results of clinical trials indicate that the method is safe and immunogenic in infants and school age children. The viral inoculum will probably need to be increased when administered to infants. From the logistical point of view, the use of the aerosol method has not been evaluated in routine immunization although feasibility of its routine implementation was proved in mass campaigns in Mexico. Cost savings will probably be demonstrated. As to licensure, its compliance with the appropriate international regulatory requirements for medical aerosol delivery devices is in process.

1
Measles Disease Burden

According to the World Health Organization (WHO) [1], immunization programs have yielded the most significant changes in child health in the last few decades. However, although some vaccines represent the most cost-effective public health intervention of all, the world does not use them enough. Measles ranks fifth among the five major childhood conditions which are responsible for 21% of all deaths in low and middle income countries [1]. For 2002, WHO estimated that 611,000 deaths due to measles occurred during that year and that the burden of disease using disability adjusted life years (DALYs) was of 21,475, 000 (sum of the years of life lost owing to premature mortality and the years lost through disability) [2].

2
New Approaches to Measles Control

Measles immunization is considered to be the most cost-effective public health intervention in the world [3]. Failure to deliver at least one dose of measles vaccine to all infants remains the primary reason for high measles morbidity and mortality. Additionally, some countries do not provide a second opportunity for measles vaccination which has the purpose of immunizing children who were not vaccinated as infants or who failed to respond to an initial dose [4]. Achievement of high measles vaccine coverage throughout populations, followed by mass campaigns, has been shown capable of interrupting transmission in the Americas where the disease is no longer endemic [3]. The Pan American Health Organization (PAHO) has recommended supplementary immunization activities to rapidly interrupt transmission of measles that have notably decreased incidence rates in the Latin American and the Caribbean countries, particularly after an initial vaccine failure [5, 6]. In other parts of the world, mass campaigns have been carried out in many countries and situations. However vaccine coverage is highly variable, estimated as low as 35% in some African countries [2]. Therefore, it is a priority to design strategies that achieve effective delivery of these interventions. Several of the advantages associated with aerosol immunization, such as public acceptance, low cost and few side effects, would contribute to extend coverage of childhood vaccination.

Another obstacle to measles eradication that is being faced by international agencies such as the United Nations Children's Fund (UNICEF) is the vaccine supply for the near future. This organization which is the single largest buyer of pediatric vaccines, has experienced in recent years temporary vaccine shortages and its administrators consider it may become a global problem [7]. In addition to the areas that are being focused by UNICEF, methods such as aerosol delivery, could potentially decrease the overall requirements for vaccine, and contribute to overcoming this obstacle.

It is recognized that unsafe injections and disposal of waste occur in both preventative and curative scenarios and place children, health staff and communities at risk for infection with blood-borne diseases. It is estimated that up to one-third of all infections administered in developing countries are unsafe [8]. Auto-disable syringes that block the plunger after a single use are the safest devices for injections because they can only be used once. However, many countries are not able to afford these new devices and continue to use glass or standard disposable syringes [9]. Other methods, such as jet injectors, have been proposed to administer vaccines through the skin without the use of conventional needles. (Dr. Ciro de Quadros discusses these methods more extensively; see his chapter in this volume.) The aerosol method would contribute to overcoming this problem by circumventing the need for needles and providing a noninvasive and safe method which would greatly reduce the need for training health personnel and would be suitable for vaccination during mass campaigns.

3
Benefits of Measles Vaccination via the Respiratory Route

In recent years, there has been a critical need to identify alternative routes of immunization for prevention of infectious diseases. The basis for this mandate derives from several sources including the requirement for more rapid, reliable, cost-effective, needle-free methods for mass immunization campaigns targeted at the global eradication of infectious diseases such as measles. Aerosol administration of measles vaccines in mass campaigns was first proposed by Dr. Albert Sabin [10]. A review of previous studies of various routes of measles immunization [11], identified several important advantages of the aerosol route. These advantages included its noninvasiveness, good serological response in seronegative children, apparently good boosting response in seropositive children, evidence of effect in young infants with maternal antibody, potential to stimulate local respiratory tract immunity and prevent re-infection and potential for administration by nonmedical personnel. Several of the advantages that had not been tested when this review was published have been confirmed though studies performed in recent years.

4
The Aerosol Method Using the Classic Mexican Device
4.1
The Classic Mexican Device

The aerosol method as used in the Classic Mexican Device was designed by Dr. Albert Sabin and adapted by Dr. Fernandez de Castro. A plastic nebulizer containing the vaccine is placed in a container with crushed ice, and aerosols are generated by connecting the nebulizer to an electric compressor. Aerosols are generated by connecting the nebulizer to an electric compressor, 40–50 psi, (Evans T045) providing approximately 0.10 to 0.18 ml of aerosol in 30-s bursts. A plastic nebulizer (AeroMist Treatment Set of IPI Medical Products catalogue No. 4107, IPI Medical Products) containing the vaccine is placed in a container with crushed ice. A plastic tube joins the nebulizer to a Teflon tube ending in a cone template through which the vaccine is administered. A paper cone is loosely fitted over the nose and month of the child and is discarded after each use (Fig. 1).

4.2
Aerosolization of Vaccine

The aerosol containing viral particles is generated by the nebulizer. A pressurized jet air stream delivered by the compressor enters through a narrow

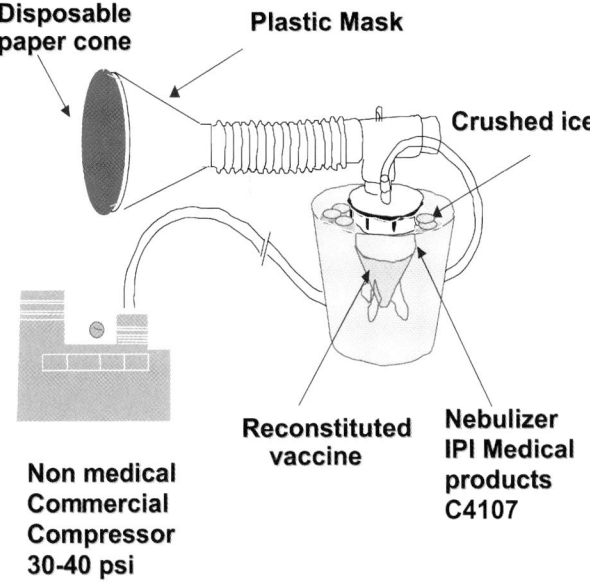

Fig. 1 Diagram of the Classic Mexican Device

tube (labeled A in Fig. 2) and is forced through a narrow opening called the venturi. The jet stream causes a pressure drop near the venturi (B). Decreased pressure creates a vacuum effect and causes liquid vaccine in the reservoir to be sucked up through the liquid feeding tube (C). The jet stream strikes the rising liquid and breaks it up into droplets (B). Large droplets fall back into the reservoir or are deflected by baffles. Small droplets (1–10 μm) are pushed by the jet stream out of the nebulizer as a fine mist that is inhaled by the subject (C) (Fig. 2)

4.3
Dose Administered by the Aerosol Method

One of the most important aspects of immunization by aerosol route is calculation of the amount of viral particles that is delivered by the nebulizer. Estimation for the dose administered by the device is based on several aspects that include vaccine potency, volume of vaccine nebulized per unit of time, total volume of aerosol produced per unit of time, average number of inspirations of the subject and tidal volume of the individual. Vaccine potency varies according to the vaccine that is used and is different for each lot. The volume of vaccine nebulized is usually calculated for 30 s. Field reports on volume of

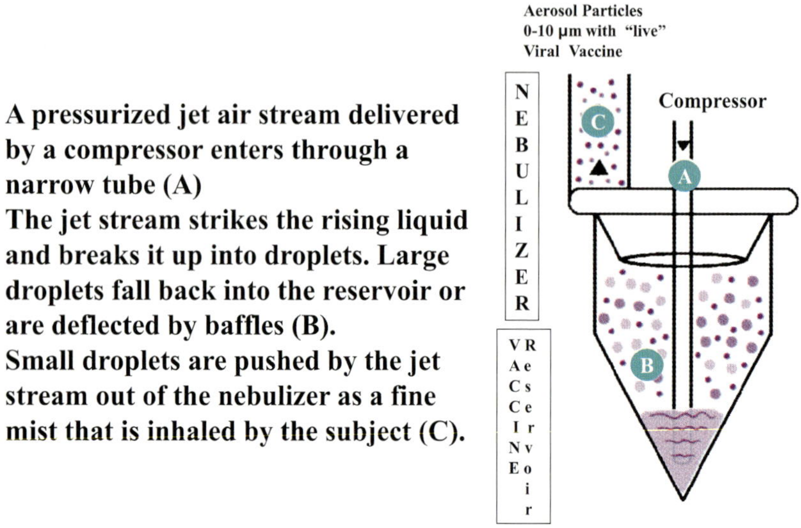
A pressurized jet air stream delivered by a compressor enters through a narrow tube (A)
The jet stream strikes the rising liquid and breaks it up into droplets. Large droplets fall back into the reservoir or are deflected by baffles (B).
Small droplets are pushed by the jet stream out of the nebulizer as a fine mist that is inhaled by the subject (C).
Aerosol Particles
0-10 μm with "live"
Viral Vaccine
NEBULIZER
VACCINE
Reservoir
Compressor
A
B
C

Fig. 2 Aerosolization of vaccine using the Classic Mexican Device

vaccine used by dose of aerosol vaccine administered have documented that 0.10–0.17 ml of vaccine is used for every 30 s of nebulization. The volume of aerosol produced every unit of time (30 s) varies according to the pressure at which the compressor is set. The compressor included in the Classic Mexican Device is of 40–50 psi. In vitro studies using this compressor and nebulizer have measured the total volume of aerosol produced in 30 s with the compressor set at 40–50 psi to be 4–7 l. The main factor that determines the average number of inspirations and tidal volume is the age of the individual. For example, for infants 9 months of age it has been estimated in 15 inspirations every 30 s and with a tidal volume per inspirations of 70 ml. Tidal volume is used because it is a conservative measure of inhaled volume. Older children may breathe more deeply on instruction, while infants breathing patterns are often erratic.

Estimation of the amount of viral particles inhaled by the individual is made by the formula shown in the upper panel of Fig. 3. The proportion of the dose delivered to the upper airway that actually deposits in the lung depends on the 'respirable fraction'. The amount of viral particles inhaled by the individual by the respirable fraction results in the amount of viral particles that are deposited in the lung (lower panel, Fig. 3).

Measles Aerosol Vaccination 171

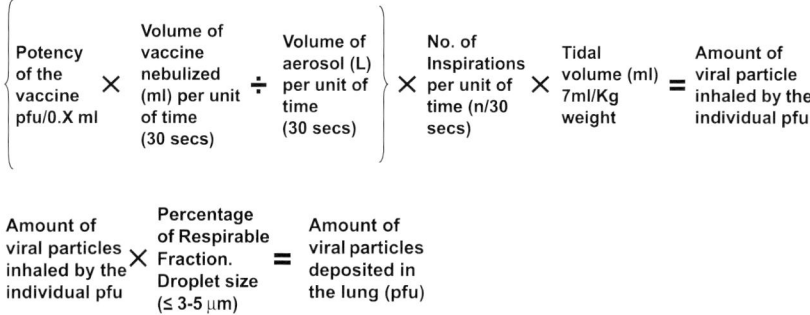

Fig. 3 The amount of viral particles inhaled by the individual and the amount of viral particles deposited in the lung are calculated by the various formulas

4.4
Dose Reaching the Lung Parenchyma

The amount of viral particles reaching the lung parenchyma is mainly dependent upon droplet size and diameter of respiratory airways. This has given rise to the concept of the 'respirable fraction' of an aerosol which is defined as the fraction of the mass of aerosol carried in particles smaller than 5 μm [12]. Existing guidelines for aerosol administration of pharmacologically active substances to the lung parenchyma recommend that devices should produce particles sizes with a median aerodynamic diameter of 1–3 μm [13]. Most probably in the case of school age children and adults respirable particles sizes necessary for immunization are mainly between 3 and 5 μm [14, 15].

4.5
Considerations on Vaccine Strain, Presentation and Manufacturer

Studies that have evaluated aerosolization of measles vaccine have used two strains: Schwarz and Edmonston-Zagreb (EZ). Results of the different studies (described in more detail below) have indicated that the EZ strain is more immunogenic when administered via the aerosol route [16–19]. Additionally in a study conducted in Mexico that evaluated different doses, results showed that the EZ strain was more immunogenic when administered subcutaneously [20, 21]. In vitro studies conducted by Drs. Bennett and Fernandez de Castro have revealed that the process of aerosolization with the Classic Mexican Device decreases vaccine potency. This effect is especially pronounced with the Schwarz vaccine which can therefore not be effectively and consistently delivered by this device.

Whether the vaccine is used in liquid or lyophilized form has also been relevant when used for aerosol immunization. Different studies have demonstrated that nonlyophilized liquid vaccine has provided the high potency that was required ($10^{4.5}$–$10^{5.0}$ pfu) [17, 18, 22, 23]. The first study to use reconstituted lyophilized vaccine (EZ strain) was conducted in 1999 in the State of Hidalgo [16, 19]. This vaccine was produced from a batch which had been produced for routine use and had a potency of $10^{4.2}$ pfu/ml. Results indicated that this vaccine was more immunogenic when administered by aerosol than the same vaccine administered by subcutaneous route as booster vaccination to school age children. Immunogenicity of this vaccine has been lower when tested in primary vaccination in children 12 months of age or younger [24, 25]. Therefore, we consider that EZ strain with a potency above $10^{4.5}$ pfu/ml should be used for aerosolization when a lyophilized vaccine is considered.

The different clinical trials have used EZ strain vaccines produced by the Mexican Institute of Virology (currently BIRMEX) [17, 18, 23, 24, 26] Swiss Serum and Vaccine Institute of Berna [16, 19], Switzerland, SmithKline Beecham [22, 27] and the Serum Institute of India [25]. Combined vaccines including measles and rubella have been proven to be safe and immunogenic [19]. A recent pilot study of MMR aerosol in adults, the first to study triple-antigen aerosol [28], yielded better serologic results after aerosol than injection for all three antigens. These initial promising findings have led to a more extensive and individually randomized Phase I study of MMR aerosol, which is currently underway in Mexico.

5
Experience in Administration of Measles Vaccine via the Respiratory Route

5.1
In Vitro Studies

Studies supported by the Measles Aerosol Project of the WHO are currently involved in determining the optimal particle size, output flow and consistency of the administration route, measurement of the size and distribution of live viral particles through the devices, and characterization of the classical Mexican aerosol device [29].

5.2
Animal Studies

The Measles Aerosol Project has also supported animal studies in Cynomologous macaques that have shown good safety and efficacy of the aerosol administration [29].

5.3
Clinical Studies

Early studies performed between 1961 and 1990 using different types of devices are described in Table 1. Table 2 presents clinical studies that have been conducted using the method developed by Dr. Albert Sabin and adapted by Dr. Fernandez de Castro. These studies are described in more detail below.

5.3.1
Initial Studies

Initial studies on aerosol administration of measles vaccine were pioneered by Dr. Sabin and collaborators who conducted small clinical trials in Mexico. In 1981 Dr. Sabin and colleagues vaccinated 4–6-month-old infants and 12–24-month-old children with and without residual maternal antibodies with high tittered human diploid cell vaccine containing the EZ strain or a chick embryo fibroblast vaccine which contained the Edmonston-Schwarz strain and ten times more virus [17, 18]. Results demonstrated the greater immunogenicity of the diploid cell vaccine using the aerosol route and that aerosolized vaccine was not blocked by maternal antibodies. Inhalation of undiluted, aerosolized measles vaccine was immunogenic in 100% of infants and older children with the human diploid cell vaccine. These initial studies demonstrated lack of reactogenicity as there were no immediate clinical reactions among participants. In 1986, in Mexico City, immunogenicity of aerosolized human diploid cell vaccine (EZ) was compared to the same vaccine administered by subcutaneous route and with chick embryo fibroblast vaccine (Schwarz) by the subcutaneous route. Results demonstrated that aerosol and subcutaneous routes were similarly immunogenic in infants and young children [23].

5.3.2
Mass Campaign

Aerosol administration of measles vaccine was used in a mass campaign in Mexico being administered both as primary and booster dose to nearly four million children as part of the control measures that were implemented during the outbreak affecting North America during 1989–1990. Efficacy of aerosol vaccination could be determined in a small community, San Juan Cosalá, of the state of Jalisco where children had been vaccinated by aerosol or subcutaneous route before the outbreak. Investigation of measles attack rate after the outbreak showed that the highest attack rate occurred in unvaccinated children (26.2% of 61 children), followed by children vaccinated subcutaneously (14.6% of 48), and lastly by children who received the vaccine by aerosol route

Table 1 Aerosol measles vaccination in infants and children, early studies

Study, year[a], site	Age	Criteria[b]	Strain and route[c]	Dose or estimated retained aerosol dose ($TCID_{50}$)	Aerosol technique	n	Sero-response (%)
Kress, 1961, USA [30]	5–7 years	Meas 0 AB 0	Edm B-a.e. Edm B-i.m.	225–375 0.3–3,000	Hand-held nebulizer directed into open mouth; 0.3–0.5 ml delivered	30 41	93 95
Okuno, 1962, Japan [31]	9 months–9 years	Meas 0 AB 0	Yr-a.e.	6–20	Hand-held nebulizer in front of nose and mouth for 30 s	49	94
McCrumb, 1961, USA [32]	1–15 years	Meas 0 AB 0	Edm B-a.e.	225–375	Hand-held nebulizer into open mouth; 0.3–0.5 ml delivered	11	100
McCrumb, 1962, USA [33]	5–10 years	Meas 0 AB 0	Edm B-a.e. Edm B-i.m.	5–200 100–3,000	As above	46 88	93 100
Okuno, 1965, Japan [35]	'Children'	Meas 0 K vacc	Biken-a.e. Biken-s.c.	20 ?	Nebulizer with compressor held in front of nose and mouth for 30 s	16 15	100 53
Ueda, 1966, Japan [34]	1–7 years	Meas 0 K vacc	Biken-a.e. Biken-s.c.	20 ?	Compressor with nebulizer for 30 s in front of nose and mouth	24 14	71 36
Terskikh, 1971, USSR (also cited by Danilov, 1973) [36,37]	1–8 years	Meas 0 AB 0	SW-a.e. SW-s.c. L-16-a.e. L-16-s.c. USSR-58-a.e. USSR-58-s.c.	40–400 1,000 40–400 1,000 40–400 1,000	Ultrasonic generator delivered aerosol into 12-m³ room for 20 min or 24-m³ room for 30 min	859 30 181 35 72 60	85 76 84 74 82 72
Whittle, 1984, Gambia [38]	4–6 years		EZ-a.e. EZ-s.c.	560–1750 39,000	Inspiron mini-neb nebulizer + mask or plastic bag; 30–60 s	51 21	94 100

Table 1 (continued)

Study, year[a], site	Age	Criteria[b]	Strain and route[c]	Dose or estimated retained aerosol dose (TCID$_{50}$)	Aerosol technique	n	Sero-response (%)
Khanum, 1987, Bangladesh [39]	4–6 years		EZ-a.e.	5,000	Nebulizer + foot pump; six strokes of pump over 10 s; infant breathed through mask	78	32 (4 weeks)
			EZ-s.c.	5,000		42	60
			SW-a.e.	6,310		59	34
			SW-s.c.	6,310		65	37
Ekunwe, 1990, Nigeria [40]	4–6 years	'Well'	SW-a.e.	250	Nebulizer, 40 strokes foot pump, mask held for 30 s while crying	51	86

[a] Studies arranged by date of publication
[b] AE 0 (seronegative prevaccinatation); URI 0 (no upper respiratory infection); M vac 0 (no previous measles vaccination); Meas 0 (no history measles); K vacc (all hand received killed measles vaccine parentally previously)
[c] Edm B (Edmonston B); SW (Schwarz); TY (Toyoshima); L-16 (Leningrad 16); a.e. (aerosol); s.c. (subcutaneous); i.m. (intramuscular)
Adapted from [11]

Table 2 Aerosol measles vaccination clinical studies: immunogenicity and adverse events

Reference/ year	Vaccine	Strain(s)	Dose in PFU or $TCID_{50}$ or $CCID_{50}$	Subjects (n)	Ages	Immunogenicity[a]	Adverse events
[18]/1981	INV (Mex)	E-Z aer	0.145 ml/30 (4.16 logs)	35	4–6 months	90% PRN seroconversion at 6 weeks	No immediate reactions
				21	12–24 months	100% PRN seroconversion at 6 wks	No significant subsequent reactions in successfully immunized children
	Sclavo	Schwarz aer	0.135 ml/30 (5.13 logs)	14	4–6 months	39% PRN seroconversion at 6 weeks	No contact infections
				25	12–36 months (no history of measles vaccine or disease)	92% PRN seroconversion at 6 weeks	
[17]/1983	INV (Mex)	E-Z aer	0.145 ml/30	17	4 and 5 months	PRN Seroconversion (6 weeks, 3 months): 47%, 82%	Significant difference between fever in chick embryo fibroblast vaccine seroconvertors (12–22 months) (40%) and the human diploid cell vaccine seroconvertors of the same age group (10%)

Table 2 (continued)

Reference/ Vaccine year	Strain(s)	Dose in PFU or $TCID_{50}$ or $CCID_{50}$	Subjects (n)	Ages	Immunogenicity[a]	Adverse events
		Undiluted: 5.04 $\log_{10}$ pfu/ml	21	12–23 months	100% at 6 weeks	Exanthem in only two seroconvertors to CEF vaccine (13 and 17 months of age)
		Diluted 1:10:	43	4 and 5 months	44%, 78%	
		4.01 $\log_{10}$ pfu/ml	28	12–23 months	100% at 6 weeks	
		Diluted 1:100	23	4 and 5 months	39%, 61%	
		3.01 $\log_{10}$ pfu/ml	18	12–23 months	72%, 79%	
Sclavo, Italy	Schwarz aer	Undiluted: 0.135 ml/30	28	4 and 5 months	36% at 6 weeks	
		6.14 $\log_{10}$ pfu/ml	27	12–23 months	93% at 6 weeks	
		Diluted 1:2 6.14 $\log_{10}$ pfu/ml	40	4 and 5 months	55%, 64%	
		Diluted 1:10 4.7 $\log_{10}$ pfu/ml	25	12–23 months	100% at 6 weeks	
		Diluted 1:100 3.7 $\log_{10}$ pfu/ml	24	12–23 monts	92%, 87%	

Table 2 (continued)

Reference/ year	Vaccine	Strain(s)	Dose in PFU or $TCID_{50}$ or $CCID_{50}$	Subjects (n)	Ages	Immunogenicity[a]	Adverse events
[23]/1984	INV (Mex)	E-Z aer	0.145 ml/30 s (5.02 log_{10} $TCID_{50}$/ml)	117	46 were 6–9 months	84.7% Seroconversion by HI 91.5%	No serious adverse effects noted. Frequency of minor events such as low grade fever and rash was the same in all groups (no data)
		E-Z sc	3.3 log_{10} $TCID_{50}$/ml	55	16 were 6–9 months	100% Seroconversion by HI 98.2%	
	Sclavo, Italy	Schwarz sc	0.135 ml/30 s (3.8 log_{10} pfu/ml)	78 (no history of measles disease or vaccine)	32 were 6–9 months	79.6% Seroconversion by HI 85.9%	
[41]/1987	INV (Mex)	E-Z aer	Estimated to be 200 PFU per child	2087 children Paired samples for 27 children with no history of measles vaccine or measles disease	27 paired samples 8–10 months: 2 1 years: 9 2–4 years: 3 5–7 years: 0 8–14 years: 13	PRN (positive $\geq$1:16) 92.3% in seronegatives (13) 75.0% in seropositives of 16–500 (4) 0% in seropositives >500 (10)	Only three of 1087 children presented rash

Table 2 (continued)

Reference/ Vaccine year	Strain(s)	Dose in PFU or $TCID_{50}$ or $CCID_{50}$	Subjects (n)	Ages	Immunogenicity[a]	Adverse events
[26]/1990 INV (Mex)	E-Z aer	Estimated to be 700 to 1000 PFU retained dose entering child	3,760,684 children	1–4 years No history of vaccine: 10.5% 6–12 years: 89.5%	152 paired samples (all >6 years) from Colima State. (PRN) 93% in seronegatives (13 children) 79% in seropositives of 26–196 titer 44% in seropositives of >200 titer	Reactions after aerosol, Aguascalientes: main reactions: Fever 29.1% Cough 12.7% Rash 10.9%
[27]/1996 SKB	AE E-Z liquid	5,000 pfu/dose	385	8.8 years	Seroresponse (ELISA) ≥fourfold: 84.7%	Reported rash 5% No differences
	Schwarz SC	14,000 pfu/dose		(5–14)		
	Lyophilized Schwarz	12,000 pfu/0.5 ml	0	9 years	Aerosolized Schwarz was not evaluated[b]	
				(5–14)	78.8%	
	EZ	10,000 pfu/0.5 ml	326 281	8.8 years (5–14)	62.6%	
[22]/1996 SKB	AE E-Z liquid Schwarz	5,000 pfu/dose 14,000 pfu			2.4 years after vaccination: seronegative HI (<1:4)	Unknown

Table 2 (continued)

Reference/ Vaccine year	Strain(s)	Dose in PFU or $TCID_{50}$ or $CCID_{50}$	Subjects (n)	Ages	Immunogenicity[a]	Adverse events
	SC Schwarz	12,000 pfu/dose			6%	
	EZ	10,000 pfu/dose			Aerosolized Schwarz was not evaluated[b] 19% 13%	
[19]/1998				Age average	Seroconversion at 4 months	Adverse events observed:
SSVIB	E-Z aer	3.9 $\log_{10}$ pfu/0.1 ml	248(31 PRN data)	6.8 years	65% (20/31)	Cough 7.5%
SSVIB	E-Z aer low dose	3.0 $\log_{10}$ pfu/0.1 ml	255(31 PRN data)	6.5 years	52% (16/31)	Rhinitis 3%
	EZ+RA27/3 aer	4.2 $\log_{10}$ pfu/0.1 mL	257(28 PRN data)	6.5 years	54% (15/28)	Fever 2.9%
	E-Z sc	3.9 $\log_{10}$ pfu/0.5 ml	275(28 PRN data)	6.8 years	4% (1/28)	Diarrhea 1.2%
	EZ+RA27/3 sc	3.9 $\log_{10}$ pfu/0.5 ml (measles)	308(30 PRN data)	6.5 years	7% (2/30)	Rash 1%
SKB	Schwarz sc	3.7 $\log_{10}$ pfu/0.5 ml	281(30 PRN data)	6.6 years	23% (7/30) GMT of each of the aerosol arm was >2400 mIU/ml, and GMT for the sc arm was 700–1000 mIU/ml	Conjunctivitis 0.7% Children who received aerosolized vaccine had less frequency of adverse events than those immunized by sc route

Table 2 (continued)

Reference/year	Vaccine	Strain(s)	Dose in PFU or $TCID_{50}$ or $CCID_{50}$	Subjects (n)	Ages	Immunogenicity[a]	Adverse events
[16]/1998	SSVIB	EZ+RA27/3 aer	3.9 $\log_{10}$ pfu/0.1 ml	255 (29 M PRN data) 125 M (ELISA data)	Age average 6.45 years	Seroconversion at 4 months M: 53.6% by PRN 98.8% by ELISA GMT 3928 by PRN	Adverse events observed (%sc, % aer): Cough (17.2, 0.4) Rhinitis (3.3, 0.4) Fever (6.5, 1.6)
		EZ+RA27/3 sc	3.9 $\log_{10}$ pfu/0.1 ml	307 (31 M PRN data) 86 M (ELISA data)	6.52 years	M: 6.5% by PRN 82.4% by ELISA GMT 865.93 by PRN	Diarrhea (1.3, 0.4) Rash (1.3, 0) Conjunctivitis (2.6, 0) Arthralgias (4.9, 0)
[28]/2000	SII	M(EZ): MMR aer	3.92 logs $TCID_{50}/0.5$ ml	50 (46 evaluable)	Adults 18–50 years	Seropositivity (ELISA) ($\geq$120mIU/ml): Baseline antibody titer $\leq$14,140 mIU/ml: 100% aerosol group	Aerosol route: $n = 46$ subjects Subcutaneous route: $n = 48$ subjects Adverse events (aer%, sc%)
		M(EZ): MMR sc	3.92 logs $TCID_{50}/0.5$ ml	50 (48 evaluable)		Baseline antibody titer >13,663 mIU/ml: 100% sc group	Post-auricular swelling (8.7/2.1) Allergy (2.2/4.2) Lethargy (6.5/0.0) Fever (2.2/4.2) Cough (0.0/2.1)

Table 2 (continued)

Reference/ year	Vaccine	Strain(s)	Dose in PFU or TCID$_{50}$ or CCID$_{50}$	Subjects (n)	Ages	Immunogenicity[a]	Adverse events
							Influenza (0.0/2.1) Rhinitis (0.0/2.1) Otitis (2.2/0.0) One or more of the above (17.4/8.3)
[42]/2000	SKB Rimevax	E-Z aer	3.2 log$_{10}$ pfu/0.1 ml in 30 s	22	6–7 years	Serum/nasal secretions collected IgG in serum and nasal secretions significantly higher with aerosol at both 1 and 3 months IgA in serum at 1 month and IgA in nasal secretions at both 1 and 3 months significantly higher with aerosol (3 months higher but not significant) S.c. dose was 5x greater than aerosol dose.	No significant differences
		E-Z sc	3.9 log$_{10}$ pfu/0.5 ml injected	27			

Table 2 (continued)

Reference/ Vaccine year	Strain(s)	Dose in PFU or $TCID_{50}$ or $CCID_{50}$	Subjects (n)	Ages	Immunogenicity[a]	Adverse events
[24]/2001 INV (Mex)					Seroconversion (>4-fold pre-vaccination antibody titer):	No significant differences for fever, rhinitis, cough, rash, diarrhea, or arthralgias. Conjunctival inflammation more common in aerosol group (57% vs 35%) No children required medical treatment
	E-Z aer	$3.6 \log_{10}$ pfu/0.1 ml	59	11–13 months	Aerosol: Seroconversion in 53 (90%) Stimulation index ≥ 3 in 43 (72%) $S.I \geq 3$ and $PRN \geq 1:120$ (86%)	
	E-Z sc	$4.27 \log_{10}$ pfu/0.5ml	55	11–13 months	SC route: Seroconversion in 55 (100%) Stimulation index ≥ 3 in 48 (87%) $SI \geq 3$ and $PRN \geq 1:120$ (100%)	
[25]/2003 SII	E-Z aer	$2.81 \log_{10}$ $TCID_{50}$/0.1 ml in 30 s	46	9 months	Seroconversion	No significant differences

Table 2 (continued)

Reference/ Vaccine year	Strain(s)	Dose in PFU or TCID$_{50}$ or CCID$_{50}$	Subjects (n)	Ages	Immunogenicity[a]	Adverse events
	E-Z sc	4.3 log$_{10}$ pfu/0.5 ml	53	9 months	Whole group 33% Whole group 92%	

Aer, Aerosol route; CCID$_{50}$, cell culture inactivated dose; E-Z, Edmonston-Zagreb vaccine strain; GMT, geometric mean titers; HI, hemagglutination inhibition; INV (Mex), Mexican Institute of Virology (currently BIRMEX); M, measles; Mos, months; pfu, plaque forming units; PRN, plaque reduction neutralization; Sc, subcutaneous route; SII, Serum Institute of India; SKB, Smith, Kline, Beecham; SSVIB, Swiss Serum and Vaccine Institute of Berne; TCID$_{50}$, tissue culture inhibiting dose

[a] Unless defined otherwise: ELISA method, measles seroconversion was defined as a change from seronegative or indeterminate to seropositive; hemagglutination inhibition (HI), seroconversion was defined as a fourfold increase over prevaccination titers. plaque reduction neutralization (PRN), measles seropositivity was defined as titers $\geq$120 IU/l; measles seroconversion was defined as a change from seronegative to seropositive status (<120 IU/l) or a fourfold increase in the level of prevaccination titers (>119 IU/l);

[b] Simulations of field aerosol conditions showed that the Schwarz vaccine had no detectable potency after two minute nebulization. Thus the authors concluded that the Schwarz vaccine had become inactivated during aerosol administration, and further antibody tests and analysis were not done on this group

(0.8% of 723). The estimated efficacy of aerosol vaccine was over 96%, considerably higher than the 44.3% of the subcutaneous vaccine [41]. However, questions have been raised in retrospect about whether the subcutaneous vaccine was properly potent, since absolute efficacy (44.3%) was unexpectedly low.

5.3.3
South African Studies

More recently, in 1996, a randomized, controlled trial of response to revaccination in 4327 South African schoolchildren showed that previously vaccinated children given aerosolized EZ vaccine (5,000 pfu/dose) had significantly better booster responses than those given comparable doses of EZ or Schwarz vaccines by injection at 1 month and 1 year after revaccination [27]. Recontact of most of these children at 2 years postvaccination demonstrated better antibody persistence in the group receiving aerosolized vaccine [22]. Additional results included the finding that as baseline titers increased, the boosting response decreased. A lower proportion of African children showed seroconversion than Indian children suggesting an effect of ethnic group. Reported illness in the month before vaccination was associated with reduced serological responses. Finally, there were no serious side effects; about 5% of children in each group had a rash within 2 weeks of vaccination.

5.3.4
Recent Mexican Studies

In 1998, a large randomized controlled study was performed in Hidalgo State in Mexico on school-aged children to investigate the immunogenicity and safety of aerosolized EZ vaccine administered as booster dose. Aerosolized EZ measles vaccine was given to three groups at different administered doses: 10^3 pfu (low-dose measles vaccine group), $10^{3.9}$ pfu (measles vaccine group) or $10^{4.2}$ pfu in a vaccine also containing RA27/3 rubella vaccine (measles–rubella vaccine group). The latter groups received doses equivalent to those normally given by injection. These groups were compared with three groups who received injected measles vaccine; two groups each received a $10^{3.9}$ pfu dose of EZ vaccine (one group was administered the vaccine as single antigen and the other combined with rubella vaccine) and a third group received $10^{3.7}$ pfu dose of subcutaneous Schwarz measles vaccine. The study involved 760 children who received aerosolized vaccine and 864 children receiving injected vaccine. Baseline seronegativity determined by ELISA was comparable for all groups, except the group that received measles–rubella vaccine subcutaneously, which had a significantly higher frequency of seronegativity.

Percentages of children seronegative by ELISA for measles antibodies by group were: Aerosolized low-dose EZ measles vaccine 15%; aerosolized EZ measles vaccine 18%, aerosolized EZ measles–rubella vaccine 18%; subcutaneous EZ measles vaccine 16%; subcutaneous Schwarz measles vaccine 20%; subcutaneous EZ measles–rubella vaccine 28%. However, there were no significant differences in seronegativity evaluated by ELISA between the two routes of administration. The superior immunogenicity of measles vaccine administered by aerosol was confirmed documenting that this advantage persisted despite aerosol doses one-fifth or less than customary injected doses. Overall, seroconversion was detected in 57% of the children in the groups that received aerosolized vaccine, but only 11% of those in the injected groups. Seroconversion was affected by baseline neutralization antibody titers, being higher among children with lowest baseline titers. The groups that received standard dose aerosolized measles and measles–rubella vaccine had symptoms significantly less frequently than any group that received injected vaccines [16]. The same researchers separately assessed reactogenicity and immunogenicity of combined measles and rubella booster vaccination via aerosol and subcutaneous routes in the 562 children who received combined antigens. Rates of measles seroconversion measured by plaque neutralization antibodies, median geometric titers and measles ELISA postvaccination seropositivity and seroconversion rate were each higher for aerosol vaccine (54%, 3928 IU/l, 99.6% and 98.8%), than for subcutaneous vaccine (7%, 866 IU/l, 92.2%, 82.4%) $P<0.01$. Reactogenicity was higher for subcutaneous vaccine ($P<0.05$) [19].

Evaluation of local immune responses of aerosol measles booster vaccination in school-aged children were evaluated in a small group of children also in Hidalgo State. A cohort of 49 children from 6 to 7 years of age were randomized to receive either aerosol or subcutaneous EZ measles vaccine. Serum and nasal secretions were collected prior to vaccination and at 1 and 3-month intervals and analyzed for immunoglobulin concentrations and measles specific Ig isotype-associated antibody by enzyme immunoassay (EIA). Serum and nasal IgG and IgA antibody responses were stimulated by either route but these responses were significantly greater by the aerosol compared to the subcutaneous route. These studies also suggested that the measurement of mucosal immune responses may serve as an important predictive marker of protective immunity to measles and lent support for aerosol immunization as an effective alternative vaccine delivery strategy for measles eradication [42].

Cellular and humoral immunity after primary immunization using the aerosol route has been studied in 9 and 12 month-old children. Results have indicated that a low dose of measles vaccine given by aerosol is effective for inducing measles-specific T-cell immunity in most children. However, results have indicated that smaller children more probably require higher doses for immunization than those that have been immunogenic for inducing a booster response in school age children. This is probably explained by their lower tidal volumes and smaller droplet size needed to reach the lung. Twelve-month-old infants were enrolled in a study conducted in the state of Morelos, Mexico [24]. This randomized controlled study involved 59 infants who received $10^{3.6}$ pfu of aerosolized EZ measles vaccine and 55 infants receiving $10^{4.27}$ pfu of subcutaneous EZ measles vaccine. Measles-specific T-cell proliferative responses with stimulation index equal or greater than three developed in 72% of children given aerosolized vaccine compared with 87% after subcutaneous vaccine. Seroconversion rates were 90% after aerosol and 100% after subcutaneous immunization and measles Geometric Mean Titers [95% confidence interval (CI)] were 237mIU (146–385) and 487 mIU (390–609) in each group, respectively. All three measurements were significantly higher for the subcutaneous immunization. Authors suggested that technical modifications, such as increasing the infectious viral inoculum or improving the aerosol delivery device, would be expected to eliminate differences in immunogenicity. Both routes were well tolerated. Episodes of conjunctival hyperemia were more frequent in the aerosol group. The need for a higher viral inoculum with the classic Mexican device was more evident when 9-month-old infants were studied. This controlled, randomized study conducted in the Queretaro State involved 46 children who received EZ measles vaccine by aerosol [$10^{2.81}$ cell culture inactivated dose $(CCID)_{50}$/dose] and 53 children who were administered the same vaccine by the subcutaneous route ($10^{4.28}$ $CCID_{50}$/dose). Measles-specific T-cell proliferative responses developed in 42% of children given aerosolized vaccine compared with 67% of those who received subcutaneous vaccine ($P = 0.01$); the mean stimulation index (SI) was 4.4±0.7 versus 6.9±1, respectively ($P = 0.05$). Seroconversion rates were 33% and 92% after aerosol or subcutaneous immunization ($P<0.001$). Among infants with serologic responses, measles geometric mean titers (GMT; 95% CI) by neutralizing antibody assay were 215mIU/ml (115–400) in aerosol vaccine recipients and 411mIU/ml (345–490) in those given subcutaneous vaccine ($P = 0.06$). There were no serious adverse reactions. Fever was more frequent in the aerosol group. The proportion of 9-month-old infants who developed cellular and/or humoral immunity to measles was lower in the aerosol vaccine group. However, among those who developed a measles-specific response, measles antibody and T-cell responses were comparable. Authors suggested that observed differences between both routes were attributable to more than 25-fold lower dose administered by aerosol route and that improvement of aerosol delivery or increasing the dose may enhance immunogenicity of primary measles vaccination by the aerosol route in this age [25].

A single study has evaluated immunogenicity and side effects of triple viral vaccine administered by the aerosol route [28]. Using a nonrandomized design these researchers vaccinated 100 adult volunteers, most of them health workers, in the state of Jalisco, Mexico with MMR vaccine: measles (EZ strain) $10^{3.917}$ 50% tissue culture inhibiting doses ($TCID_{50}$) per dose; rubella (RA27/3 strain) $10^{3.950}$ $TCID_{50}$ per dose; and mumps (L-Zagreb strain) $10^{4.833}$ $TCID_{50}$ per dose. The aerosol route was superior for measles, mumps and rubella when baseline titers were controlled for in multivariate analysis. Since most of the participants had high baseline measles antibody levels, there were few seroconversions, which raised considerable uncertainty about the true magnitude by which the response to the measles component of aerosolized MMR exceeded that for injected MMR. Investigation of adverse effects was limited by the fact that associated events were self-reported. Although side effects did not differ by vaccination route, an unexpected higher frequency of postauricular swelling (8.7% of 46 individuals in the aerosol group versus 2.1% of 48 individuals in the subcutaneous group) and lethargy (6.5% of 46 individuals in the aerosol group versus 0% of 48 individuals in the subcutaneous group) were observed, which was speculated to most likely derive from the mumps component.

6
Future Challenges

There are several concerns regarding aerosol immunization that will need to be solved before this method can be globally implemented: (1) the dose that interacts with the individual needs to be precisely determined; (2) experience of studies in South Africa have shown that there may be loss of potency in some vaccine strains. Therefore, it is necessary to determine the vaccine strains that can be aerosolized and maintain adequate potency; (3) available equipments are cumbersome and noisy. It is necessary to test other devices that are more practical for use in the field and in small health centers; (4) another concern regards the potential environmental effects. Aerosol administration may expose vaccinators or household contacts of vaccinated children to measles vaccine. Until now, no contacts of children vaccinated with aerosolized measles vaccine have developed a measles-like illness. Of greater concern are the potential risks associated with exposure of immunocompromised individuals to vaccine virus if it is effectively shed by persons vaccinated via the aerosol method. This is of greater concern in regions where HIV/AIDS is prevalent since attenuated measles vaccine virus has caused fatal disease in one severely immunosuppresed HIV-infected patient [43]; (5) researchers have questioned whether measles vaccine might reach the brain of aerosol vaccinees by retrograde transport via the olfactory nerve fibers. Experience of mass administration or clinical trials has provided no evidence that indicates central nervous system symptoms after vaccination; (6) finally it is necessary to conduct clinical trials that study immunogenicity and safety in asthmatic and HIV infected individuals.

7
The Measles Aerosol Project

The WHO has recognized the need of extending the coverage of measles vaccine through implementation of novel methods of administration among which is included the aerosol route. In 2002, in view of the results of several studies on the administration of measles vaccine through the aerosol route, WHO, in collaboration with other organizations, established the Measles Aerosol Project, with the purpose of conducting the necessary studies to achieve the licensure of a product (device and vaccine) administered through this route [44]. A multidisciplinary group of experts was invited to provide advice and guidance on the project.

The goal of the WHO's Measles Aerosol Project is to license at least one method for respiratory delivery of currently licensed measles vaccines. During 2004 and 2005 preclinical studies, economic analyses and phase I and phase II studies are being planned and initiated [44].

8
Conclusions

Measles aerosol studies have used some of the vaccine strains that are recommended for subcutaneous use. The EZ strain has been proved to be stable in these studies. Future studies will need to evaluate stability of other strains. Animal studies have been performed that indicate that measles aerosol immunization is safe and immunogenic when administered to macaques. These results have been confirmed in clinical trials that indicate that the method is safe in school age children and infants. Immunogenicity results in school age children have shown that the aerosol route is immunogenic when the vaccine is administered as booster dose. Seroconversion was affected by baseline neutralization antibody titers, being higher among children with lowest baseline titers. As to infants, data indicate that the vaccine administered as primary immunization is immunogenic but that viral concentration will probably need

Table 3 Summary of immunogenicity of EZ measles aerosol vaccination. Median seroresponse and range in various studies

		Infants	Children	
Potency of vaccine $\log_{10}$ (pfu or $CCID_{50}$) 1ml	Dose aerosol vaccine (ml)	Presumably seronegative % (range) [Reference]	Presumably seronegative % (range) [Reference]	Presumably seropositive % (range) [Reference]
≥ 5.0	0.145	97% (91–100) [17, 23]	–	–
4.0–4.9	0.12–0.17	97% (90–100) [18]	89% (85–93) [26, 27]	79% (79) [26]
≤ 3.9	0.10–0.17	61% (33–79) [24, 25]	92% (92%) [41]	76% (53–100) [16, 19, 28, 42]

to be increased. These studies have indicated that potency of the vaccine will probably need to be at least $10^{4.5}$ pfu when administered as primary dose to infants or as booster dose to children with baseline antibody titers (Table 3). From the logistical point of view, the use of the aerosol method has not been evaluated in routine immunization although feasibility of its implementation was proved in the mass campaign implemented in Mexico during the outbreak of 1990. During this campaign, it was found to be simple and easy to use, that it could operate for many hours, with minimal need for cleaning and sterilization and that could undergo replacement of parts for maintenance. However, the involved devices have not been evaluated as to their portability or weight. Cost savings will probably be demonstrated. As to licensure, its compliance with the appropriate international regulatory requirements for medical aerosol delivery devices is in process.

References

1. WHO (1999) The World Health Report, 1999. Making a difference. World Health Organization, Geneva
2. WHO (2004) The World Health Report, 2004. Changing history. World Health Organization, Geneva, 2004
3. De Quadros CA (2004) Can measles be eradicated globally? Bull World Health Org 82:134–138

4. WHO, World Health Organization. Measles. Mortality reduction and regional elimination. Strategic Plan 2001–2005. [electronic resource] Geneva: World Health Organization; 2001. [cited 2005 Jan 19]. Available from: http://www.who.int/vaccines-documents/DocsPDF01/www573.pdf
5. De Quadros CA, Izurieta H, Carrasco P, Brana M, Tambini G (2003) Progress toward measles eradication in the region of the Americas. J Infect Dis 187 (Suppl.1): S102–S110
6. de Quadros CA, Izurieta H, Venczel L, Carrasco P (2004) Measles eradication in the Americas: progress to date. J Infect Dis 189 (Suppl. 1):S227–S235
7. Tomich N (ed) (2002) The Global Vaccine Shortage: The threat to children and what to do about it. Proceedings of the Albert B. Sabin Vaccine Institute. Ninth Annual Vaccine Colloquium. Cold Spring Harbor, New York, 23–25 October 2002. [cited 2005 Jan 25]. Available from: http://www.sabin.org/PDF/entiredoc.pdf search='vaccine%20shortage%20unicef'
8. WHO, UNICEF. State of the world's vaccines and immunization. Geneva, Switzerland, WHO/GPV/96.04, 1–159
9. UNICEF (2005) Fact sheet. [cited 2005 Jan 25]. Available from: http://www.unicef.org/immunization/23245_safety.html
10. Sabin AB (1992) My last will and testament on rapid elimination and ultimate global eradication of poliomyelitis and measles. Pediatrics 90:162–169
11. Cutts FT, Clements CJ, Bennett JV (1997) Alternative routes of measles immunization: a review. Biologicals 25:323–338
12. Coates AL (2005) Aerosol delivery of medication to children with acute asthma Ceska Iniciativa pro Astma [cited 2005 Jan 25]. Available from: http://www.cipa.cz/abstracts/abstr69.html
13. AARC, American Association for Respiratory Care. Clinical Practice Guideline. (1996) Selection of a Device for Delivery of Aerosol to the Lung Parenchyma. Respir Care 41:647–653
14. Brand P, Haussinger K, Meyer T, Scheuch G, Schulz H, Selzer T, Heyder J (1999) Intrapulmonary distribution of deposited particles. J Aerosol Med 12:275–284
15. Gerrity TR, Lee PS, Hass FJ, Marinelli A, Werner P, Lourenco RV (1979) Calculated deposition of inhaled particles in the airway generations of normal subjects. J Appl Physiol 47:867–873
16. Bennett JV, Fernandez de Castro J, Valdespino-Gomez JL, Garcia-Garcia ML, Islas-Romero R, Echaniz-Aviles G, Jimenez-Corona A, Sepulveda-Amor J (2002) Aerosolized measles and measles-rubella vaccines induce better measles antibody booster responses than injected vaccines: randomized trials in Mexican schoolchildren. Bull World Health Org 80:806–812
17. Sabin AB, Flores Arechiga A, Fernandez de Castro J, Albrecht P, Sever JL, Shekarchi I (1984) Successful immunization of infants with and without maternal antibody by aerosolized measles vaccine. II. Vaccine comparisons and evidence for multiple antibody response. JAMA 251:2363–2371
18. Sabin AB, Flores Arechiga A, Fernandez de Castro J, Sever JL, Madden DL, Shekarchi I, Albrecht P (1983) Successful immunization of children with and without maternal antibody by aerosolized measles vaccine. I. Different results with undiluted human diploid cell and chick embryo fibroblast vaccines. JAMA 249:2651–2662

19. Sepulveda-Amor J, Valdespino-Gomez JL, Garcia-Garcia ML, Bennett J, Islas-Romero R, Echaniz-Aviles G, de Castro JF (2002) A randomized trial demonstrating successful boosting responses following simultaneous aerosols of measles and rubella (MR) vaccines in school age children. Vaccine 20:2790–2795
20. Cutts FT, Grabowsky M, Markowitz LE (1995) The effect of dose and strain of live attenuated measles vaccines on serological responses in young infants. Biologicals 23:95–106
21. Markowitz LE, Sepulveda J, Diaz-Ortega JL, Valdespino JL, Albrecht P, Zell ER, Stewart J, Zarate ML, Bernier RH (1990) Immunization of six-month-old infants with different doses of Edmonston-Zagreb and Schwarz measles vaccines. N Engl J Med 322:580–587
22. Dilraj A, Cutts FT, Bennett JV, Fernandez de Castro J, Cohen B, Coovadia HM (2000) Persistence of measles antibody two years after revaccination by aerosol or subcutaneous routes. Pediatr Infect Dis J 19:1211–1213
23. Fernandez de Castro J, Valdespino Gomez JL, Diaz Ortega JL, Zarate Aquino ML (1986) Diploid cell measles vaccine. JAMA 256:714
24. Wong-Chew RM, Islas-Romero R, Garcia-Garcia ML, Beeler AJ, Audet S, Santos PJ, Gans H, Lew YL, Maldonado Y, Arvin AM, Valdespino Gomez JL (2004) Comparison of cellular and humoral immune response to measles vaccine administered by aerosol and subcutaneous route in 12 month old children. J Infect Dis 189:254–257
25. Wong-Chew RM, Islas-Romero R, Garcia-Garcia ML, Beeler J, Audet S, Santos JI, Gans H, Lew YL, Maldonado Y, Arvin AM and Valdespino Gomez JL (2006) Immunogenicity of Aerosolized versus Subcutaneous Edmonston-Zagreb Measles Vaccine given as a Primary Dose to 9 Month Old Mexican Children. Vaccine 24:683–690
26. Fernandez-de Castro J, Kumate-Rodriguez J, Sepulveda J, Ramirez-Isunza JM, Valdespino-Gomez JL (1997) [Measles vaccination by the aerosol method in Mexico]. Salud Publica Mex 39:53–60
27. Dilraj A, Cutts FT, de Castro JF, Wheeler JG, Brown D, Roth C, Coovadia HM, Bennett JV (2000) Response to different measles vaccine strains given by aerosol and subcutaneous routes to schoolchildren: a randomised trial. Lancet 355:798–803
28. Fernandez de Castro J, Bennett J, Gallardo Rincon H, Alvarez y Muñoz MT, Partida Sanchez LA, Santos JI (2005) Evaluation of immunogenicity and side effects of triple viral vaccine (MMR) in adults, given by two routes: subcutaneous and respiratory (aerosol). Vaccine 23:1079–1084
29. WHO (2004) Proceedings of the Fourth Global Vaccine Research Forum. WHO/IVB/04.09.[electronic resource] World Health Organization, Geneva. [cited 2005 Jan 19]. Available from: http://www.who.int/vaccines-documents
30. Kress S, Schluederberg A, Hornick R (1961) Studies with live attenuated measles-virus vaccine. Am J Dis Child 101:57–63
31. Okuno Y (1962) Vaccination with egg passage measles virus by inhalation. Am J Dis Child 103:211–214
32. McCrumb F (1961) Studies with live attenuated measles virus vaccine: clinical and immunologic responses in institutionalized children. Am J Dis Child 101:45–56
33. McCrumb F, Bulkeley J, Hornick R (1962) Clinical trials with living attenuated measles virus vaccines. Am J Public Health 52:11–15

34. Okuno Y, Ueda S, Hosai H, Kitawaki T, Nakamura K, Chiang TP, Okabe S, Onaka M, Toyoshima K (1965) Studies on the combined use of killed and live measles vaccines. II. Advantages of the inhalation method. Biken J 8:81–85
35. Ueda S, Hosai H, Minekawa Y, Okuno Y (1966) Studies on the combined use of killed and live measles vaccines. 3. Conditions for the "take" of live vaccine. Biken J 9:97–101
36. Terskikh A, Danolov A, Sheltchkov G (1971) Theoretical substantiation and effectiveness of immunization with aerosols of liquid measles vaccine. Vestn Akad Med Nauk SSSR 26:84–90
37. Danilov A (1973) The basis for vaccination against measles by aerosols of live vaccine. In Hers JFP, Winkler KC (eds) Airbone transmission and airborne infection. John Wiley and Sons, New York, pp 344–345
38. Whittle HC, Rowland MG, Mann GF, Lamb WH, Lewis RA (1984) Immunisation of 4–6 month old Gambian infants with Edmonston-Zagreb measles vaccine. Lancet 2:834–837
39. Khanum S, Uddin N, Garelick H, Mann G, Tomkins A (1987) Comparison of Edmonston-Zagreb and Schwarz strains of measles vaccine given by aerosol or subcutaneous injection. Lancet 1:150–153
40. Ekunwe EO (1990) Immunization by inhalation of aerosolized measles vaccine. Ann Trop Paediatr 10:145–149
41. Fernandez de Castro J, Kumate-Rodriguez J (1990) La vacunación contra el sarampión en México y America; avances en el metodo de inmunización por aerosol. Bol Med Hosp Inf Mex 47:449–461
42. Bellanti JA, Zeligs BJ, Mendez-Inocencio J, Garcia-Garcia ML, Islas-Romero R, Omidvar B, Omidvar J, Kim G, Fernandez De Castro J, Sepulveda Amor J, Walls L, Bellini WJ, Valdespino-Gomez JL (2004) Immunologic studies of specific mucosal and systemic immune responses in Mexican school children after booster aerosol or subcutaneous immunization with measles vaccine. Vaccine 22:1214–1220
43. CDC, Centers for Disease Control and Prevention (1996) Measles pneumonitis following measles-mumps-rubella vaccination of a patient with HIV infection: 1993 MMWR Morb Mortal Wkly Rep 45:603–606
44. WHO, World Health Organization. Initiative for Vaccine Research. 2004–2005. Strategic Plan. WHO7IVB704.13. [electronic resource] Geneva: World Health Organization; 2004. [cited 2005 Jan 31]. Available from: http://www.who.int/vaccines-documents

Mass Vaccination Campaigns for Polio Eradication: An Essential Strategy for Success

R. W. Sutter (✉) · C. Maher

Polio Eradication Initiative, World Health Organization, Geneva, Switzerland
sutterr@who.int

1	Introduction	196
2	**Early Polio Control Efforts**	197
2.1	Industrialized World	197
2.2	Developing World	197
3	**Oral Poliovirus Vaccine**	198
3.1	Immunogenicity	198
3.2	OPV Modifications to Improve Immunogenicity and Potency at the Point of Use	199
3.3	Effectiveness of OPV in Mass Campaigns	200
3.4	Vaccine-Associated Paralytic Poliomyelitis in Campaigns	203
4	**Mass Vaccination in the Polio Eradication Era**	203
4.1	Strategies	203
5	**Programmatic Aspects of Mass Campaigns**	205
5.1	Campaign Scope and Strategies for Delivering Immunization	205
5.2	Planning, Operational, and Logistical Issues for SIAs— Lessons Learned During the Polio Eradication Initiative	206
5.3	Improvement in Quality of SIAs	210
5.4	Effect of Mass Campaigns: Progress in Polio Eradication	210
6	**The Future: OPV Use in Campaigns Post-Polio Eradication**	214
7	**Conclusions**	215
References		216

Abstract Effective vaccines against poliomyelitis became available in the mid-1950s and early 1960s. Mass campaigns were an integral part of early control efforts. Thereafter, polio vaccines were used largely in routine childhood programs. The resolution in 1988 to eradicate polio globally led to the development of appropriate strategies to achieve this goal, including mass vaccination campaigns (i.e., national immunization days, sub-national immunization days and mop-up activities), to achieve the highest possible coverage in the shortest possible time. Unlike other vaccines, mass campaign use of oral poliovirus vaccine enhances the immunogenicity of this vaccine, primarily due to: (1) the decrease in the prevalence of other enteroviruses that potentially interfere with seroconversion; and (2) the secondary spread of vaccine virus from vaccinees to close contacts, resulting in seroconversion of some unvaccinated contacts. To reach the highest possible coverage, detailed planning, meticulous execution, careful supervision and standardized monitoring are critical. A number of innovative approaches to improve the quality and/or coverage have become the 'standard' of supplemental immunization activities. These mass campaigns have led to dramatic decreases in the incidence of polio. This chapter reviews the scientific, operational and programmatic data on mass campaign use of polio vaccines, and summarize the lessons learnt from implementing the mass vaccination strategies used to eradicate poliomyelitis globally.

1
Introduction

Mass campaigns have been an essential strategy for polio control since effective vaccines were first licensed, starting with inactivated poliovirus vaccine (IPV) in 1955, and oral poliovirus vaccine (OPV) in 1961 [1]. While both vaccines provide individual protection against paralytic disease, OPV has attributes which made it the vaccine of choice for the global eradication initiative, and which make it very suitable for campaign use: (1) it can be administered by volunteers after basic training (health professionals are not essential for all immunization activities) [2]; (2) it induces mucosal immunity which decreases the community transmission of polioviruses; and (3) it is associated with secondary spread from vaccines to close contacts, thereby immunizing some of these contacts.

In 1988, the World Health Assembly (WHA) resolved to eradicate polio by 2000 [3]. The polio eradication initiative designed and implemented eradication strategies for all polio-endemic countries, including the use of mass campaigns with OPV to rapidly raise population immunity and interrupt the circulation of wild poliovirus [4].

To make the most of the attributes of OPV, and achieve the maximum benefit of OPV in campaigns, it is essential to reach a very high proportion of the target population with potent vaccines, and to do that consistently with each immunization round. Operational planning and effective management are essential to ensuring the quality of campaigns, and to achieving consistent high coverage. Effective implementation of mass campaigns with OPV has been instrumental in interrupting wild poliovirus circulation in many countries, and campaigns will continue to be a critical strategy for the final achievement of polio eradication globally.

This chapter focuses on OPV use through mass campaigns for polio prevention and interruption of poliovirus transmission.

2
Early Polio Control Efforts

2.1
Industrialized World

Following licensure of IPV of Salk in 1955, the industrialized world put in place aggressive immunization programs, which boosted population immunity levels, and led to dramatic decreases in the incidence of poliomyelitis [1]. For example, in the US, the number of reported cases fell from 18,308 in 1954 to 2,525 in 1960, the last year where IPV was used exclusively. Despite the need for trained health professionals to inject IPV, campaigns were an integral part of these control efforts. These campaigns were usually not large-scale, but instead focused on schools, churches, and work places (see polio pioneers [5]). To induce immunity, three to four doses of IPV were needed; the first three considered priming doses, and the last as boosting dose.

Pioneering work on OPV, conducted in the Soviet Union, demonstrated the effectiveness and established the safety profile of OPV, and provided much of the scientific base for eventual licensure in the US [6, 7]. Between 1961 and 1962, monovalent OPV (mOPV) 1, 2, and finally 3, of Sabin, were licensed in the US, and then used extensively in mass campaigns. These campaigns were called SOS (Sabin Oral Saturday or Sunday), and administered mOPV1, mOPV3, and mOPV2 sequentially, with an interval of 4 weeks between the monovalent vaccines [8, 9].

In 1963, trivalent OPV (tOPV) was licensed in the US [1]. This vaccine was developed primarily on programmatic grounds (a single vaccine greatly facilitated stock keeping and recording in vaccination sites), and contained 'a balanced formulation' of the three Sabin strains [10]. Three doses were needed for a primary immunization schedule. This vaccine soon became the mainstay of polio control efforts in most of the industrialized world, until the 1990s when progress toward polio eradication dramatically reduced the risk of wild poliovirus importation in these countries, and the burden of vaccine-associated paralytic poliomyelitis (VAPP), the only serious side effect of OPV, became increasingly unacceptable. Sequential use of IPV, or exclusive IPV use, replace tOPV, as many industrialized countries [1, 11, 12].

2.2
Developing World

In the 1950s and 1960s, few individuals in the tropical developing world profited from polio vaccines, whether IPV, mOPVs, or tOPV. The vaccines were not used widely, primarily due to two reasons: (1) at the time, there was a widespread perception that poliomyelitis was not a public health problem in these tropical developing settings (only the lameness surveys in the 1960s and 1970s dispelled the myth [13, 14]); and (2) the operational capacity in these countries to reach a large proportion of the population with vaccines was limited. There was, however, one noticeable exception. The national campaigns with OPV in 1962 in Cuba rapidly eliminated wild poliovirus transmission [15–17].

The establishment of WHO's Expanded Program on Immunization (EPI) in 1977 focused attention on [18]: (1) the burden of vaccine-preventable diseases; (2) the need for control strategies; (3) the supply of affordable vaccines; and (4) the need for adequate funding. The Universal Childhood Immunization Initiative (UCI) in the mid-1980s, promoted the vision of 80% global coverage with routine immunization, to be achieved by 1990 [19]. The vaccine of choice for polio control in the EPI program was OPV. The EPI and UCI initiatives were successful in initiating and strengthening vaccine program infrastructure and capacities, and were an effective tool to draw attention to immunization as one of the most cost-effective public health control interventions [20]. However, after 1990 when UCI ended, attention and funding focused on other health priorities. During the 1990s, routine coverage levels stagnated in many developing countries [21].

The impact of the early polio immunization efforts were variable. If one assumes that 1 in 200 children susceptible to poliomyelitis will develop paralytic disease after exposure to wild poliovirus, approximately 600,000 paralytic cases would have occurred in the absence of vaccination in the world in 1988, the year that global polio eradication was resolved by the WHA. The polio eradication initiative estimated that in 1988, 350,000 cases occurred in the world, or a 42% reduction [1]. But, 58% of paralytic cases were still occurring–most totally preventable through vaccination–and almost all residing exclusively in the developing world.

3
Oral Poliovirus Vaccine

3.1
Immunogenicity

In industrialized countries, three doses of OPV induce immunity in >90% of vaccinees against all three poliovirus serotypes [22, 23]. In contrast, OPV is less immunogenic in developing, especially tropical, countries. A review of studies in developing countries reported that three doses of OPV induced median seroconversion levels in 72%, 95%, and 65% of vaccinees to poliovirus types

1, 2, and 3, respectively [24]. There are a number of reasons for the lower immunogenicity of OPV in developing countries, including interference between Sabin strains, interference with concurrent nonpolio enterovirus infections, diarrhea, and other nonspecific factors [24, 25]. To partly compensate for the lower immunogenicity of OPV in developing countries, WHO recommended since the 1980s that polio-endemic countries use four doses of OPV in the routine immunization programs [26]. The first OPV dose is customarily given at birth (or shortly thereafter, and if that is not feasible, administered as fourth dose together with measles vaccine at 9 months of age).

3.2
OPV Modifications to Improve Immunogenicity and Potency at the Point of Use

Several changes were made to OPV over the past 40 years, the most significant being: (1) the change in type 3 seed strain from Sabin Original (SO) to Pfizer RSO (a seed virus change); (2) the change in formulation (increasing the potency of the type 3 component); and (3) the addition of vaccine-vial monitor (VVMs) (allowing evaluation of vaccine potency at point of use).

The change in seed strain from Sabin SO to Pfizer RSO is important because it probably decreased the neurovirulence of the vaccine. The immediate grounds for the change were the relatively high proportion (~10%) of type 3 bulks that did not pass the release criteria for regulatory approval, and this change increased the predictability that type 3 bulks would pass the neurovirulence testing requirements before release [27, 28].

A change in OPV formulation was implemented following a type 3 outbreak in northeastern Brazil [29]. The formulation changed from a 10:1:3 to 10:1:6 to boost the immunogenicity of the type 3 component of the vaccine from 300,000 median tissue culture infective dose ($TCID_{50}$) to 600,000 $TCID_{50}$. Nevertheless, even with these changes, the immunogenicity of OPV in developing countries remains substantially lower than in industrialized countries. It has been estimated that six to seven doses of OPV are needed to induce immunity to type 1 in >90% of vaccinees, and that 11–13 doses of OPV are needed to induce immunity in >90% of vaccinees to type 3 [30].

Substantial efforts to develop a more thermostable OPV with the use deuterium as a stabilizer were ongoing in the 1990s [31]. However, the development and introduction of VVMs in the late 1990s (requirement for procurement of this vaccine by United Nations' agencies), allowing assessment of OPV vaccine potency at any point in the cold chain [32]. VVMs allowed vaccinators to take the vaccine out of the cold chain in selected circumstances (i.e., fast chain) and be confident that the vaccine is potent, if so indicated by the VVM, at the point of administration.

3.3
Effectiveness of OPV in Mass Campaigns

OPV has distinct operational advantages for administration in mass campaigns, because the oral administration could be done by volunteers, limiting the number of trained health professionals required. However, OPV had additional attributes which increased the impact of use in campaign settings, and which became apparent as campaigns were conducted, particularly in developing country settings. OPV administered in mass campaign appears to be considerably more immunogenic than if administered during routine immunization activities [7, 8] (Table 1). The effectiveness of OPV administered as a routine vaccine in infancy and childhood in reducing the burden of poliomyelitis, including in developing countries, has been well

Table 1 Operational and scientific rationale for using OPV in mass campaigns

Attribute	Operational consequences	Impact
Administration	Can be administered by volunteers (non-health care professionals); allowing the mobilization of large numbers of volunteers	Making higher coverage possible
Cold chain	Use of OPV in short campaigns (3–5 days) permitted novel approaches to cold chain ('fast-chain'), which was strengthened by vaccine-vial monitors (VVMs) in the late 1990s; allowing vaccinators at point of administration to determine the effectiveness of OPV	More effective vaccines could be administered
Secondary spread from vaccines to close contacts	Inherent characteristic of OPV, but accentuated in campaigns with a high proportion of the target age group vaccinated in a short period of time	Reaching unvaccinated contacts, and inducing immunity in some (the magnitude of this effect is hightlighted in Figure 2)
Mucosal immunity	Inherent characteristic of OPV, but accentuated because of less interference with OPV-take due to decreases of nonpoliovirus enterovirus (NPEV) transmission after mass campaigns	Providing a more effective barrier to community spread and transmission of wild polioviruses
OPV immunogenicity	Higher during campaigns because of administration of effective vaccines (cold chain), and the combined secondary spread from vaccines, and mucosal immunity	OPV substantially more immunogenic when administered during mass campaigns

documented [1, 33]; however, the use of OPV in massive campaigns demonstrated dramatic, immediate impact [34, 35]. Two factors appear to be largely responsible for the enhanced effectiveness of OPV during campaign use: (1) substantially-increased coverage with campaign use, even in countries with no or suboptimal health systems [36, 37]; and (2) significantly-enhanced immunogenicity of OPV when administered in campaigns. The latter effect is likely composed of several elements: (1) vaccine quality may be less compromised than during routine use (the introduction of VVMs, and the use of 'fast chain' distribution procedures are among the elements helping to ensure viable vaccine during campaigns); (2) secondary exposure of close contacts to vaccines appears to be massive; and (3) reduction of interference with other nonpolio enteroviruses during and after the campaigns [38]. The developer of OPV, Dr. Albert Sabin, always believed that the best way to use his vaccine would be in mass vaccination campaigns [8].

A landmark study of large-scale OPV use in Mexico in 1959–1960 demonstrated an additional benefit of OPV, the temporary displacement of other enteric pathogens, especially nonpolio enteroviruses [38], in the vaccinated population, therefore decreasing the interference of such agents with OPV take. OPV gained further prominence after Brazil demonstrated in 1980 that OPV use in large-scale mass vaccination campaigns in a developing tropical country could dramatically decrease the incidence of poliomyelitis (Fig. 1) [39]. The experiences in Brazil were instrumental in motivating the public health community to call for better polio control in the developing world [40]. The state of the art of large scale, nationwide immunization activities were defined [41].

While it has been known that vaccine viruses can be transmitted from vaccines to close contacts from the beginning of OPV use, the magnitude of this effect is difficult to estimate. The spread of mOPV2 virus from vaccines to siblings and extra-familial contacts was demonstrated during the winter 1960 in Houston, at a time when conditions are typically not favorable for polioviruses transmission [42]. The magnitude of secondary exposure in industrialized countries to OPV poliovirus administered in routine vaccination programs were further elaborated for the US [43] and England [44].

In the developing world, several reports suggest that OPV administered in campaigns spread to nonimmunized children. The report from the Magreb Immunization Days in Morocco documented the relatively high proportion of children not reached during the campaign that did seroconvert [45]. In Oman a trial of IPV and OPV allowed the evaluation of OPV secondary transmission to the IPV vaccinated group, following a large mass campaign with OPV. While the study district was excluded from the OPV campaign, study participants in the IPV arm could be stratified by exposure to the campaign [46]. Figure 2

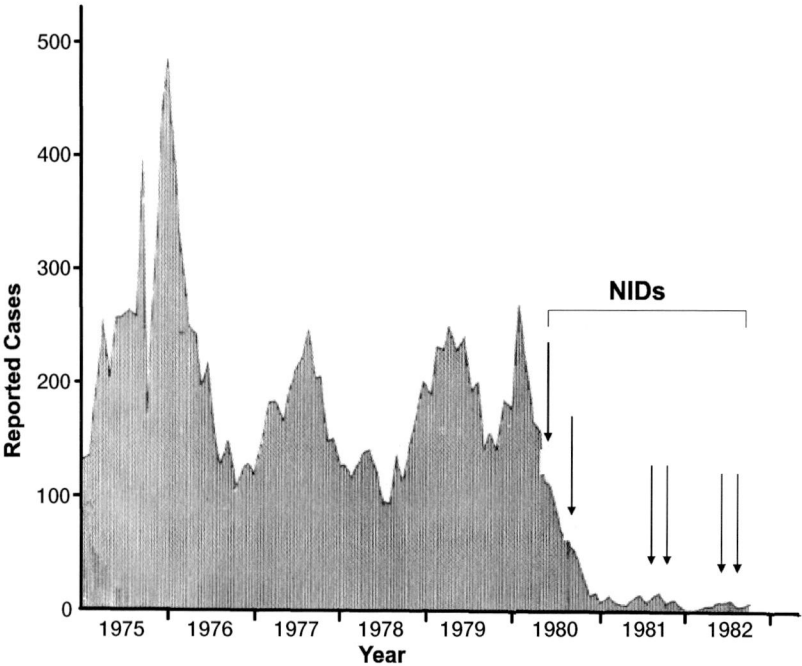

Fig. 1 Impact of national immunization campaigns on incidence of poliomyelitis, Brazil. (From [39])

shows seroconversion in the IPV study arm (participants had received a single dose of IPV at 6 weeks of age) between birth and 10 weeks by exposure. Seroconversion rates increased from 28% to 64% for poliovirus type 1, 40% to 82% for poliovirus type 2, and remained relatively stable at 37% and 41% for poliovirus type 3, for participants without or with campaign exposure, respectively. The magnitude of secondary exposure and infection was estimated to be very high for types 1 and 2 (~80–90%), but much lower for type 3.

A study from Jordan also showed very high seroconversion rates following OPV administration during two rounds of national immunization days (NIDs) [47]. As expected, the effect of two rounds of NID was most pronounced in those who the fewest previous doses of OPV.

However, the mass campaigns are usually conducted during the low transmission season, when interference with other nonpolio enteroviruses on OPV take should be minimized. There is a suggestion that the effectiveness of OPV is higher during the low transmission season [48], at a period when incidence of diarrheal diseases would be lowest [49].

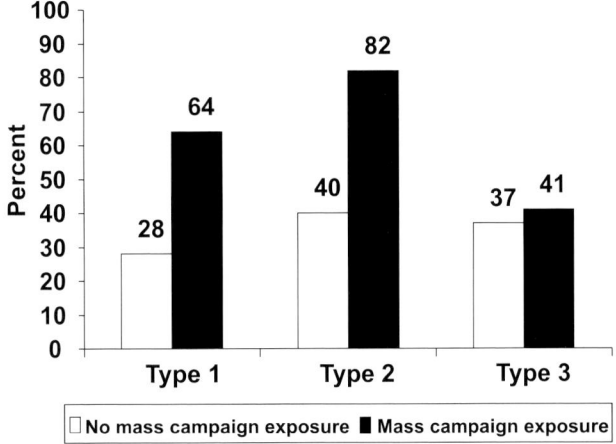

Fig. 2 Seroconversion between birth and 10 weeks of age to poliovirus types 1, 2, and 3, among infants receiving a single dose of IPV vaccine at 6 weeks of age, stratified by potential exposure to mass campaign, Oman. (Constructed from data in [46])

3.4
Vaccine-Associated Paralytic Poliomyelitis in Campaigns

Soon after widespread use of OPV began in 1961, it was found that OPV could on rare instances cause exactly the disease they were designed to prevent [50–55]. VAPP was found in both vaccine recipients and contacts. Studies in the US found an overall risk of VAPP of one case per 2.5 million doses of OPV administered [56–59]. Immunodeficient individuals were found to be at substantially higher risk for VAPP [60]. However, it does not appear that the mass campaign use of OPV is associated with a higher risk of VAPP in developing countries [53–55].

4
Mass Vaccination in the Polio Eradication Era

4.1
Strategies

With the beginning of the elimination efforts in the Western Hemisphere in the 1980s, the polio eradication strategies were defined first for the Americas, and then for the world [4, 61, 62]: (1) achieve and maintain the highest levels of routine immunization coverage with OPV; (2) establish sensitive surveillance to detect all cases of acute flaccid paralysis (AFP); (3) conduct supplemental immunization activities (SIAs) with OPV, first as NIDs or subnational immunization days (SNIDs) to reduce widespread poliovirus transmission; and (4) carry-out focused campaigns (mop-up campaigns) to eliminate the last foci of transmission.

Mass vaccination campaigns used in the polio eradication program can be classified as: (1) NIDs, national campaigns, usually targeting all children less than 5 years of age, regardless of previous vaccination status, administering two rounds of OPV, separated by 4–6 weeks; these campaigns initially were health facility and boot-based; (2) SNIDs, same target age group and operational approaches, but campaigns limited to subnational levels; and (3) mop-up activities, targeting the same age group (or determined by epidemiology of remaining cases) but in a limited geographic area (a district or multiple districts), and administering OPV by vaccination teams going house-to-house to achieve the highest possible coverage. In the early phases of polio eradication, outbreak response immunization activities were used, usually providing a single dose of OPV to children in close contact with a confirmed polio case. These activities were usually small-scale, with hundreds of doses administered. The impact of the mass campaigns were dramatic as the experiences from the Americas and the Western Pacific Region indicated [63, 64].

By the end of 1999, fewer than 20 polio-endemic countries remained, and the program intensified to address the remaining challenges in these polio-endemic countries. The intensification addressed both the frequency and quality of the mass vaccination campaigns. In many areas, more than two rounds of NID were carried out, often using a house-to-house method of administration, or a combination fixed facility and house-to-house use. Simi-

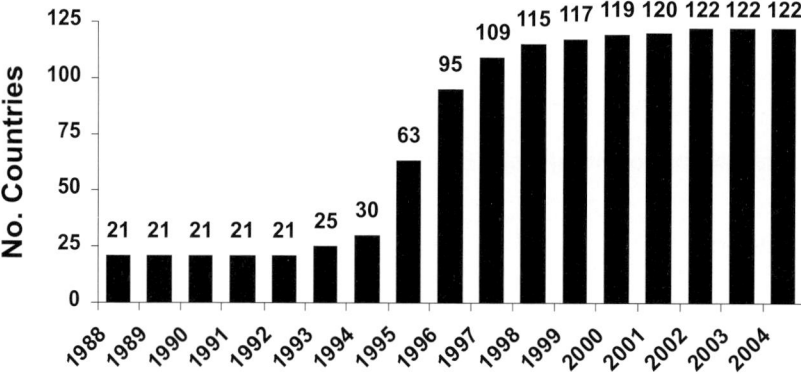

Fig. 3 Cumulative number of countries conducting national immunization days, 1988–2004. (WHO unpublished data)

larly, mop-up campaigns were extended to cover epidemiologically important areas. Figure 3 shows the cumulative number of countries that conducted NIDs from 1988 to 2004.

5
Programmatic Aspects of Mass Campaigns

The capacity of campaigns to consistently reach and vaccinate a very high proportion of children depends on how well they are prepared for, and how they are conducted. The key to success is careful planning, uniform execution, strong monitoring and supervision, and finally evaluation to identify problems to be addressed prior to the next round. The WHO Polio Field Guide outlines in detail the basic processes for planning, carrying-out, and evaluating campaigns [65].

5.1
Campaign Scope and Strategies for Delivering Immunization

The operational objective of campaigns using OPV is to reach all children in the target age group (usually all children below 5 years of age) in the area selected for the campaign, with potent vaccine. While this objective has never varied, campaigns have been carried out in different ways at different times and in different places during the period of the global polio eradication initiative. As noted above, campaigns using OPV are referred to generally as SIAs, and they can be roughly divided into three groups: (1) those that were national in scope; (2) large subnational campaigns, usually targeting areas of known higher risk of transmission; and (3) mop-ups, intense activities intended to interrupt the last chains of transmission in particular areas or as response to importations of wild poliovirus, that varied in geographic extent.

A characteristic of polio SIAs is the need for multiple rounds in order to achieve a significant impact. SIA rounds are typically 4–6 weeks apart, and a minimum of two rounds are usually conducted. In the most intensely endemic areas of the Americas and the Western Pacific Region, and later in particular in the critical reservoir countries (India, Pakistan, Nigeria), multiple rounds have often been conducted in an attempt to maximize impact.

Two basic methods have been used to deliver vaccine to children during SIAs. The first is based on delivering immunization from fixed sites or posts in communities, to which children are brought by parents or caregivers. This method was most commonly used during the earlier years of the polio eradication era, and in particular in countries with a better developed health delivery system; for example, this method was widely used in countries in the Americas and in the Western Pacific Region [63, 64]. To be effective, campaigns based on fixed sites required very strong planning, and particularly strong communications and social mobilization activities to ensure that families were aware of the immunization activity and of the importance of bringing their children to the immunization post.

The second method is most commonly known as house-to-house immunization (effectively family-to-family or child-to-child). This involves teams of vaccinators visiting each dwelling or each household to identify and immunize children in the target age group. This was pioneered in the Americas in the later stages of eradication in that Region, was subsequently adopted in the final stages of eradication in the Western Pacific and European Regions, and has ultimately become the standard approach for all SIAs in the South East Asian, Eastern Mediterranean, and African Regions. It is certainly the method of choice for all mop-up activities. House-to-house activities take considerably longer than pure fixed post rounds, typically lasting several days as opposed to 1 or 2 days.

Both of the broad methods described above have often been supplemented by additional strategies such as immunization teams covering transit points such as railway stations, congregation points such as markets, and other places where target age children may be found, and mobile immunization teams targeting areas where families live in nonformal dwellings. In practice the methods used have not been exclusive, and the highest quality SIAs have made use of a flexible mixture of strategies to ensure good access to all children in the target group. In India for example, current SIAs employ a mixture of fixed post activities (typically the first day of the round), followed by several days of house-to-house activity, supplemented by teams covering transit points (i.e., railway or bus stations, highways, roads, etc.) and other areas where children congregate.

5.2
Planning, Operational, and Logistical Issues for SIAs—Lessons Learned During the Polio Eradication Initiative

Whatever the extent of the campaign or the delivery strategies used, in practice, achieving high coverage of a very large target population (often more than 15% of the total population of any given country or area), with potent vaccine, is extremely difficult and challenging. Even more challenging is achieving this same high coverage consistently round after round. Experience has shown that different aspects of planning, preparation, conduct, and evaluation have been critical to the success of campaigns. Some critical aspects are outlined below, although this is not an exhaustive list.

1. National Interagency Coordinating Committee (ICC). In many countries, the presence of a strong ICC at national level, involving different government sectors and other national and international agencies and usually chaired by the Ministry of Health, has been of major benefit in the process of national planning and preparation. These committees have frequently had responsibility for approving overall plans and budgets and coordinating the technical and resource inputs of various government sectors and other agencies. In several instances these committees have raised considerable resources from nongovernment sectors.

2. Engaging local government. At subnational level, the engagement of local (district level) government has been critical to ensuring operational quality. The development of district management teams or district task forces, which are multi-sectoral in nature (usually chaired by the senior government official in the district), and which can engage nongovernment community groups at local level, has been a consistent feature of successful activities. In the most difficult areas for eradication (such as the western districts of Uttar Pradesh in India, and in Pakistan), the engagement of local government has been the major factor in the improvement in quality of SIAs.

3. Detailed microplanning from district to community level, on all aspects of operations and logistics. The development of plans at district and even community level is the step that moves planning from the theoretical to the practical. In areas conducting the best quality SIAs, microplans include not only the details of local logistics requirements, but also the details of immunization teams, the areas they are supposed to cover (including maps of these areas on a day-by-day basis), the supervisors and their responsibilities, local community leaders and influencers, and basic social mobilization activities.

4. Identification of high risk areas and groups for special attention. In many polio-endemic areas, certain population groups have been at higher risk of polio, and of sustaining wild poliovirus transmission even when the general population is largely free of polio. These groups have tended to be ethnic or religious minorities, particular social classes or groups, or mobile populations—all somewhat outside the orbit of general society and the provision of regular government services. The identification of these groups and development of specific plans for ensuring special attention to them during SIAs has proven critical to reaching them effectively; everything from communications and social mobilization strategies through to the make up of the immunization team can have a direct impact on reaching children.

5. Communications and social mobilization. Two aspects of communications and social mobilization strategy have been of great importance. The first is the general strategy of broad communication to the general community to ensure awareness of the SIA activity, and mobilization of mainstream community groups to hopefully achieve a high level of active community participation. The second is specific communications and mobilization strategies for the highest risk groups referred to above. On several occasions during the polio eradication era, failure to recognize high risk groups with particular communications needs has resulted in setbacks for the program (the most recent examples are western UP in northern India, and most spectacularly northern Nigeria, where immunization activities actually stopped in several states due to community concerns over vaccine safety). Reaching these communities has required specific and extensive communications activities, designed to address community concerns and engage influential figures.

6. A flexible mixture of strategies. As noted above, there is no 'one size fits all' as far as reaching the maximum proportion of children is concerned, particularly where health infrastructure is weak. The core strategy for immunization delivery, whether it is fixed site or house-to-house or a combination of the two, must be supplemented by other strategies. The switch from fixed site to house-to-house as a standard strategy in part of India and in Pakistan early in this decade led to immediate increases in the number of children covered; subsequently, however, the need for at least some fixed sites, and for special activities to cover transit points, have been recognized, and the addition of these strategies have led to further improvements in access to children. In the Mekong Delta area of Cambodia and Vietnam, the use of mobile teams on boats commencing in 1996 provided access to boat-dwelling communities who regularly moved up and down the waterways, and who could be reached in no other way.

7. Training of supervisors and immunization teams and selection of the correct team members. Once the planning has been done and the logistics put in place, everything rests on the work of immunization teams and supervisors. The selection of these teams, and their training and motivation, has long been recognized as critical to the success or failure to reach children during campaigns. In situations where health infrastructure is weak, the emphasis placed on selection and training becomes even more critical. Selection of appropriate team members where particular high risk groups exist has been noted above to strongly influence the acceptance of the activity by communities; it has been noted that for traditional communities in Pakistan, for example, the presence of a woman on the

immunization team greatly facilitates entry to multi-household dwelling compounds, and therefore the chance of finding particularly the youngest children and immunizing them.

8. Technical support from partner agencies available at the district level. This aspect has been most important in countries, or areas of countries, with weaker health infrastructure and less local trained human resources. WHO and UNICEF in particular have supported district teams in several countries through the deployment of national or international staff. The partner agency staff support local district teams in microplanning, selection and training of immunization teams and supervisors, local communications and social mobilization activities, monitoring of immunization activities, and evaluation following rounds. The deployment of partner agency staff has to be carefully planned to ensure maximum benefit; these staff numbers are generally limited and usually have to be concentrated in areas where the quality of SIAs has been weakest.

9. Intensive monitoring using standard indicators for immediate feedback and action on problems. Over time, in most countries conducting SIAs a process of monitoring immunization activities during immunization rounds has developed, using monitors independent of the immunization activity where possible. The indicators monitored are simple but critical, including outcome indicators by area monitored such as the proportion of children found by the monitor who have not been immunized during the round, and the proportion of houses/households found that have not been visited or reached, as well as process indicators such as whether immunization team members encountered have received training, whether supervisory visits are being conducted, etc. Monitoring has proved extremely useful in two ways, firstly by allowing immediate feedback to responsible district officers in evening meetings during each day of SIA activities to enable action to be taken to address problems during the round, and secondly by providing an independent assessment of quality of activities for use in evaluation.

10. Review of lessons learned after each round and identification of actions needed to improve quality in subsequent rounds. Using monitoring data and other indicators, in many countries a review of the overall quality of activities is held immediately following a round, including the impact of various tactics used to improve access to children by immunization teams. This has proven extremely helpful in identifying actions that can be undertaken to improve subsequent rounds. This kind of review process is now standard in all remaining endemic countries.

5.3
Improvement in Quality of SIAs

The quality of SIAs, in terms of the proportion of children reached with potent vaccines, has varied dramatically in different countries or areas of countries, and at different times during the polio eradication process. In general, as the program has evolved in different places the quality of SIAs has gradually improved. Many innovative approaches were adapted over the years (Table 2). Occasionally a deterioration of quality has occurred (for example, in India in 2001 and early 2002, when polio appeared to be on the way out), which has usually been rapidly punished by a resurgence of disease. Despite these variations, the operational capacity to conduct high quality campaigns now exists virtually everywhere wild poliovirus still circulates; in some areas, such as northern India, parts of Pakistan, and Afghanistan, campaign quality is truly excellent despite extremely difficult conditions. Indeed in these areas it is possible to see 'state of the art' activities, where all of the critical components mentioned above are being addressed more or less effectively.

SIAs have been carried out over the past two decades in countries with widely different circumstances. Countries like Afghanistan, Somalia, Angola, Cambodia, and Democratic Republic of Congo, which carried out years of campaigns while in the grip of complex emergencies, and which at the time of writing are either polio-free or extremely close to becoming polio-free. India, China, Vietnam, Egypt, Brazil, Bangladesh, and Pakistan coped with massive population size, extremely high population density in different areas, and a wide variety on internal geography and social organization to conduct increasingly high quality activities; all those except Afghanistan, India, and Pakistan are polio free, and these countries are very close to achieving the goal.

5.4
Effect of Mass Campaigns: Progress in Polio Eradication

In 1980, Brazil conducted national immunization campaigns with OPV for the first time, and demonstrated a dramatic impact in this developing tropical country (Fig. 1). The number of reported cases decreased from 1,290 in 1980 to 122 in 1981 [28]. The experiences from Brazil, and elsewhere, were critical in promoting more ambitious control and elimination targets. In 1985, the Pan American Sanitary Conference adopted the goal of elimination of poliomyelitis in the hemisphere by 1990 [66]. Progress was remarkable, and by 1988, the WHA resolved to eradicate poliomyelitis globally by the year 2000 [3]. The last case of poliomyelitis in the Americas was reported in 1991,

Table 2 Some operational and programmatic innovations in SIA implementation, 1988–2005

Intervention	First extensive use in SIAs	Advantage
Mobile teams/ transit teams	Widely used in the Americas and Western Pacific Region in early SIAs, now very important in India and Pakistan	Reaches children who are moving during the SIA round and who will not be reached by either fixed posts or house to house; reaches children living on the streets
House-to-house (child to child) vaccination	First used nationally in Cuba in the 1960s, used extensively in mop-ups in the Americas from 1989, and in the Western Pacific Region (including rural China) from the mid 1990s. Since 2000 this has been the preferred strategy in all polio-endemic countries	Increases coverage of children particularly in areas with less well developed health infrastructure; allows use of a geographical target area rather than a numerical target
House marking	Introduced following wide adoption of house-to-house approach in SIAs from 2000, firstly in India. Currently highly developed in India and Pakistan	Permits supervisors and monitors to rapidly check on the quality of work of vaccination teams
Finger marking with indelible ink of each vaccinated child	Gentian violet marking used frequently in Western Pacific, African, and South East Asian Regions; in 2000, silver nitrate marker pens first used in India	Permits rapid assessment of vaccination status of target children (without having to rely on parental recall); particularly useful in transit points, markets, etc., and in monitoring quality of work
Formal monitoring process using standard indicators	Early monitoring processes in WPR and the Americas; subsequently in other regions. Extensive monitoring using standard indicators adopted in India in 2002, now in general use	Allows for immediate feedback on quality based on indicators during SIA rounds, so that corrective actions can be quickly taken; provides the basis for evaluation of SIA quality
Identification of high risk areas and groups for special attention	Recognized as important from the late 1980s in the Americas; integral part of SIA planning in WPR and European Region; currently standard approach in SEAR and EMR countries, and increasingly used in AFR countries	Ensures development of plans to specifically target these groups and increase the likelihood of reaching children; targets communications and social mobilization activities

and in 1994 the hemisphere was certified by an international commission as polio free [67].

Progress in the other WHO regions followed. The Western Pacific Region and the European Region were certified as polio free in 2000, and 2001, respectively [68, 69]. Between 1988 and 2004, the number of polio cases has decreased from an estimated more than 350,000 cases to a reported 1,263 cases (data as of 29 March 2005) (Fig. 4), and the number of polio-endemic countries has declined from more than 125 to six. However, due to a resurgence of polio in Africa between 2003–2005, 18 previously polio-free countries in West, Central and East Africa, as well as the Middle East and Indonesia, imported poliovirus. Currently, polio transmission is occurring in three WHO regions (African Region, Eastern Mediterranean Region, and South Asia Region) (Fig. 5). Figure 6 shows the incidence of poliomyelitis in India during 1998 to 2005, and demonstrates the intensity (number and type) of SIAs needed to control, and hopefully, eliminate wild poliovirus transmission under the most difficult circumstances (high population density, high population movements, and low hygiene and sanitation).

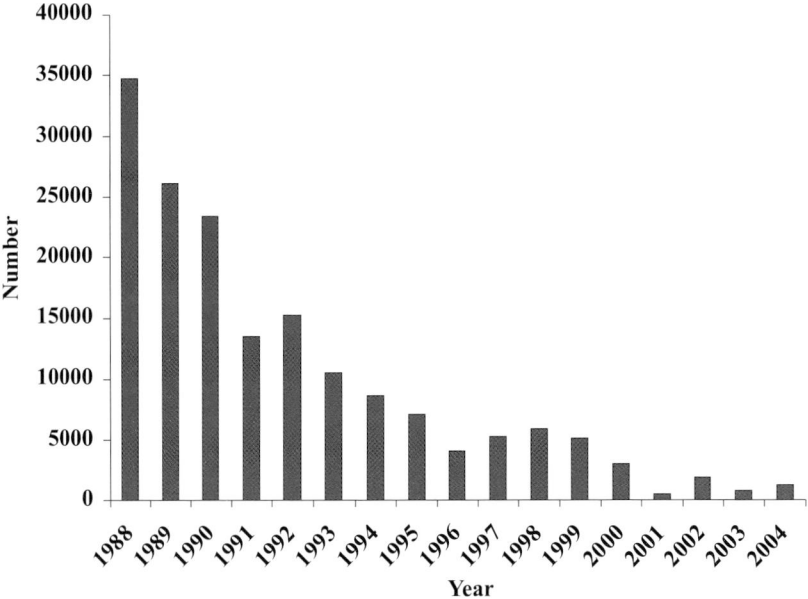

Fig. 4 Reported number of poliomyelitis cases, worldwide, 1988–2004. (WHO unpublished data)

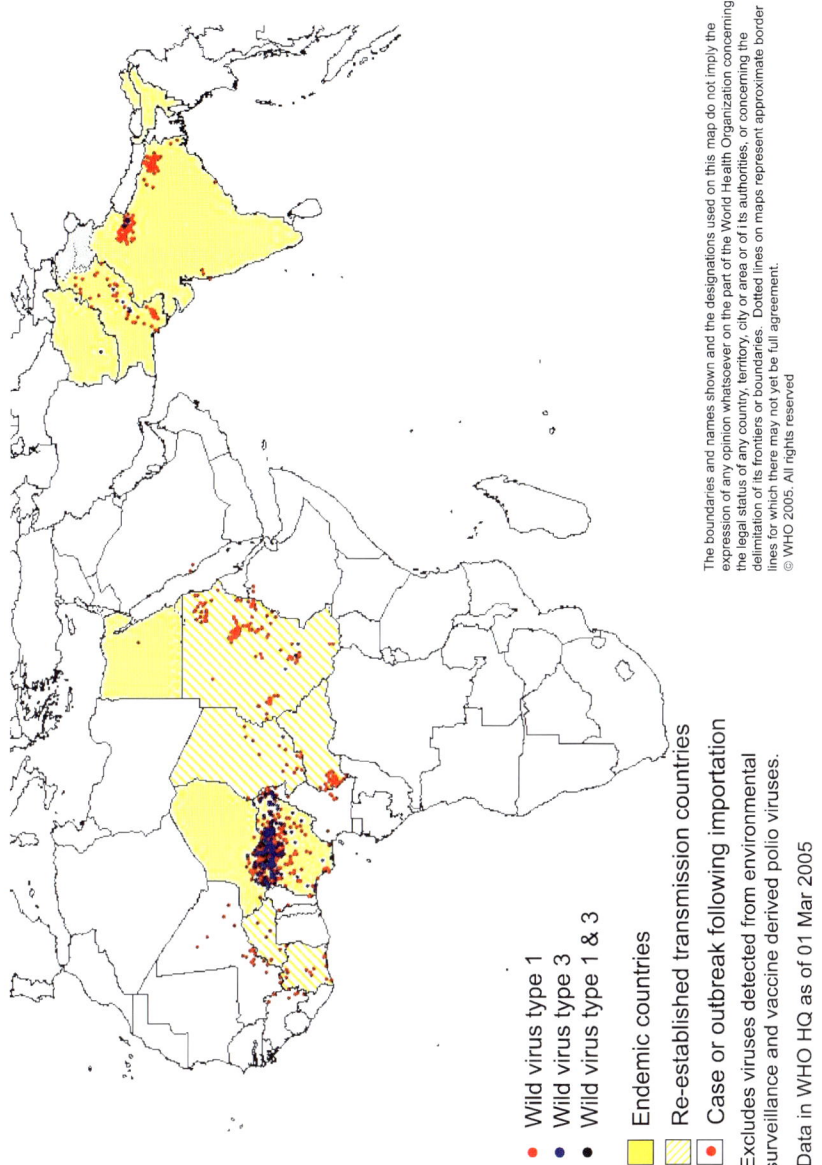

Fig. 5 Polio-endemic and countries with re-established poliovirus circulation, 2004. (WHO unpublished data)

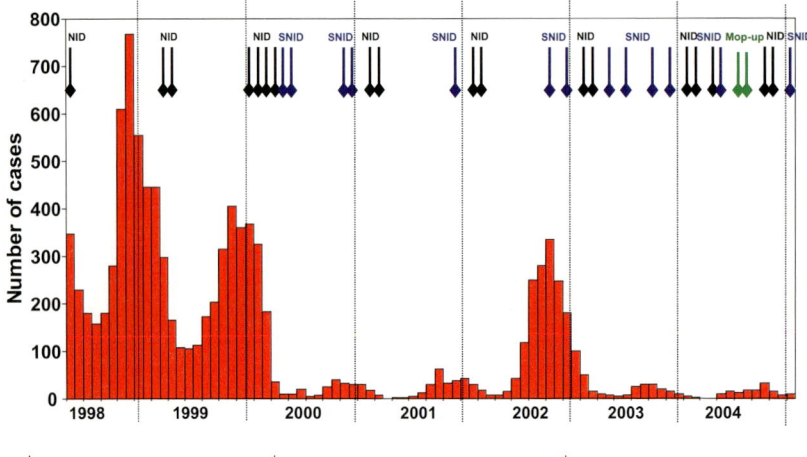

Fig. 6 Reported number of poliomyelitis cases, and national and subnational vaccination campaigns, India, 1998–2005

6
The Future: OPV Use in Campaigns Post-Polio Eradication

There is now a growing consent that OPV use must be discontinued some interval after interruption of wild poliovirus transmission has been accomplished [70, 71]. OPV use must be discontinued because of the well-known risks for paralytic poliomyelitis associated with its continued use; but the overriding objective is to remove all forms of polioviruses from human populations, and ensure that the achievements of polio eradication will be permanent. Continued use of OPV will almost certainly lead to reversion of vaccine viruses to assume the neurovirulence and transmission characteristics of wild poliovirus, circulate, and re-establish poliovirus circulation, thus negating the achievements of polio eradication.

Six prerequisites must be fulfilled to discontinue OPV: (1) confirmation of interruption of wild poliovirus transmission in all WHO Regions; (2) biocontainment of all poliovirus laboratory stocks and production facilities; (3) polio vaccine stockpile and response capacity; (4) detection and response capacity; (5) concurrence for synchronous OPV cessation; and (6) national immunization policies in place. It is likely that industrialized countries will continue using IPV (in combination vaccine preparations); however, it is less apparent what developing countries will do. It may be anticipated that some countries will switch to IPV, while many others may discontinue all polio vaccination. In those countries that decide to discontinue all polio vaccination, future birth cohorts would remain susceptible to poliomyelitis.

In the post-OPV cessation era, the use of OPV would be highly restricted through international consensus and agreement. In this period OPV would only be used (most likely, in the form of monovalent OPV types 1, 2, and 3, respectively) for emergency control activities, should poliovirus be re-introduced and circulate in human populations. The ensuing campaigns would likely to be large-scale and aimed at controlling (and, if possible, eliminating) re-introduced poliovirus, or at a minimum, decreasing the paralytic burden, until routine immunization could again be re-introduced.

7
Conclusions

The record with polio vaccines is extensive. These vaccines have been used over the past 50 years, in all countries of the world, and have had a substantial and predictable impact on the incidence of paralytic disease due to polioviruses. With the global consensus to eradicate poliomyelitis globally, vaccine use increased several-fold in the past decade.

Polio vaccines were administered through the routine program, and in campaigns. During the past decade more than 122 countries conducted NIDs, SNIDs and mop-up operations. The impact of the massive use of OPV has been dramatic, at the beginning of 2006, only four countries were polio-endemic (and even within these countries poliovirus transmission was highly focal). Suspension of vaccination in Kano State, Nigeria, for more than a year, however, was followed by importation of virus into 18 countries, primarily West and Central Africa, but also to the Horn of Africa, the Arabian peninsula, and as distant as Indonesia. In response, massive synchronized immunization campaigns have been put in place to rapidly eliminate virus transmission.

There is a synergistic effect of OPV attributes which make the vaccine almost ideally suited for mass campaign use; both with the effect in the individual (individual protection against paralysis; decreased shedding following subsequent exposure) and effect in the community (establishing a barrier; and mass secondary spread immunizing some unvaccinated individuals). However, the future of OPV appears to be grim, just like the disease, this vaccine must be relegated to history once wild poliovirus transmission has been interrupted globally.

References

1. Sutter RW, Kew OM, Cochi SL (2003) Poliovirus vaccine – live. In: Plotkin SA, Orenstein WA (eds), 4th edn. Vaccines. W.B. Saunders Company, Philadelphia, 25:651–705.
2. Majiyagbe J (2004) The volunteers' contribution to polio eradication. Bull WHO 82:2
3. World Health Assembly (1988) Polio eradication by the year 2000. Resolutions of the 41th World Health Assembly. Geneva: World Health Organization, 1988 (WHA resolution no. 41.28)
4. Hull H, Ward NA, Hull B, Milstien JB, de Quadros C (1994) Paralytic poliomyelitis: seasoned strategies, disappearing disease. Lancet 343:1331–1337
5. Smith J (1990) Patenting the Sun. Polio and the Salk Vaccine. William Morrow & Company, New York
6. Chumakov MP, Voroshilova MK, Drozdov SG, et al. (1961) Some results of the work on mass immunization in the Soviet Union with live poliovirus vaccine prepared from Sabin strains. Bull WIIO 25:79–91
7. Agol VI, Drozdov SG (1993) Russian contribution to OPV. Biologicals 21:321–325
8. Sabin AB (1985) Oral poliovirus vaccine: history of its development and use and current challenge to eliminate poliomyelitis from the world. J Infect Dis 151:420–436
9. Sabin AB (1984) Strategies for elimination of poliomyelitis in different parts of the world with use of oral poliovirus vaccine. Rev Infect Dis 6(Suppl 2):S391–S396
10. Robertson HE, Acker MS, Dillenberg HO, et al. (1962) Community-wide use of a "balanced" trivalent oral poliovirus vaccine (Sabin): a report of the 1961 trial at Prince Albert, Saskatchewan. Can Public Health J 53:179–191
11. CDC. Poliomyelitis Prevention in the United States (1997) Introduction of a sequential vaccination schedule of inactivated poliovirus vaccine followed by oral poliovirus vaccine. Updated Recommendations of the Advisory Committee on Immunization Practices (ACIP). MMWR Morb Mortal Wkly Rep 46(RR-3)
12. CDC (2000) Poliomyelitis Prevention in the United States. Updated Recommendations of the Advisory Committee on Immunization Practices (ACIP). MMWR Morb Mortal Wkly Rep 49(RR-5)
13. Ofusu-Amahh S, Kratzer JH, Nicholas DD (1977) Is poliomyelitis a serious problem in developing countries? – lameness in Ghanaian schools. Brit Med J i:1012–1014
14. Bernier RH (1984) Some observations on poliomyelitis lameness surveys. Rev Infect Dis 6(Suppl.2):S371–S375
15. Cruz RR (1984) Cuba: mass polio vaccination program, 1962–1982. Rev Infect Dis 6(Suppl.2):S408–S412
16. Mas Lago P, Ramon Bravo J, Andrus JK, Comellas MM, Galindo MA, de Quadros CA, Bell E (1994) Lessons from Cuba: mass campaign administration of trivalent oral poliovirus vaccine and seroprevalence of poliovirus neutralizing antibodies. Bull WHO 72:221–225
17. Mas Lago P (1999) Eradication of poliomyelitis in Cuba: a historical perspective. Bull WHO 77:681–687

18. Henderson RH (1984) The Expanded Programme on Immunization of the World Health Organization. Rev Infect Dis 6(Suppl.2):S475–S479
19. Grant JP (1991) Reaching the unreached: a miracle in the making. Asia Pac J Public Health 5:154–162
20. Murray C, Kreuser J, Whang W (1994) Cost-effectiveness analysis and policy choices: investing in health systems. Bull WHO 72:663–674
21. Vaccine and Biologicals Department (2003) WHO vaccine-preventable diseases: Monitoring system. 2003 global summary. Geneva: World Health Organization, (WHO/V&B/03.20)
22. McBean AM, Thoms ML, Albrecht P, et al. (1988) Serologic response to oral polio vaccine and enhanced-potency inactivated polio vaccine. Am J Epidemiol 128:615–628
23. Faden H, Modlin JF, Thoms ML, McBean AM, Ferdon MB, Ogra PL (1990). Comparative evaluation of immunization with live attenuated and enhanced-potency inactivated trivalent poliovirus vaccines in childhood: systemic and local immune responses. J Infect Dis 162:1291–1297
24. Patriarca PA, Wright PF, John TJ (1991) Factors affecting the immunogenicity of oral poliovirus vaccine in developing countries: review. Rev Infect Dis 13:926–939
25. Domök I, Balayan MS, Fayinka OA, Skrtic N, Soneji AD, Harland PS (1974) Factors affecting the efficacy of live poliovirus vaccine in warm climates. Efficacy of type 1 Sabin vaccine administered together with antihuman gamma-globulin horse serum to breast-fed and artificially fed infants in Uganda. Bull WHO 51:333–347
26. Expanded Program on Immunization (1989) Global Advisory Group (1988). Wkly Epidemiol Rec 64:5–10
27. Rezapkin GV, Norwood LP, Taffs RE, et al. (1995) Microevaluation of type 3 Sabin strain of poliovirus in cell cultures and its implications for oral poliovirus vaccine quality control. Virology 211:377–384
28. Nathanson N, Horn SD (1992) Neurovirulence tests of type 3 oral poliovirus vaccine manufactured by Lederle Laboratories, 1964–1988. Vaccine 10:469–474
29. Patriarca PA, Laender F, Palmeira G, et al. (1988) Randomized trial of alternative formulations of orla poliovaccine in Brazil. Lancet i:429–433
30. Patriarca PA, Linkins RW, Sutter RW, Orenstein WA (1993) Optimal schedule for the administration of oral poliovirus vaccine. In Kurstak E (ed). Measles and poliomyelitis—vaccines and immunization. Springer, New York, Chapter 24 pp 303–313
31. Milstien JB, Lemon SM, Wright PF (1997) Development of a more thermostable poliovirus vaccine. J Infect Dis 175(Suppl.1):S247–S253
32. Anonymous (1996) Vaccine vial monitors take guesswork out of immunization. Vaccine Immun News 1:7–8
33. Heymann DL, Murphy K, Brigaud M, et al. (1987) Oral poliovirus vaccine in tropical Africa: greater impact on incidence of paralytic disease than expected from coverage surveys and seroconversion rates. Bull WHO 65:495–501
34. Olivé J-M, Risi JB Jr, de Quadros CA (1977) National immunization days: Experience in Latin America. J Infect Dis 175(Suppl.1):S189–S193
35. Bilous J, Maher C, Tangermann RH, Aylward RB, et al. (1997) The experience of countries in the Western Pacific Region in conducting national immunization days for polio eradication. J Infect Dis 175(Suppl.1):S194–S197

36. Tangermann RH; Hull HF, Jafari H, Nkowane B, Everts H, Aylward BR (2000) Eradication of poliomyelitis in countries affected by conflict. Bull WHO 78:330–338
37. CDC (1999) Progress toward poliomyelitis eradication during armed conflict—Somalia and Southern Sudan, January 1998-June 1999. MMWR Morb Mortal Wkly Rep 48:633–637
38. Benyesh-Melnick M, Melnick JL, Rawls WE, et al. (1967) Studies on the immongenicity, communicability, and genetic stability of oral poliovaccine administered during the winter. Am J Epidemiol 86:112–136
39. Risi JB (1984) The control of poliomyelitis in Brazil. Rev Infect Dis 6(Suppl 2):S400–S403
40. Hinman AR, Foege WH, de Quadros CA, Patriarca PA, Orenstein WA, Brink EW (1987) The case for global eradication of poliomyelitis. Bull WHO 65:835–840
41. Birmingham ME, Aylward BR, Cochi SL, Hull HF (1977) National immunization days: State of the art. J Infect Dis 175(Suppl.1):S183–S188
42. Benyesh-Melnick M, Melnick JL, Rawls WE, et al. (1967) Studies on the immongenicity, communicability, and genetic stability of oral poliovaccine administered during the winter. Am J Epidemiol 86:112–136
43. Chen RT, Hausinger S, Dajani AS, et al. (1996) Seroprevalence of antibody against poliovirus in innercity preschool children: implications for vaccination policy in the United States. JAMA 275:1639–1645
44. Ramsey ME, Begg NT, Ghandi J, Brown D (1994) Antibody response and viral excretion after live polio vaccine or a combined schedule of live and inactivated polio vaccines. Pediatr Infect Dis J 13:1117–1121
45. Richardson G, Linkins RW, Eames MA, Wood DJ, Minor PD, Patriarca PA (1995) Immunogenicity of oral polio vaccine administered in mass campaigns versus routine immunization programs. Bull WHO 73:769–777
46. WHO Collaborative Study Group on Oral and Inactivated Poliovirus Vaccines (1997) Combined immunization of infants with oral and inactivated poliovirus vaccines: Results of a randomized trial in the Gambia, Oman, and Thailand. J Infect Dis 175(Suppl.1):S215–S227
47. Reichler MR, Kharabshah S, Rhodes P, Otoum H, BLoch S, Majid MA, et al. (1997) Increased immunogenicity of oral poliovirus vaccine administered in mass vaccination campaigns compared with the routine vaccination program in Jordan. J Infect Dis 175(Suppl.1):S198–S204
48. Deming MS, Linkins RW, Jaiteh KO, Hull HF (1997) The clinical efficacy of trivalent oral polio vaccine in The Gambia by season of vaccine administration. J Infect Dis 175(Suppl.1):S254–S257
49. Posey DL, Linkins RW, Couto Oliveira MJ, Monteiro D, Patriarca PA (1997) The effect of diarrea on oral poliovirus vaccine failure in Brazil. J Infect Dis 175(Suppl.1):S258–S263
50. Terry L (1962) The Association of Cases of Poliomyelitis with the Use of Type 3 Oral Poliomyelitis Vaccines. US Department of Health, Education and Welfare, Washington DC
51. Anonymous (1964) Oral poliomyelitis vaccine. Report of the Special Advisory Committee on Oral Poliomyelitis Vaccines to the Surgeon General of the Public Health Service. JAMA 190:161–163

52. Henderson DA, Witte JJ, Morris L, Langmuir AD (1964) Paralytic disease associated with oral polio vaccines. JAMA 190:41–48
53. Andrus JA, Strebel PM, de Quadros CA, Olive JM (1995) Risk of vaccine-associated paralytic poliomyelitis in the America, 1989–1991. Bull WHO 73:33–40
54. Kohler KA, Banerjee K, Hlady WG, Andrus JK, Sutter RW (2002) Vaccine-associated paralytic poliomyelitis in India, 1999: decreased risk despite massive use of oral polio vaccine. Bull WHO 80:210–216
55. Kohler KA, Banerjee K, Sutter RW (2002) Further clarity on vaccine-associated paralytic polio in India (letter). Bull WHO 80:987
56. Schonberger LB, McGowan JE Jr, Gregg MB (1976) Vaccine-associated poliomyelitis in the United States, 1961–1972. Am J Epidemiol 104:202–211
57. Nkowane BM, Wassilak SGF, Orenstein WA, et al. (1987) Vaccine-associated paralytic poliomyelitis: United States, 1973 through 1984. JAMA 257:1335–1340
58. Strebel PM, Sutter RW, Cochi SL, Biellik RJ, Brink EW, Kew OM, Pallansch MA, Orenstein WA, Hinman AR (1992) Epidemiology of poliomyelitis in the United States: One decade after the last reported case of indigenous wild virus-associated disease. Clin Infect Dis 14:568–579
59. Alexander LN, Seward JF, Santibanez TA, Pallansch MA, Kew OM, Prevots DR, Strebel PM, Cono J, Wharton M, Orenstein WA, Sutter RW (2004) Vaccine policy changes and epidemiology of poliomyelitis in the United States. JAMA 292:1696–1701
60. Sutter RW, Prevots DR (1994) Vaccine-associated paralytic poliomyelitis among immunodeficient persons. Infect Med 11:426,429–430,435–438
61. de Quadros CA, Andrus JK, Olive J-M, Da Silveira CM, Eikhof RM, Carrasco P, Fitzsimmons JW, Pinheiro FP (1991) Eradication of poliomyelitis: progress in the Americas. Pediatr Infect Dis J 10:222–229
62. Wright PF, Kim-Farley RJ, de Quadros CA, Robertson SE, Scott RM, Ward NA, Henderson RH (1992) Strategies for the global eradication of poliomyelitis by the year 2000. N Engl J Med 325:1774–1779
63. Olivé J-M, Risi JB Jr, de Quadros CA (1977) National immunization days: Experience in Latin America. J Infect Dis 175(Suppl.1):S189–S193
64. Bilous J, Maher C, Tangermann RH, Aylward RB, et al. (1997) The experience of countries in the Western Pacific Region in conducting national immunization days for polio eradication. J Infect Dis 175(Suppl.1):S194–S197
65. WHO (1996) Expanded Program on Immunization. Field Guide for Supplementary Activities Aimed at Achieving Polio Eradication. World Health Organization, Geneva (WHO document WHO/EPI/GEN/95.01 REV.1)
66. Pan American Health Organization (1985) Director announces campaign to eradicate poliomyelitis from the Americas by 1990. Bull Pan American Health Org 19:213–215
67. CDC (1994) Certification of polio eradication – the Americas, 1994. MMWR Morb Mortal Wkly Rep 43:720–722
68. CDC (2001) Certification of polio eradication – Western Pacific Region, 2000. MMWR Morbid Mortal Wkly Rep 50:1–3
69. WHO (2002) Certification of poliomyelitis eradication, European Region, June 2002. Wkly Epidemiol Rec 77:221–223

70. WHO (2004) Progress towards global poliomyelitis eradication: preparation for the oral poliovirus vaccine cessation era. Wkly Epidemiol Rec 79:349–355
71. WHO (2004) Conclusions and recommendations of the Ad Hoc Advisory Committee on Poliomyelitis Eradication, Geneva, 21–22 September 2004. Wkly Epidemiol Rec 79:401–407

Rubella Mass Campaigns

S. Reef (✉)

CDC, 1600 Clifton Road NE, Atlanta, GA 30333, USA
ser2@cdc.gov

1	Introduction	221
2	Other Regions	225
2.1	European Region	225
2.2	Eastern Mediterranean Region	226
2.3	South Eastern Region	226
2.4	African Region	226
2.5	Western Pacific Region	226
3	Rubella Campaigns	227
3.1	Issues and Components to Mass Campaigns	227
3.1.1	Safety Issues	228
4	Conclusions	229
	References	229

Abstract The availability of vaccines that contain both measles and rubella components allows for the elimination of both diseases. Although routine infant vaccination with rubella vaccine has had profound effects on the incidence of both acquired and congenital rubella, mass vaccination rapidly stops circulation of the virus and prevents paradoxical increases in susceptibility of women that might result from decreased exposure in childhood. Whereas routine rubella vaccination has eliminated the infection from many developed countries, mass vaccination has rapidly accomplished the same goal in Latin America and the Caribbean, and is being applied in other developing country areas.

1
Introduction

Rubella, once thought to be a benign illness, gained public health importance when Dr. Norman Gregg associated the risk of rubella in pregnant women and congenital birth defects [1]. In the early 1960s, the ability to isolate the virus was achieved by two separate groups [2, 3]. A worldwide rubella epidemic that began in 1962 in Europe led to the 1964–1965 rubella epidemics in the US. The US epidemic alone involved an estimated 12.5 million cases of rubella including 2,000 cases of encephalitis, 11,250 abortions, 2,100 neonatal deaths, and 20,000 infants born with congenital rubella syndrome (CRS). The financial cost of the epidemic was estimated at $1.5 billion. The morbidity and mortality of the epidemic spurred development of rubella vaccines, and emphasized the need for control strategies for rubella to prevent a recurrence of this devastating epidemic [4]. In 1969, three rubella vaccines were licensed in the US, ultimately reduced to one (RA 27/3).

In light of the pending licensure of the rubella vaccines, there was considerable debate on the best approach for implementing the vaccination program. The goal of a rubella vaccination program is the prevention of congenital rubella infections. Because the rubella vaccine is a live-attenuated vaccine, there were initial concern of vaccination of women who were later found to be pregnant might result in fetal infection and deformities. This concern resulted in two different strategies that were used by various industrialized countries [5, 6]. These strategies included vaccination of children-resulting in herd immunity and known as the indirect approach-and vaccination of women of childbearing age-providing individual protection and known as the direct approach. The rational for the direct approach was that as rubella incidence was greatest in preschool and elementary school children, it was reasoned that vaccination of this age group would decrease or interrupt the circulation of the virus; susceptible pregnant women would be protected indirectly by virtually eliminating the risk of exposure. The risk of giving a potentially teratogenic live virus vaccine to young women of childbearing age was undefined. The direct approach would provide individual immunity and decrease the risk of CRS; however, would not interrupt rubella virus circulation.

In the US, to increase the immunity among children aged 1 year to puberty several mass campaigns were undertaken. These campaigns ranged from local to statewide [7].

With over two decades of experience with the initial vaccination programs, the best options were to target both children and women of child-bearing age. The US and UK started with two different approaches but now vaccinate both children and women of childbearing age [8].

Another vaccination strategy that is now being used widely for rubella is the Mass Immunization Campaign (MIC). MICs have played a significant role in the eradication of polio and control/elimination of measles [9].

In the 1990s, MICs were part of the strategy used for measles elimination by PAHO that was subsequently adapted in other parts of the World Health Organization (WHO) regions. The strategy used for measles control included:

catch-up, mop-up, keep-up, and follow-up [10]. The initial catch-up campaign for measles was to conduct a MIC in the highest risk group—children less than 15 years of age. This target group comprised the highest group of susceptibles. This was followed by keep-up to maintain high coverage in children less than 5 years of age.

With the successful control of measles, the public health importance of rubella became apparent. Approximately 30% of the suspected measles cases were rubella (PAHO). Even though there are limited data available on the burden of CRS, several countries (Brazil, US, Canada, Mexico, Barbados, Jamaica, Cuba and Belize) have documented cases of CRS or fetal infection. It has been estimated that in the Western Hemisphere more than 20,000 infants with CRS were born annually in the pre-vaccine era [11].

As part of the measles elimination strategy, countries in the Western Hemisphere were already conducting MICs in children aged 1–14 years. Rubella vaccine is available as a single antigen or in combinations of measles-rubella (MR) or measles-rubella-mumps (MMR) vaccine, so it is straightforward to incorporate a rubella-containing vaccine into the existing measles vaccination program. With no rubella control goal in the Western Hemisphere, and the extensive previous experience with established vaccination programs, the question of what would be the most appropriate strategy was raised. Introduction of rubella vaccine into childhood programs would decrease the circulation of rubella virus; however, it would not have an immediate impact on CRS. However, a complete rubella vaccination program would include individual protection by vaccination of women of childbearing age and of children to interrupt rubella virus transmission. It was recommended that countries add a rubella-containing vaccine to their routine childhood program, and as part of the follow-up campaign in children aged 1–4 years also and to conduct a one-time mass campaign among adults. Countries that would like to accelerate their control of rubella and CRS should rapidly introduce rubella-containing vaccine into the adult population in addition to the routine childhood program. To accelerate CRS prevention, countries are advised to conduct a one-time mass campaign that targets all females from ages 5 to 39 years [12]. Countries wanting to control/prevent rubella and CRS are advised to conduct a one-time mass campaign that targets both males and females from ages 5 to 39 years [12].

The Caribbean subregion was the first to establish a rubella elimination goal in the Western Hemisphere. As part of the measles eradication resolution adopted in 1991, measles surveillance was established. Rubella vaccine had been introduced in the late 1970s and early 1980 in several countries in the Caribbean. The vaccination strategy was to target adolescent girls; however, the coverage was less than 80%. Rubella continued to circulate throughout the Caribbean with increased recognized rubella activities in 1986, 1988 and 1990. As part of the catch-up campaigns, 11 of the 18 countries included rubella-containing vaccine. To understand the financial impact of CRS and rubella, a costing study was conducted. It was estimated that without the current vaccination strategies, it would cost more than $60,000,000; however, the cost to conduct mass adult campaigns to eliminate rubella and CRS would be only $4.3 million. From this exercise it became apparent that mass immunization campaigns were a very cost-effective strategy. In 1998, after reviewing the available epidemiology, serologic and cost data, CARICOM Council for Human and Social Development passed a resolution to eliminate rubella and CRS by 2000. Between 1998 and 2001, 18 of the 19 countries conducted adult mass campaigns. Since 2001 and 1999, no rubella or CRS cases have been confirmed. One of the lessons learned from the Caribbean experience is that the mass campaigns must be completed within 1 month. Numerous campaigns lasting over several months resulted in fatigue of health care staff and interruption of the routine health care system.

Because of the widespread circulation of rubella in the Western Hemisphere and the potential for rubella epidemics, the Technical Advisory group for PAHO recommended in 1997 that strengthening of rubella and CRS prevention efforts. The vaccination strategies included: incorporation of rubella-containing vaccine into the routine childhood program at 12 months of age, and as part of the complementary follow-up campaigns (part of the measles elimination strategy) targeting children aged 1–4 years every 4 years depending on the routine coverage. Countries that wish to accelerate their control of rubella and CRS should introduce rubella-containing vaccine rapidly into the adult population in addition to the routine childhood program. In 1999, at the TAG meeting in Canada, TAG recommended that countries conduct a one-time mass campaign targeting all females aged 5–39 years. This strategy rapidly decreases the number of CRS cases; however, men remain susceptible and rubella virus could continue to circulate. With the success of the accelerated rubella control and CRS prevention, in 2003, all the PAHO member countries passed a resolution calling for the elimination of rubella and CRS by 2010. To achieve this goal, countries must have the political will and financial commitment to sustain a program involving both sexes.

After the success in the Caribbean, countries in Latin America embarked on adult mass vaccination campaigns (Table 1). In 1999, Chile conducted a mass campaign, but vaccinated only women up to the age 29 years. In 2001, Costa Rica embarked on a mass campaign in adults (males and females) after a large rubella outbreak in 1998–1999. The highest incidence was among persons aged 25–34 years followed by the 35–44 year-old group. Several lessons were learned as part of this campaign including the importance

Table 1 Countries that have conducted adult mass campaigns[a]

Countries	Year of campaign	Type of campaign	Number vaccinated
Sri Lanka	1996	Female only	
English-speaking Caribbean	1997–2001 18 Countries	Adult 17/18 Female/male 1 Female only	2.16 million
Chile	1999	Female only	2.5 million
Costa Rica	2001	Male/female	1.6 million
Brazil	2001–2002	Females only	29 million
Kyrgyzstan	2001	Females only	
Honduras	2002	Male/female	3.3 million
Iran	2003	Male/female	33.0 million
El Salvador	2004	Male/female	2.8 million
Ecuador	2004	Male/female	4.8 million
Libya	2004	Male/female	2.75 million

[a] Albania did not do a mass campaign—conducted in routine program

of integration of partners into the process, the importance of social mobilization/communication, effective microplanning and supervision and safety issues. Since the campaign the last case of rubella and CRS both occurred in 2001. As noted in Table 1, several countries in Latin America have conducted campaigns, each building on the previous experience of other countries. To achieve the rubella goal by 2010, eight countries are planning to conduct adult MICs in 2005. The remaining countries plan to conduct adult mass campaigns in 2006.

2
Other Regions

2.1
European Region

The EURO region of WHO has established a goal of measles and rubella elimination by 2010 and prevention of congenital rubella infection (CRI) (CRS (<1/100,000 live births by 2010) [13]. To accomplish the measles and rubella elimination goal and the CRI prevention goal, the recommended strategies include: achieve and maintain high coverage (95%) with two doses of measles-containing vaccine and at least one dose of rubella vaccine through routine services; provide a second opportunity through supplementary immunization activities (SIAs); provide rubella vaccination opportunities including the opportunity provided by the SIAs to target all rubella-susceptible populations including children, adolescents and women of childbearing age. Between 1990 and 2004, nine SIAs were conducted, six of which used rubella-containing vaccine. In addition, three countries simultaneously offered rubella-containing vaccine to women of childbearing age.

2.2
Eastern Mediterranean Region

The WHO Eastern Mediterranean Region has established a goal for elimination of CRS by 2010. Several of member countries have conducted campaigns using rubella-containing vaccine. Of the 23 countries, 10 countries, particularly the Arab/Gulf states, have conducted catch-up campaigns using rubella-containing vaccine. Only two countries have vaccinated women of childbearing age above 18 years of age. In 2003, Iran conducted a MIC using MMR targeting both males and females between 5 and 25 years of age. In 2004, Libya conducted a mass campaign in males/females between ages 9 months to 20 years.

2.3
South Eastern Region

This region has not established a rubella/CRS goal. However, several countries have been interested in understanding the burden of CRS in their countries. In 1996, Sri Lanka established a goal for the prevention of CRS. In 1996, a rubella immunization day targeting girls and women aged 11–44 years. During 2001 and 2004, the coverage in women aged 11–44 years ranged from 72% to 82%.

2.4
African Region

This region has not established a rubella/CRS goal. Several countries have been assessing their burden of rubella/CRS; however, no country has conducted adult mass campaigns.

2.5
Western Pacific Region

This region has not established a rubella/CRS goal. However, two countries in the South Pacific have conducted mass campaigns in response to outbreaks.

In 2002, the kingdom of Tonga experienced a rubella outbreak. With many of the cases occurring among adults and documented high susceptibility (20%) in women, a mass campaign was undertaken for all children aged 9 months to 14 years and for women aged 15–44 years. The coverage in both groups was 95%. In addition, measles vaccine was replaced with MR vaccine in the routine childhood schedule. In 2003, a rubella outbreak occurred in Samoa. Like Tonga, rubella vaccine had not been introduced into their national program. In response to the outbreak, a mass campaign was conducted.

3
Rubella Campaigns

3.1
Issues and Components to Mass Campaigns

To plan a successful campaign, several aspects must be included. These include political commitment at all levels of the government along with the necessary financial support; intersectorial participation of various department of the government (e.g., labor, education). After the target population for vaccination has been identified, development of the vaccination strategy is necessary. Different vaccination approaches may be based on the situation in each area, such as access to existing services, availability of resources and previous experience with similar activities. Several tactics that have been previously used included mobile posts, a call to gather at strategic locations, the use of brigades, house-to-house vaccination, and flexible hours.

For adult campaigns, social mobilization was critical. Development of a strong and comprehensive social mobilization plan may include the participation of political, union and religious leaders, national personalities, community associations, presidents of professional societies, representatives of education, artists, entrepreneurs, local non-government organizations, and the media.

To ensure that the goal of the vaccination campaign is met, organization, planning, training and supervision at all levels of government are critical components. To adequately prepare for a campaign, the minimum time needed is 6 months with 9 months being preferable. Each level of the government must know what their role and responsibilities are. Microplanning to the lowest level is critical. This will ensure that the proposed strategy is implemented as planned. To ensure that staff understand the plan, training at all levels is critical for the success of the campaign. This has been realized time after time with each campaign. Even with the best planning, supervision at all levels is a critical component. Monitoring the progress of the campaign ensures that goals are being achieved and corrective measures taken. To ensure that the target population has been vaccinated, rapid monitoring of vaccination coverage must be conducted. If unvaccinated populations are identified, then strategic corrective measures should be undertaken. Unlike childhood campaigns, adult campaigns are more challenging. The two areas that required additional planning includes pregnant women and blood banks.

3.1.1
Safety Issues

Vaccination of Unknowingly Pregnant Women   Prior to the licensure of the rubella vaccines in 1969, vaccine virus strains were shown to cross the placenta and asymptomatically infect the fetus [11, 12]. Because of the theoretical risk, it is recommended that pregnancy be a contraindication to rubella vaccination. Since that time, data from several countries including the US, Germany, and the UK have shown that a small percentage of infants will be infected; however, no infant has been born with CRS. If considering the highest risk period for CRS (mothers vaccinated 1–2 weeks before to 4–6 weeks after conception, the maximum theoretical risk is 1.3%). This risk is substantially less than the >20% risk for CRS associated with maternal infection during the first 20 weeks of pregnancy.

Additional data were obtained during the mass campaigns in Costa Rica and Brazil. Follow-up of these more than 1,000 pregnancies has provided more information on the safety of rubella-containing vaccine. Even though 3.6% of the infants had rubella antibodies, no cases of CRS were identified. These data show a further decrease in the known theoretical risk of CRS due to vaccination of unknowingly pregnant women.

Blood Bank   After receipt of rubella-containing vaccine, persons are not eligible to donate blood for 1 month. In many countries, the targeted age-group may account for a majority of the blood donors in a country. In Costa Rica, the campaign was expected to decrease the blood supply in the country, and the national blood bank observed a 52% decrease in blood donations compared with previous months. To maintain the blood supply, several strategies can be used including targeted awareness and motivational campaigns to persons aged 40 and older, who were not targeted for vaccination and donation of blood just prior to the campaign of the targeted age-group.

4
Conclusions

The use of adult rubella mass campaigns have resulted the significant reduction of rubella and CRS cases, particularly in the Western Hemisphere. However, their role in the other parts of the world remains to be evaluated and the overall cost-effectiveness of conducting these mass campaigns needs to be determined. Initial calculations document the financial savings of these campaigns; however, thorough evaluation of the cost–benefit and cost effectiveness is currently underway.

References

1. Gregg NM (1941) Congenital cataract following German measles in the mother. Trans Ophthalmol Soc Aust 3:35–46
2. Weller TH, Neva FA (1962) Propagation in tissue culture of cytopathic agents from patients with rubella-like illness. Proc Soc Exp Bio Med 111:215–225
3. Parkman PD, Beuscher EL, Artenstein MS (1962) Recover of rubella virus from army recruits. Proc Soc Exp Bio Med 111:225–230
4. Cooper LZ (1975) Congenital rubella in the United States. In: Krugman S, Gershon A (eds). Symposium on infections of the fetus and newborn infant. Alan R. Liss, New York
5. Centers for Disease Control and Prevention (1969) Prelicensing statement on rubella virus vaccine: Recommendation of the Public Health Service Advisory committee on Immunization Practices. MMWR 18
6. Tobin JO, Sheppard S, Smithells RW, Milton A, Noach N, Reid D (1985) Rubella in the United Kingdom, 1970–1983. Rev Infect Dis 7:S47–S52
7. Irons B, Lewis MJ, Dahl-Regis M, Castillio-Soloranzo Carrasco P, deQuadro C (2000) Strategies to eradicate rubella in the English-speaking Caribbean. Am J Public Health 90:1545–1549
8. Vyse AJ, Gay NJ, White JM, et al. (2002) Evolution of surveillance of measles, mumps, and rubella in England and Wales: providing the platform for evidence-based vaccination policy. Epidemiol Rev 24(2):125–136.
9. Castillo-Solorzano C, Carrasco P, Tambini G, et al. (2003) New horizons in the control of rubella and prevention of congenital rubella syndrome in the Americas. J Infect Dis 187 Suppl 1:S146–152.
10. de Quadros CA, Izurieta H, Venczel L, Carrasco P (2003) Measles eradication in the Americas: progress to date. J Infect Dis 189 Suppl 1:S227"235.
11. Hinman AR, Hersh BS, deQuadros C (1998) Rationale use of Rubella vaccine for the prevention of congenital rubella syndrome in the Americas. Rev Panam Salud Publica 4:156–160
12. World Health Organization (2000) Rubella vaccine: WHO position paper. Wky Epidemiol Rec 75(20):161–166.
13. WHO Weekly Epidemiologic Record (2005) Progress towards elimination of measles and prevention of congenital rubella infection in the WHO European Region 1990–2004. WHO WER 80:66–71

Mass Vaccination to Control Epidemic and Endemic Typhoid Fever

M. M. Levine (✉)

Center for Vaccine Development, University of Maryland School of Medicine, 685 West Baltimore St., Baltimore, MD 21201, USA
mlevine@medicine.umaryland.edu

1	Introduction	231
1.1	Typhoid Fever: Clinical Disease and Epidemiologic Behavior	231
1.2	Typhoid Vaccines	233
1.2.1	Killed Whole Cell Parenteral Vaccine	233
1.2.2	Ty21a	234
1.2.3	Vi	234
1.2.4	Strategies to Deliver Typhoid Vaccines	235
2	**Mass Vaccination with Typhoid Vaccines**	235
2.1	Experience with Killed Whole Cell Parenteral Vaccine	235
2.1.1	Early Experiences with Poorly Standardized Killed Whole Cell Vaccines in Military Populations	235
2.1.2	Early Experiences with Poorly Standardized Killed Whole Cell Vaccines in Civilian Populations	238
2.1.3	Modern Experiences With Mass Vaccination Using Killed Whole Cell Parenteral Vaccine	238
2.2	Experiences with Ty21a Live Oral Typhoid Vaccine	239
2.3	Experiences with Parenteral Vi Vaccine	241
	References	243

1 Introduction

1.1
Typhoid Fever: Clinical Disease and Epidemiologic Behavior

Typhoid fever is a generalized infection of the reticuloendothelial system (spleen, liver, bone marrow), gut-associated lymphoid tissue and gall bladder caused by the highly human host restricted pathogen *Salmonella enterica* serovar Typhi (*S. Typhi*). The propensity with which this pathogen causes disease in populations is closely correlated with the adequacy of sanitation and availability of protected drinking water. School age children (5–19 years of age) and young adults bear the brunt of the clinical disease burden in endemic areas in developing countries. Typhoid fever also constitutes a risk for travelers from industrialized countries who visit developing countries where typhoid is endemic or epidemic (Steinberg et al. 2004).

In endemic areas, chronic gall bladder carriers (usually adult females who excrete large numbers of typhoid bacilli) constitute an important long-term reservoir of infection (Levine et al. 1982). Where sanitation is deficient, fecal contamination from inapparent carriers (chronic or temporary) and clinically ill patients can contaminate water supplies. If treatment of water sources is inadequate or unavailable, water can serve as an important vehicle of transmission (Mermin et al. 1999).

Consumption of contaminated water and food vehicles by susceptible subjects results in either clinical or subclinical infection, depending on the dose ingested, the nature of the contaminated vehicle that conveys the typhoid bacilli and the susceptibility of the host (Hornick et al. 1970). Onset of clinical disease ensues after a fairly long incubation period (8–14 days) that follows the ingestion of typhoid bacilli. The typical typhoid clinical syndrome in older children and adults includes fever (that increases in step-wise fashion and persists for weeks if improperly treated), headache and abdominal discomfort. A wide array of clinical complications may occur, since typhoid bacilli reach many organs. However, the intestinal complications (perforation or hemorrhage that occur in ~1%–2% of patients) are particularly common and feared. It is not well appreciated but in the pre-antibiotic era the case fatality of typhoid fever was circa 15%. Thus, the demonstration in the late 1940s that chloramphenicol could successfully treat typhoid fever, decreasing the case fatality to <1%, constituted a benchmark advance in public health. Over the next few decades, mortality due to typhoid fever decreased in many endemic countries because of early therapy of suspected cases with oral chloramphenicol, a practical and inexpensive intervention. Nevertheless, in ensuing years, typhoid fatality remained a problem whenever relevant antibiotic therapy was delayed or unavailable, or when inappropriate antibiotics were administered. With this background providing context, one appreciates how the emergence of antibiotic-resistant *S. Typhi* greatly diminishes the role that antibiotics can play as a control measure (Butler et al. 1973; Gilman et al. 1975). Since 1990 the world has entered a hallmark era in the history of typhoid fever because of the emergence, dissemination and persistence in Asia and Africa of *S. Typhi* strains that carry resistance to most of the clinically relevant antibiotics (Gupta, 1994; Mermin et al. 1998, 1999; Mikhail et al. 1989; Rowe et al. 1997).

Since typhoid bacilli may reach many organs, a wide array of clinical complications can ensue. However, because the gut-associated lymphoid tissue (in particular Peyer's patches in the ileum) constitutes the most overt site of gross pathology, intestinal complications such as perforation or hemorrhage (which occur in around 1%–2% of patients) are particularly well recognized and feared.

Most large and protracted epidemics of typhoid fever are due to contamination of water supplies. Contamination of food vehicles usually leads to less extensive epidemics than water-borne outbreaks. In areas of high endemicity epidemics of typhoid fever can also occur. Interest in mass vaccination to control endemic typhoid typically occurs when prevalent strains become resistant to the most clinically relevant antibiotics resulting in an increase in hospitalizations, cases with severe complications and fatalities.

1.2
Typhoid Vaccines

Currently, three types of licensed vaccines to prevent typhoid fever are available in various countries. These include the venerable heat-inactivated, phenol-preserved parenteral whole cell vaccine, Ty21a attenuated live oral vaccine, and purified Vi capsular polysaccharide parenteral vaccine. Over the years, each of these vaccines has been used in mass vaccinations to control either endemic or epidemic typhoid fever.

1.2.1
Killed Whole Cell Parenteral Vaccine

The heat-inactivated, phenol-preserved whole cell parenteral vaccine developed at the end of the nineteenth century was the first bacterial vaccine of any kind to be widely used in humans (Pfeiffer and Kolle 1896; Wright and Semple 1897). From its earliest days, the killed whole cell parenteral vaccine gained infamy because of the frequent and severe adverse reactions that it invoked, including high fever, malaise and headache. In the 1950s and 1960s, controlled field trials carried out under the sponsorship of the World Health Organization in Eastern Europe and South America assessed the safety and the efficacy of the killed whole cell vaccine (Ashcroft et al. 1967; Hefjec et al. 1969; Yugoslav Typhoid Commission 1962; Yugoslav Typhoid Commission 1964). The heat-inactivated, phenol-preserved vaccine was shown to confer a moderate (51%–66%) level of efficacy. However, it was highly reactogenic, causing notable adverse reactions in circa 25% of vaccinees (Ashcroft et al. 1964; Hejfec et al. 1966; Yugoslav Typhoid Commission 1964). Whereas the heat-inactivated phenol-preserved whole cell typhoid vaccine was once manufactured by many public health institutes and a few private sector manufacturers, only a few public health institutes in the developing world still produce this vaccine.

1.2.2
Ty21a

Attenuated *S. Typhi* strain Ty21a, which serves as a live oral vaccine, was derived by chemical mutagenesis from wild type strain Ty2 (Germanier and Furer 1975). Among the multiple mutations contributing to the attenuation of this strain is the inability of Ty21a to express the Vi capsular polysaccharide (Germanier and Furer 1975). Ty21a was the first vaccine to be well tolerated yet to provide a level of protection that equals or surpasses that conferred by the heat-inactivated, phenol-preserved whole cell parenteral vaccine. Thus, upon its licensure by many countries, Ty21a provided an alternative that vastly improved the ability to prevent typhoid fever (Levine et al. 1989c).

An enormous evidence base generated in controlled trials and post-licensure surveillance has established that Ty21a is well tolerated and safe and confers a moderate to high level of protection, depending on the formulation administered. In a controlled field trial in Santiago, Chile, three doses of Ty21a in an enteric-coated capsule formulation given on an every other day schedule conferred 67% efficacy against typhoid fever over 3 years of follow-up (Levine et al. 1987, 1999); continued surveillance documented 62% efficacy over 7 years of follow-up. In another controlled field trial in Santiago, three doses of a liquid (reconstituted lyophilate) formulation were found to confer 78% protection over 5 years of follow-up (Levine et al. 1990, 1999). Ty21a is administered as a three-dose regimen (a dose every other day); an exception is the USA where a four-dose regimen is recommended. There is evidence that large-scale immunization with Ty21a led to a herd immunity effect (Levine et al. 1989a).

1.2.3
Vi

S. Typhi expresses on its surface a capsular polysaccharide referred to as Vi (for 'virulence') (Robbins and Robbins 1984). Parenteral immunization with purified Vi polysaccharide elicits serum Vi antibodies and confers protection. Vi polysaccharide vaccine is given as just a single (usually 25 or 30 µg) parenteral dose because as a polysaccharide it does not elicit immunologic memory and the serologic responses elicited are not boostable by administering additional doses (Keitel et al. 1994). In controlled field trials, a single 25-µg

(Nepal and South Africa) or 30-µg (China) dose of purified Vi polysaccharide administered as a parenteral (subcutaneous or intramuscular) vaccine was shown to be both well tolerated and to confer a moderate level of protection.

A controlled field trial in South Africa demonstrated that Vi confers 64% efficacy over 21 months of follow-up and 55% over 3 years of surveillance (Klugman et al. 1987, 1996), while another field trial in Nepal demonstrated 72% efficacy over 17 months of follow-up (Acharya et al. 1987).

In Guangxi, China, 131,271 subjects 3–50 years of age were randomly allocated to receive a 30-µg subcutaneous dose of Vi polysaccharide prepared by the Shanghai Institute of Biological Products (n = 65,287) or saline placebo (n = 65,984); subjects were followed for 19 months thereafter to detect cases of typhoid fever (Yang et al. 2001b). The Shanghai Vi vaccine conferred 69% efficacy against culture-confirmed typhoid fever (Yang et al. 2001b).

Thus, data from multiple controlled trials with several different sources of Vi vaccine have generated a robust evidence base demonstrating that Vi vaccine confers ~70% efficacy against typhoid fever for at least 2 years. In all of the above-mentioned controlled trials Vi vaccine was well tolerated. It thus constitutes another alternative to the reactogenic killed whole cell vaccine.

1.2.4
Strategies to Deliver Typhoid Vaccines

The main strategy to deliver the existing licensed typhoid vaccines to high risk populations in endemic areas is via school-based immunization programs or mass vaccination campaigns rather than by vaccination of infants through the Expanded Program on Immunization. The reasons include the fact that the main burden of typhoid fever falls among school age children 5–19 years of age and the current vaccines are not readily amenable to use in infants either because of reactogenicity (killed whole cell parenteral vaccine), poor immunogenicity (Vi polysaccharide) or lack of data (Ty21a).

2
Mass Vaccination with Typhoid Vaccines
2.1
Experience with Killed Whole Cell Parenteral Vaccine
2.1.1
Early Experiences with Poorly Standardized Killed Whole Cell Vaccines in Military Populations

Prior to the 1960s, most killed whole cell parenteral vaccines manufactured globally were poorly standardized. Nevertheless, several reports of mass immunization with killed whole cell parenteral typhoid vaccine carried out in the first decades of the twentieth century provide useful information, as summarized below.

In 1898, consequent to the Spanish American War, the troop strength of the US Army increased rapidly from a standing army of 25,280 troops (mean annual strength, 1893–1897) to a wartime army of 147,795. During the Spanish-American War (1898), 20,926 cases of typhoid and paratyphoid fever were admitted to 'sick report' and 2192 died; ~73% of the enteric fever cases were typhoid and 27% paratyphoid (Siler et al. 1941).

During the first decade of the twentieth century, typhoid fever remained highly endemic among soldiers in the US Army, including those assigned to its bases throughout the USA. The mean annual incidence rate of typhoid fever admissions in the US Army for the years 1901–1905 was 521.0 cases per 10^5 troops and for the period 1906–1910 it was 361.28 cases per 100,000 troops. Approximately 10%–15% of soldiers who contracted typhoid fever in this era died (Siler et al. 1941).

In an attempt to control the typhoid problem, the US Army introduced the use of typhoid vaccine (Siler et al. 1941). In March 1909, vaccine was offered on a voluntary basis and fewer than 1000 of the 84,077 soldiers in the Army elected to receive it. Vaccination remained voluntary through 1910. In March 1911, a division of troops (15,000 soldiers constituting ~18% of all men in the US Army) was mobilized in Texas and for the first time the administration of typhoid vaccine was made compulsory. Because of the low incidence of typhoid among troops in the Texas Division, beginning on 30 September 1911, vaccination with heat-inactivated, phenol-preserved whole cell vaccine was instituted by the US Army as a compulsory preventive measure for all soldiers. Thereafter, the reported incidence of typhoid fever in the US Army plummeted by >90%, from a mean of 361.28 cases per 10^5 troops annually in the period 1906–1910 to an annual mean of 25.05 cases per 10^5 troops in the period 1911–1915 (Siler et al. 1941). The diagnosis of cases of typhoid fever among US soldiers in this era was surprisingly specific as most cases on bases within the USA were diagnosed by isolation of typhoid bacilli from blood, urine or stool or by serology (Widal test) (Siler et al. 1941). The striking diminution in the incidence of typhoid fever documented by the US military following systematic use of the killed whole cell vaccine provides a strong indication that the vaccine was effective.

The vaccine used by the US Army in the period 1909 through 1916 was a heat-inactivated (56°C for 60 min), phenol-preserved whole cell vaccine containing 10^9 'Rawlings strain' killed typhoid bacilli per ml (Siler et al. 1941). Three doses were given with a 1-week interval between doses. The first dose contained 5×10^8 inactivated bacilli and the second and third doses each contained 10^9 killed bacilli. A booster dose was administered 3 years after initial immunization. The heat-inactivated phenol-preserved typhoid vaccine was licensed by the USA in 1914. Among the various nations whose armies were major combatants in World War I, troops of the US Army had the lowest reported incidence of typhoid fever (Batson 1949). It is presumed that the routine use of typhoid vaccine contributed to this low incidence.

During the Boer War (1899–1902), typhoid fever was a major health problem faced by the 208,000 British troops in South Africa (Cockburn 1955), 10% annually being admitted as cases and 1.5% each year dying of this disease. Indeed, more British soldiers died of typhoid fever (8225 deaths) than of wounds from battle (7582 deaths). Approximately 100,000 British soldiers participating in the Boer War received a heat-inactivated phenol-preserved vaccine prepared by Wright and Leishman. However, it was not possible to derive a clear effect of the vaccine. Therefore, in the period between 1904 and 1908, following the Boer War, the British Army undertook a somewhat more systematic evaluation of the effect of typhoid vaccine in more than 10,000 soldiers who volunteered to be vaccinated before being deployed abroad (Cockburn 1955); 9,000 unvaccinated subjects in the same units served as 'controls'. Twenty-four units, mainly deployed in India, participated in this evaluation of the typhoid vaccine and were followed up for 4–24 months after their arrival at their foreign duty stations (Cockburn 1955). A Typhoid Commission concluded that vaccination with typhoid vaccine diminished by sixfold the risk of development of typhoid fever (Cockburn 1955). However, a more detailed and stringent analysis was also carried out in which the denominators consisted of all soldiers present at the initiation of the deployment (Greenwood and Yule 1915). In this analysis, it was shown that soldiers in units 1–7 who had received an 'old-type' vaccine (in which the bacteria were inactivated at a higher temperature) did not have a lower attack rate of typhoid fever than nonvaccinated soldiers (Greenwood and Yule 1915). In contrast, soldiers in units inoculated with the 'new-type' typhoid vaccine had a fourfold (units 8–14) or threefold (units 15–23) lower incidence of typhoid than the unvaccinated solders in their units. As the solders who volunteered to be vaccinated may have differed in other ways from those who did not, their exposure risk may have been different. Therefore, one must be cautious in concluding that the difference in attack rate between vaccinated and unvaccinated soldiers was entirely due to the protective effect of vaccine.

2.1.2
Early Experiences with Poorly Standardized Killed Whole Cell Vaccines in Civilian Populations

The first instance of compulsive mass vaccination of a civilian population against typhoid fever was instituted by the Belgian government during the First World War. In April 1915, the Belgian government made typhoid vaccination compulsory for 14,836 civilians residing in Ypres and its environs (Goodall 1937); anyone refusing vaccination was threatened with expulsion. The typhoid vaccinations were carried out by a unit of the Red Cross. One decade later in Hamburg, Germany, in response to a typhoid epidemic that resulted in 2200 cases, a mass vaccination was rapidly organized and 117,000 residents of the city were vaccinated (Hahn 1927; Tarr et al. 1999).

In the USA during the first three decades of the twentieth century, the control of endemic typhoid was overwhelmingly accomplished by the provision of treated water supplies (Wolman and Gorman 1931). However, on several occasions small mass vaccinations with killed whole cell typhoid vaccine were carried out in response to epidemics of typhoid (Batson 1949). One rural geographic locale in the USA where typhoid vaccination was widely practiced to control endemic typhoid fever was Williamson, County, Tennessee (Williams and Bishop 1936). In two highly endemic districts of Williamson, County where 87% of the population had received typhoid vaccine, the disease was virtually eliminated in the period 1927–1931. In a comparator control district in the county during this period that had a similar size population and socioeconomic level but where only 41.5% of the population had been vaccinated, the incidence of disease did not decline (Williams and Bishop 1936).

2.1.3
Modern Experiences With Mass Vaccination Using Killed Whole Cell Parenteral Vaccine

Typhoid fever was endemic in Thailand, including Bangkok, in the 1960s and early 1970s. In the period 1974–1976, the incidence of typhoid fever increased sharply in Bangkok. Accordingly, the Thai Ministry of Health initiated a national immunization program against typhoid fever among schoolchildren 7–12 years of age using a locally manufactured heat inactivated, phenol preserved whole cell parenteral vaccine containing 10^9 organisms per ml (Bodhidatta et al. 1987). At the peak of the vaccination campaign in the late 1970s and early 1980s, more than 80% of Thai schoolchildren 7–12 years of age received annual inoculations with 0.25 ml of typhoid vaccine (Bodhidatta et al. 1987).

The reported incidence of typhoid fever in Bangkok dropped following initiation of the mass vaccinations (Bodhidatta et al. 1987). Thai epidemiologists reviewed blood culture data at the four main teaching hospitals in Bangkok for school age children to assess the impact of the immunization campaign. Since the typhoid vaccination campaign would be expected to have a protective effect against *S. Typhi* infections but not likely against *S. Paratyphi* A infections (which were also endemic in Thailand), the ratio of *S. Typhi* to *S. Paratyphi* A isolations in blood cultures was calculated for the pre-campaign years and during the years of mass vaccination. The ratio of *S. Typhi* to *S. Paratyphi* isolations dropped from 4.1:1 in the period 1970–1973 to 1.2:1 in 1980–1985, after several years of mass vaccination of school children (Bodhidatta et al. 1987).

A mass vaccination was carried out of residents of a refugee camp in Phnom-Penh, Cambodia in response to a typhoid epidemic. In total, 172 2–5 year olds, 362 6–14 year olds and 455 adults constituted the target population for mass vaccination with a combination vaccine prepared by the Cambodian Pasteur Institute that contained inactivated typhoid and paratyphoid bacilli and tetanus toxoid (Bollag 1980). Children were targeted to receive four parenteral immunizations and adults three, with a 1-week interval between doses. Considerable publicity about the impending campaign preceded its initiation. Febrile adverse responses were observed commonly, including in 86 of 415 children (20.7%) and 37 of 315 adults (11.7%). Presumably because of these frequent adverse reactions, only 20% of residents returned for their final dose in the immunization schedule.

2.2
Experiences with Ty21a Live Oral Typhoid Vaccine

In the late 1980s, Ty21a in the enteric-coated capsule formulation was licensed in many countries following the reports of the successful field trial in Santiago, Chile of a three-dose regimen with vaccine administered at an interval of 48 hours between doses (Levine et al. 1987). Chile also licensed this formulation of Ty21a. At the time (mid-1980s), typhoid fever was endemic among school age children in Santiago; approximately two-thirds of all reported cases of typhoid fever occurred among children 5–19 years of age (Levine et al. 1986). This is the typical epidemiologic age-specific pattern of endemic typhoid fever.

To determine the practicality of mass school-based immunization with different regimens of Ty21a in the enteric-coated capsule formulation, more than 225,000 schoolchildren (>80% of age-eligible children) attending schools in the Area Sur and Area Central Health Services of Santiago were enrolled in a post-licensure effectiveness trial (Ferreccio et al. 1989). The design of the effectiveness trial was to compare practicality, logistics and typhoid incidence among schoolchildren 6–19 years of age who were given either a two-dose, a three-dose or a four-dose regimen of Ty21a. Since two of the regimens (two-dose and four-dose) differed from the three-dose recommended schedule for licensed Ty21a, parental consent was obtained for participation (Ferreccio et al. 1989). Classes in the government schools were randomly allocated to receive two, three or four doses of Ty21a in enteric-coated capsules. In total, 216,692 of the children for whom parental consent was obtained received at least one dose of Ty21a vaccine. Of these, 189,819 children (84%) received the complete assigned regimen. Failure to receive the full number of assigned doses was due to school absenteeism or difficulty among young children in swallowing the capsule; approximately 8% of children 5–7 years of age could not ingest a capsule. Impressively, 93% of children allocated to receive two doses, 84% assigned to get three doses and 76% intended to receive four doses successfully completed the oral vaccination regimen. Particularly among adolescents and teenagers, it was logistically simple and practical with this oral vaccine to rapidly immunize large numbers of classes in each school.

Surveillance to detect cases of typhoid fever was maintained for 3 years. Two blood cultures were drawn from suspect cases and cases were considered confirmed only if *S. Typhi* was isolated. Table 1 summarizes the results of both the 'per protocol' and 'intent-to-treat' analyses. Children who received a four-dose regimen exhibited a significantly lower incidence of typhoid fever than the three-dose or two-dose regimens. These data influenced the US FDA to license a four-dose regimen, whereas in other countries a three-dose immunization schedule with Ty21a is followed (Levine et al. 1989c).

Between 1980 and 1990, four large-scale field evaluations were carried out in the different health services of Santiago, Chile, encompassing ~500,000 schoolchildren, 5–19 years of age, approximately 80% of whom received Ty21a vaccine in one or another formulation or immunization schedule (Black et al. 1990; Ferreccio et al. 1989; Levine et al. 1987, 1990, 1999). Over the course of the decade during which these trials were undertaken there was strong evidence that mass immunization with Ty21a conferred indirect protection to unimmunized persons in the community. As summarized in Table 2, this was observed by continuing to measure the incidence rate in the control group in the first vaccine trial site, Area Norte. In the first year of that trial (and in several preceding years), the incidence of typhoid fever in the unimmunized control children was ~225 cases/10^5 schoolchildren. Each time a field trial was initiated in another part of Santiago, the incidence in the control group in Area Norte fell (Table 2). The one year (1985) when no new trial was initiated, the incidence rose (Levine et al. 1989b).

Table 1 The incidence of typhoid fever in children vaccinated with two, three of four doses of Ty21a in a large-scale effectiveness trial in Area Sur and Area Central, Santiago, Chile

Allocated regimen	Per protocol analysis			Intent to treat analysis		
	Number of school-children	Number of typhoid cases	Incidence of typhoid per 100,000 children	Number of school-children	Number of typhoid cases	Incidence of typhoid per 100,000 children
2-dose	66,615	123	184.6	71,754	149	207.6
3-dose	64,783	104	160.5	77,246	143	185.1
4-dose	58,421	56	95.8	76,998	97	126

The incidence of typhoid fever was significantly lower in recipients of four doses compared to children who received three or two doses ($P < 0.01$)

Table 2 Herd immunity indirect protective effect on unimmunized school children in Area Norte, Santiago, Chile consequent to the widespread use of Ty21a vaccine in other Areas of Santiago

Year of follow-up	Typhoid incidence in the control group in the Area Norte trial (cases/10^5)	Site of new field trial	Impact of new trial on typhoid incidence in the control group in Area Norte
1982	227	–	–
1983	139	Occidente	↓ 39%
1984	70	Sur and Central	↓ 39%
1985	103	None	↑ 32%
1986	62	Suroriente & Norte	↓ 40%

Following the Gulf War of 1991, a large-scale mass vaccination of 12,000 Kurdish refugees in a refugee camp in southern Iran was carried out with oral Ty21a to control an epidemic of typhoid fever (Reisinger et al. 1994). Before the mass vaccination the incidence of typhoid fever was 12 cases per week. Following the mass vaccination, the incidence fell to 2 cases per week.

2.3
Experiences with Parenteral Vi Vaccine

An advantage of Vi polysaccharide is that the immunization schedule requires only a single intramuscular or subcutaneous dose. This makes it amenable to use in mass campaigns. There are two reports on the use of Vi vaccine in mass immunizations to control epidemic disease or endemic typhoid, both from Asia.

During the massive and prolonged epidemic of multiply antibiotic-resistant typhoid fever in Tajikistan in the 1990s (Mermin et al. 1999; Tarr et al. 1999), a Russian Vi polysaccharide vaccine was given to 18,362 Russian Border guards 18–21 years of age stationed in Dushanbe, Tajikistan in March 1997 (Tarr et al. 1999). During January and February 1997, 174 cases and two deaths from typhoid fever were recorded among the Russian troops in Dushanbe, prompting a mass vaccination in March with the Vi vaccine (Tarr et al. 1999). Thereafter, from April through December only 51 cases of typhoid were observed among the troops, suggesting that the vaccine was responsible for the decrease.

Based on the positive safety and efficacy results of two field trials of Vi vaccine in Jiangsu and Guangxi Provinces in China (Wang et al. 1997) and evidence of effectiveness from an outbreak investigation in an area where Vi was used among school children (Yang et al. 2001a), Vi vaccine has been used widely in China since July 1996. More than 10 million doses were administered in 1997, with 800,000 doses being given in Guangxi Province. The general strategy in China has been to vaccinate school children. In reactive vaccination in response to typhoid outbreaks in China, a broader age range is targeted that extends well into adulthood.

In 1995, public health officials in 40 counties of Guangxi Province, China introduced immunization with a Vi vaccine manufactured by the Wuhan Institute of Biological Products (Yang et al. 2001a) as a measure to control endemic typhoid fever. A single 30-μg subcutaneous dose was given. From 1996 through 1999 in Xing-An county, 61,303 doses of the Wuhan Vi vaccine were administered, including, as of 1998, in school based immunization programs. During May 1999, an outbreak of typhoid fever occurred in Xing-An, thereby providing an opportunity to carry out a field evaluation of vaccine effectiveness by means of a epidemiologic investigation. Immunization records of school children were compared with confirmed cases to calculate attack rates and assess effectiveness. For 1701 school children immunized in 1998 or 1999, the outbreak investigation estimated that the Vi vaccine conferred 71% protection against typhoid fever (Yang et al. 2001a).

Some individuals have voiced concern that widespread use of Vi polysaccharide vaccine may lead to the emergence of disease caused by Vi-negative strains of *S. Typhi* (Arya, 2000, 2002). Although *S. Typhi* strains lacking Vi are rare among clinical isolates and tend to be less virulent, they are nevertheless capable of causing typhoid fever (Hornick et al. 1970). To address this concern, it will be important to maintain adequate surveillance in typhoid-endemic areas and populations where Vi vaccine is being used on a large-scale. Such surveillance is also likely to demonstrate that, as was observed in Bangkok when killed whole cell vaccine was introduced programmatically, the ratio of *S. Typhi* to *S. Paratyphi* isolations will probably change notably as the incidence of typhoid diminishes (Bodhidatta et al. 1987).

References

Acharya VI, Lowe CU, Thapa R, Gurubacharya VL, Shrestha MB, Cadoz M, Schulz D, Armand J, Bryla DA, Trollfors B, Cramton T, Schneerson R, Robbins JB (1987) Prevention of typhoid fever in Nepal with the Vi capsular polysaccharide of *Salmonella typhi*. A preliminary report. N Engl J Med 317:1101–1104

Arya SC (2000) Salmonella typhi Vi antigen-negative isolates in India and prophylactic typhoid immunization. Natl Med J India 13:220

Arya SC (2002) Field effectiveness of Vi polysaccharide typhoid vaccine in the People's Republic of China. J Infect Dis 185:845–846

Ashcroft MT, Morrison-Ritchie J, Nicholson CC (1964) Controlled field trial in British Guyana schoolchildren of heat-killed-phenolized and acetone-killed lyophilized typhoid vaccines. Am J Hyg 79:196–206

Ashcroft MT, Nicholson CC, Balwant S, Ritchie JM, Sorvan E, William F (1967) A seven-year field trial of two typhoid vaccines in Guiana. Lancet 2:1056–1060

Batson HC. 1949. Typhoid fever prophylaxis by active immunization. Pub Health Rep supplement 212:1–34

Black RE, Levine MM, Ferreccio C, Clements ML, Lanata C, Rooney J, Germanier R (1990) Efficacy of one or two doses of Ty21a *Salmonella typhi* vaccine in enteric-coated capsules in a controlled field trial. Chilean Typhoid Committee. Vaccine 8:81–84

Bodhidatta L, Taylor DN, Thisyakorn U, Echeverria P (1987) Control of typhoid fever in Bangkok, Thailand, by annual immunization of school children with parenteral typhoid fever. Rev Infect Dis 9:841–845

Bollag U (1980) Practical evaluation of a pilot immunization campaign against typhoid fever in a Cambodian refugee camp. Int J Epidemiol 9:121–122

Butler T, Linh NN, Arnold K, Pollack M (1973) Chloramphenicol-resistant typhoid fever in Vietnam associated with R factor. Lancet 2:983–985

Cockburn WC (1955) The early history of typhoid vaccination. J Royal Army Medical Corps 101:171–185

Ferreccio C, Levine MM, Rodriguez H, Contreras R (1989) Comparative efficacy of two, three, or four doses of Ty21a live oral typhoid vaccine in enteric-coated capsules: a field trial in an endemic area. J Infect Dis 159:766–769

Germanier R, Furer E (1975) Isolation and characterization of gal E mutant Ty21a of *Salmonella typhi*: A candidate strain for a live oral typhoid vaccine. J Infect Dis 141:553–558

Gilman RH, Terminel M, Levine MM, Hernandez Mendosa P, Calderone E, Vasquez V, Martinez E, Snyder MJ, Hornick RB (1975) Comparison of trimethoprim-sulfamethoxazole and amoxicillin in therapy of chloramphenicol-resistant and chloramphenicol-sensitive typhoid fever. J Infect Dis 132:630–636

Goodall EW (1937) Immunization against typhoid. BMJ 1197

Greenwood M, Yule GU. 1915. The statistics of anti-typhoid and anti-cholera inoculations and the interpretation of such statistics in general. Proc Roy Soc Med 8:113–194

Gupta A (1994) Multidrug-resistant typhoid fever in children: epidemiology and therapeutic approach. Pediatr Infect Dis 13:124–140

Hahn M (1927) Mitteilungen zur Typhusendemie in Hannover. Med Klin 27:1009–1012

Hefjec LB, Levina LA, Kuz'minova ML, et al. (1969) A controlled field trial to evaluate the protective capacity of a single dose of acetone-killed agar-grown and heat-killed broth-grown tphoid vaccines. Bull WHO 40:903–907

Hejfec LB, Salmin LV, Lejtman MZ, Kuzminova ML, Vasileva AV, Levina LA, Bencianova TG, Pavlova EA, Antonova AA (1966) A controlled field trial and laboratory study of five typhoid vaccines in the USSR. Bull WHO 34:321–339

Hornick RB, Greisman SE, Woodward TE, DuPont HL, Dawkins AT, Snyder MJ (1970) Typhoid fever; pathogenesis and immunologic control. N Eng J Med 283:686–691, 739–746

Keitel WA, Bond NL, Zahradnik JM, Cramton TA, Robbins JB (1994) Clinical and serological responses following primary and booster immunization with *Salmonella typhi* Vi capsular polysaccharide vaccines. Vaccine 12:195–199

Klugman K, Gilbertson IT, Kornhoff HJ, Robbins JB, Schneerson R, Schulz D, Cadoz M, Armand J (1987) Protective activity of Vi polysaccharide vaccine against typhoid fever. Lancet 2:1165–1169

Klugman KP, Koornhof HJ, Robbins JB, Le Cam NN (1996) Immunogenicity, efficacy and serological correlate of protection of *Salmonella typhi* Vi capsular polysaccharide vaccine three years after immunization. Vaccine 14:435–438

Levine MM, Black RE, Ferreccio C, Clements ML, Lanata C, Sears S, Morris JG, Cisneros L, Germanier R, Chilean TYphoid Commission (1986) Interventions to control endemic typhoid fever: Field studies in Santiago, Chile. In: Washington, D.C.:PAHO Copublication Series No. 1. p. 37–53

Levine MM, Black RE, Lanata C, Chilean Typhoid Committee (1982) Precise estimation of the numbers of chronic carriers of *Salmonella typhi* in Santiago, Chile, an endemic area. J Infect Dis 146:724–726

Levine MM, Ferreccio C, Abrego P, Martin OS, Ortiz E, Cryz S (1999) Duration of efficacy of ty21a, attenuated salmonella typhi live oral vaccine. Vaccine 17 Suppl 2:S22-S27

Levine MM, Ferreccio C, Black RE, Germanier R, Chilean Typhoid Committee (1987) Large-scale field trial of Ty21a live oral typhoid vaccine in enteric-coated capsule formulation. Lancet 1:1049–1052

Levine MM, Ferreccio C, Black RE, Tacket CO, Germanier R (1989a) Progress in vaccines against typhoid fever. Rev Infect Dis 11 Suppl 3:S552–S567

Levine MM, Ferreccio C, Black RE, Tacket CO, Germanier R, Chilean Typhoid Committee (1989b) Progress in vaccines to prevent typhoid fever. Rev Infect Dis 11:S552–S567

Levine MM, Ferreccio C, Cryz S, Ortiz E (1990) Comparison of enteric-coated capsules and liquid formulation of Ty21a typhoid vaccine in randomised controlled field trial. Lancet 336:891–894

Levine MM, Taylor DN, Ferreccio C (1989c) Typhoid vaccines come of age. Pediatr Infect Dis J 8:374–381

Mermin JH, Townes JM, Gerber M, Dolan N, Mintz ED, Tauxe RV (1998) Typhoid fever in the United States, 1985–1994: changing risks of international travel and increasing antimicrobial resistance. Arch Intern Med 158:633–638

Mermin JH, Villar R, Carpenter J, Roberts L, Samaridden A, Gasanova L, Lomakina S, Bopp C, Hutwagner L, Mead P, Ross B, Mintz ED (1999) A massive epidemic of multidrug-resistant typhoid fever in Tajikistan associated with consumption of municipal water. J Infect Dis 179:1416–1422

Mikhail IA, Haberberger RL, Farid Z, Girgis NI, Woody JN (1989) Antibiotic-multiresistant *Salmonella typhi* in Egypt. Trans R Soc Trop Med Hyg 83:120

Pfeiffer R, Kolle W (1896) Experimentelle Untersuchunger zur Frage der Schutzimpfung des Menschen gegen Typhus abdominalis. Dtsch Med Wocheschr 22:735–737

Reisinger EC, Grasmug E, Krejs GJ (1994) Antibody response after vaccination against typhoid fever in Kurdish refugee camp. Lancet 343:918–919

Robbins J, Robbins J (1984) Reexamination of the protective role of the capsular polysaccharide Vi antigen of *Salmonella typhi*. J Infect Dis 150:436–449

Rowe B, Ward LR, Threlfall EJ (1997) Multidrug-resistant *Salmonella typhi*: a worldwide epidemic. Clin Infect Dis 24 Suppl 1:S106–109

Siler JF, Dunham GC, Longfellow D, Luippold GF (1941) Immunization to typhoid fever. [17], pp. 1–276. 1941. Baltimore, Johns Hopkins Press. Am J Hygiene monographic series. Ref Type: Serial (Book,Monograph)

Steinberg EB, Bishop R, Haber P, Dempsey AF, Hoekstra RM, Nelson JM, Ackers M, Calugar A, Mintz ED (2004) Typhoid fever in travelers: who should be targeted for prevention? Clin Infect Dis 39:186–191

Tarr PE, Kuppens L, Jones TC, Ivanoff B, Aparin PG, Heymann DL (1999) Considerations regarding mass vaccination against typhoid fever as an adjunct to sanitation and public health measures: potential use in an epidemic in Tajikistan. Am J Trop Med Hyg 61:163–170

Wang ZG, Zhou WZ, Shi J (1997) [Efficacy and side effects following immunization with *Salmonella typhi* Vi capsular polysaccharide vaccine]. Zhonghua Liu Xing Bing Xue Za Zhi 18:26–29

Williams WC, Bishop EL (1936) The typhoid control program and results of 13 years' work in Williamson County, Tennessee, 1922–35. Pub Health Rep 51:1–27

Wolman A, Gorman A (1931) The significance of waterborne typhoid fever outbreaks. Baltimore: Williams & Wilkins

Wright AE, Semple D (1897) Remarks on vaccination against typhoid fever. BMJ 1:256–258

Yang HH, Kilgore PE, Yang LH, Park JK, Pan YF, Kim Y, Lee YJ, Xu ZY, Clemens JD (2001a) An outbreak of typhoid fever, Xing-An County, People's Republic of China, 1999: estimation of the field effectiveness of Vi polysaccharide typhoid vaccine. J Infect Dis 183:1775–1780

Yang HH, Wu CG, Xie GZ, Gu QW, Wang BR, Wang LY, Wang HF, Ding ZS, Yang Y, Tan WS, Wang WY, Wang XC, Qin M, Wang JH, Tang HA, Jiang XM, Li YH, Wang ML, Zhang SL, Li GL (2001b) Efficacy trial of Vi polysaccharide vaccine against typhoid fever in south-western China. Bull WHO 79:625–631

Yugoslav Typhoid Commission (1962) A controlled field trial of the effectiveness of phenol and alcohol typhoid vaccines. Bull WHO 26:357–369

Yugoslav Typhoid Commission (1964) A controlled field trial of the effectiveness of acetone-dried and inactivated and heat-phenol-inactivated typhoid vaccines in Yugoslavia. Bull WHO 30:623–630

Mass Vaccination: Solutions in the Skin

G. M. Glenn (✉) · R. T. Kenney

Iomai Corporation, 20 Firstfield Road, Suite 250, Gaithersburg, MD 20878, USA
gglenn@iomai.com

1	Introduction	248
2	Structure of the Skin	249
3	The Skin as the Best Site for Vaccination	251
3.1	Overview of Skin Immunization Techniques	251
3.2	Dose-Sparing Techniques	252
3.3	Barriers to Passive Skin Immunization	252
3.4	TCI Techniques	253
3.5	Animal Models for Skin Delivery of Vaccines	254
4	The Safety and Immunogenicity of an Adjuvant on the Skin	256
4.1	Preclinical Safety	256
4.2	Clinical Safety	257
4.3	Immune Response to Transcutaneous Immunization	258
4.4	Transcutaneous Immunization Induces Functional Antibodies	260
4.5	Dose-Sparing and Immune Enhancement via a Universal Adjuvant Patch	261
5	Mass Vaccination: Logistics of an Anthrax Patch	263
6	Conclusions	264
	References	264

Abstract The skin is populated with Langerhans cells, thought to be efficient, potent antigen-presenting cells, that are capable of inducing protective immunity by targeting antigen delivery to the skin. Delivery to the skin may be accomplished by active delivery such as intradermal injection, use of patches or a combination of a universal adjuvant patch with injections. The robust immunity induced by skin targeting can lead to dose sparing, novel vaccines and immune enhancement in populations with poorly responsive immune systems, such as the elderly. Vaccine delivery with patches (transcutaneous immunization), may allow self-administration, ambient temperature stabilization and ease of storage for stockpiling, leading to a new level of efficient vaccine distribution in times of crisis such as a bioterror event or pandemic influenza outbreak. The use of an adjuvant (immunostimulant) patch with injected vaccines has been shown in clinical studies to enhance the immune response to an injected vaccine. This can be used for dose sparing in pandemic influenza vaccines in critically short supply or immune enhancement for poor responders to flu vaccines such as the elderly. Transcutaneous immunization offers a unique safety profile, as adjuvants are sequestered in the skin and only delivered systemically by Langerhans cells. This results in an excellent safety profile and allows use of extremely potent adjuvants. The combination of the skin immune system, safe use of potent adjuvants and ease of delivery suggests that skin delivery of vaccines can address multiple unmet needs for mass vaccination scenarios.

1
Introduction

The skin is well equipped to deal with the hostile microbial world. It is regularly challenged with frequent exposure to microbes through micro-trauma and disruption of its protective barriers. The skin is populated with dendritic cells, whose role is to provide effective surveillance and immune responses to infectious challenges coming through the skin. These cells are thought to be efficient and potent antigen-presenting cells for induction of protective immunity. In comparison to skeletal muscle, which is the target of intramuscular (IM) injections, the skin is a far more attractive immune environment and thus has great potential to address the unmet needs of mass vaccination, such as dose-sparing and ease of delivery. One may ask 'why has the skin been overlooked as a vaccine target, and why is it of interest now?' We would suggest that one contributing factor is that many of the long-held established maxims regarding delivery to the skin were erroneous and should be modified based on new preclinical and clinical data. There is a great deal of new data on skin delivery with over 100 publications on the subject in the past 7 years. This has created a major new research paradigm in vaccine development. The interest is well placed from a historical perspective, considering that the most successful mass vaccination campaign ever conducted used a crudely delivered and simply prepared dried vaccine, and fully eradicated smallpox by means of skin immunization. Vaccines delivered to the skin have recently been shown to induce robust immune responses, leading to improved efficacy markers and enhanced antibody responses to new candidate vaccine antigens. These and other data, and the new delivery systems under development, have caused vaccinologists to reexamine the advantages of the skin as a target for new vaccines for both improved efficacy and ease of use.

In this chapter we review the skin anatomy and immune system from a practical point of view. We also look at strategies for immune manipulation that may address needle free vaccination, dose-sparing, enhancement of the immune responses in the senescent immune system, and improved initial responses to a first dose in the immune naïve population. We then look forward and suggest avenues of further development that should be considered to address the unmet needs of mass vaccination.

2
Structure of the Skin

Mammalian skin is composed of three primary layers (Fig. 1). The stratum corneum (SC), the outermost layer of the skin, is composed of 10–20 layers of quiescent, cornified epidermal skin cells called keratinocytes that are continuously shed. During the formation of the SC, the keratinocytes secrete lipids that form a type of mortar encasing the dead and dying cells. The human SC is organized in a 10–20-μm-thick 'bricks-and-mortar' format and represents an effective but fragile barrier to microbes, fluids, and foreign material. The thickness of the SC varies based on anatomic site (on the extremities, palms

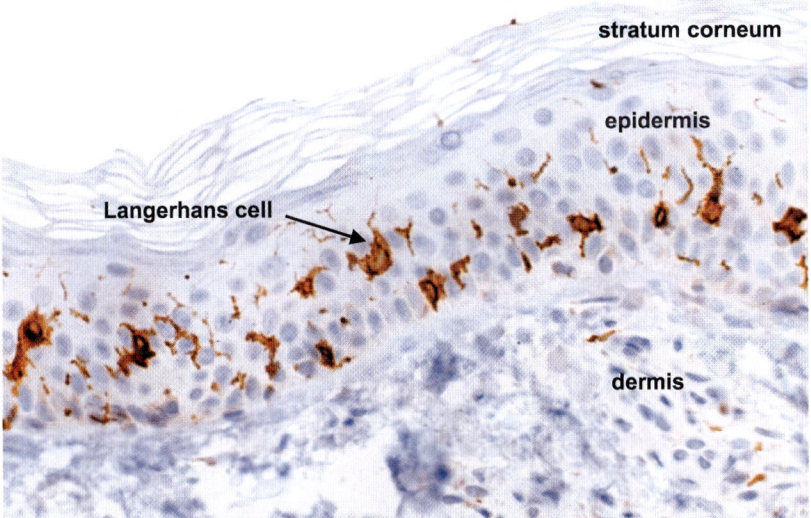

Fig. 1 Structure of human skin. The skin is composed of three principal layers: the dermis, epidermis, and stratum corneum. Existing vaccine delivery involves perforation through the skin, bypassing the immune-rich layers of the skin. New technologies targeting the skin take advantage of the skin immune system elements, such as epidermal Langerhans cells, shown here stained with anti-CD1a. (Adapted from Glenn et al. 2000, with permission)

and soles), pigmentation (thicker with darker skin), smoking history (thinner in smokers), and different phenotypes (dry vs. moist skin) (Sandby-Moller et al. 2003). Although the question of whether skin vaccination techniques will be influenced by these variations is important, the initial data from Phase 2 clinical trials suggests a minor role for skin types at best. Scarification as a delivery method, used with the smallpox vaccine, clearly paid little attention to skin types, with the exception of avoidance of diseased skin. Similarly, transdermal delivery of other drugs demonstrates that patch application can be quite flexible and effective over the range of skin types and ages. For patch vaccine delivery techniques, the SC is the primary barrier, as it is for transdermal drug delivery and, as discussed below, methods for its disruption lead to improved efficiency of vaccine delivery. If SC disruption accompanies vaccine delivery, the technique will need to overcome any individual variability.

The epidermis underlies the SC and is composed of keratinocytes and other skin elements in a continuous growing layer of epithelium. The final layer of the skin, the dermis, supports the epidermis with connective tissue, contains the blood vessels (generally the target for transdermal drug delivery), nerves, and lymphatics, and provides a foundation for the epidermal appendages such as hair and sweat glands. The epidermis is also a dynamic immune environment, with active traffic of immune cells in and out of the epidermis. The primary antigen-presenting cell (APC) found in the epidermis is the Langerhans cell (LC), a dendritic cell that migrates from the bone marrow into the skin and plays the dual role of immune surveillance and antigen presentation (Jakob and Udey 1999). Confocal microscopy in human skin demonstrated that LCs cover 25% of the total skin surface area, although they account for approximately only 1%–3% of the epidermis cells (Yu et al. 1994). There is some suggestion that a homeostasis exists that maintains immune health through constant challenge with skin and gut pathogens. Beyond this basal activity, the skin immune system is sensitive to 'spikes' in the danger signals presented by microbes that trigger effective immune responses. LC density, accessibility, and antigen presentation function create an ideal target for vaccine delivery.

The dermis also contains dendritic cells and LC in transit, but the density of APC in the dermis does not match that of the epidermis (Udey 1997) although hair follicles, which extend into the dermis, have their own unique microenvironment of immune cells (Christoph et al. 2000). The normal practice of vaccine delivery by needle perforates the skin to deliver antigens below the skin, bypassing the highly attractive skin immune system and it is the object of this review to point out the merits of delivery into the skin.

3
The Skin as the Best Site for Vaccination

3.1
Overview of Skin Immunization Techniques

The gold standard skin immunization technique was developed in the 1700's (or earlier) for smallpox. The modern technique involves intradermal inoculation with a bifurcated needle. Specifically, the needle is dipped into a vial of vaccine and a small volume of vaccine (0.0025 ml), adherent by capillary action between the tines of the needle, is applied by stroking the skin 15 times so that a trace of blood appears at the vaccination site. The vaccine take can readily be observed, since the local infection leaves an eschar. The most recent embodiment uses a dried, stabilized antigen on a bifurcated needle and the US stockpile vaccine utilized this type of product. This seemingly crude technique results in very high levels of vaccine uptake and is in large part responsible for eradication of smallpox worldwide (Henderson et al. 2004). As a skin delivery scenario, bifurcated delivery has the merits of efficacy and is the only safe means by which this live viral vaccine can be delivered. However, adverse reaction rates are high and the systemic infection triggered by the use of this live virus would not be acceptable for the general population except in a crisis scenario.

Intradermal (ID) delivery using a small-gauge needle and small volume of material ($\leq$ 100 µl) is commonly used in the US and other countries for TB testing. ID injections are also used for infant BCG immunization in most countries of the world, as well as for post-exposure rabies prophylaxis. Studies with hepatitis B, rabies, and influenza vaccines suggest the potential for greater immunogenicity and dose-sparing (Briggs et al. 2000; Bryan et al. 1992; Kenney et al 2004b; Redfield et al. 1985). Some of the data using hepatitis B suggested that ID injection resulted in inconsistent immunogenicity, which has led to a widely held perception that ID delivery is inconsistent and difficult to perform. However, the dose in these studies was one-tenth the normal human dose, therefore incomplete seroconversion might be expected. A thorough dose study may yield a clearer picture of the ID dose response. Technological advances in needle design have improved the utility of the ID approach. ID vaccination can be performed effectively using a 27-gauge, 1/2-inch detachable needle, such as the BD Precisionglide™ slip tip with an ID bevel, to deliver 100 µl from a 1-ml syringe (calibrated in hundredths) (Kenney et al. 2004b). Trained medical personnel can readily and reliably perform this technique.

Transcutaneous immunization and similar techniques (discussed below) specifically target the skin for delivery. In the simplest embodiment, the vaccine is placed in a patch and the antigen is delivered passively into the skin. Active delivery techniques using patches are also being investigated. Gas-powered gun devices have been used for decades but skin targeting has only recently been refined. Gas-powered guns for delivering antigen into the skin could theoretically be used with dry, stabilized formulations, but scale-up for mass immunization or even a common vaccine product is not feasible.

3.2
Dose-Sparing Techniques

ID immunization is a long-standing delivery technique that can be used in attempts to dose-spare. We recently conducted a controlled trial in which subjects were immunized with a licensed trivalent influenza vaccine (egg-based, purified hemagglutinin antigen) either by the intramuscular (IM) route or via the ID route using one-fifth the dose (100 µl) of the standard vaccine (Kenney et al. 2004b). The immune responses to the ID injection were similar or superior compared to responses in the IM group. The data were published concurrently with the recent US vaccine supply crisis of 2004 and clearly suggested a simple dose-sparing strategy might be implemented using such a technique (La Montagne and Fauci 2004).

Other important issues, such as the paucity of multi-dose vialing, lack of 100-µl filling capacity, and ID syringe validation data, are barriers to ready implementation of dose-sparing. Many public health thinkers seem to be of the view that ID immunization is cumbersome or complex to administer, and unsuitable for mass vaccination. We believe that this impression may need to be reevaluated in the context of influenza with the recent improvements in the syringes and needles designed for ID use. In the hands of skilled health care workers, ID immunization may be reliably administered to a large number of subjects in a reasonable time frame. In the context of influenza, where hemagglutination inhibition (HAI) titers can be reasonably assumed to be the protective correlates, the 'efficacy' of ID influenza can be evaluated in trials of sufficient size and appropriate populations (e.g., the elderly) to confidently use ID vaccination in settings where dose-sparing would meet a crisis need. In particular, in the setting of an annual 'flu vaccine shortage and severe influenza epidemics, or in the event of a pandemic, such a technique could be critical to achieving full coverage of at-risk populations or to compensate for supply shortfalls due to manufacturing limitations.

3.3
Barriers to Passive Skin Immunization

The SC is an effective but fragile barrier to the direct penetration of fluids, large molecules, particles and microbes. Long-held maxims of skin penetration have stated that even with use of skin penetration techniques, delivery of drugs and bioactive molecules greater than 500 Da is not possible. However, it has become clear that these maxims were often based on transdermal delivery of drugs to the blood vessels in the dermis or due to the failure to deliver larger moieties such as insulin through the combined barrier created by the SC, epidermis, and dermis. By contrast, vaccine antigens and adjuvants targeting the skin, defined here as transcutaneous immunization (TCI), merely require delivery into the skin, where they can be carried to the draining node to induce a response by the resident immune cells.

3.4
TCI Techniques

The superficial nature of anatomical targets for antigen delivery suggests that few restrictions for antigen size apply to TCI. In human skin, which is the most relevant setting for testing vaccine delivery concepts, we have shown that with crude patches and minimal SC disruption, very large recombinant antigens in the order of 1,500,000 Da can be delivered to elicit strong systemic immune responses (Güereña-Burgueño et al. 2002). This study followed initial observations that the heat-labile enterotoxin of *Escherichia coli* (LT) (86,000 Da) was effectively delivered through human skin by simply applying LT in wet gauze to the skin without any other manipulation (Glenn et al. 2000). Most currently licensed vaccine antigens fall within this size range, (e.g., tetanus toxoid ~160,000 Da). Extensive animal data has shown that whole viruses (Hammond et al. 2000), recombinants (Yu et al 2002), and even whole bacterial cells (L.R. Ellingsworth, unpublished observations) can be effectively delivered to the skin immune system. These observations suggest that the delivery of a range of antigens and adjuvants is feasible.

Disruption of the SC is important for efficient delivery and lends itself to relatively simple techniques. Occlusion, wetting of the skin, and other methods lead to hydration of the SC. Hydration of the SC results in swelling of the keratinocytes and pooling of fluid in the intercellular spaces, leading to dramatic microscopic changes in the SC structure (Richter et al 2004; Roberts and Walker 1993) that have no lasting effect once the skin is allowed to dry. Simple hydration using a saline-wetted patch results in hydrated SC that clearly allows antigens to pass through the skin (Glenn et al. 2000). The transit pathways utilized by antigens (as well as transdermal drugs) to traverse the SC are not well characterized. Transdermal drug delivery of polar small molecule drugs is thought to occur through aqueous intercellular channels formed between the keratinocytes in hydrated skin, and it is possible that similar pathways are engaged for antigen delivery by TCI (Roberts and Walker 1993).

Physical and chemical penetration enhancement techniques that disrupt the integrity of the SC have also been described (Chen et al. 2001; Glenn and Alving 1999a; Glenn et al. 2003; Guebre-Xabier et al. 2004; Mikszta et al. 2002). We have tested concepts with clinical relevance to patch delivery in model systems and subsequently applied them to human skin where penetration enhancement appears to represent an improvement over simple hydration of the skin. For product development, we have focused on the use of simple, inexpensive materials with clinical utility in other settings, and simple methods of use and application that lead to consistent, heightened immune responses. Device-based techniques also disrupt the SC and use various means for delivery of antigens and adjuvants into the epidermis; however, with the exception of gas-powered gun delivery, these techniques have not been proven to work in the clinic to date and only limited animal immunization data exist. Disruption of the SC using mild abrasive materials is a technique used clinically for enhancing conductivity of electrical fields through the skin to record EKGs. The same materials used in conjunction with hydrating solutions improve antigen delivery, creating a single, simple pretreatment swab for use prior to patch placement. Studies in our laboratory have explored this concept and demonstrated its feasibility and effect on the delivery of both an antigen and adjuvant. In preclinical studies, the optimized application of a simple, wet patch compares well with the efficiency of adjuvanted, injected antigen.

3.5
Animal Models for Skin Delivery of Vaccines

Animal modeling for skin delivery of vaccines is under continuous refinement in several settings, but needs clinical data with which it may be correlated. Preliminary TCI studies in mice often predict the general response to coadministered antigens, but their skin anatomy is quite different from human skin, which makes dose comparisons difficult. The guinea pig's SC and epidermal thickness is similar to human skin (Panchagnula et al. 1997) and this represents a convenient and immunologically responsive model. Shaved hairy and hairless guinea pigs can be used to examine the effect of mild abrasives or devices for stratum corneum disruption. Biopsy of skin treated to disrupt the SC suggested that this method might aid in efficiency of antigen delivery and allow optimization and testing of agents to disrupt the SC (Glenn et al. 2003). Simple topical immunization studies with wet patches and no pretreatment will yield little useful information (Mikszta et al. 2002). It has been suggested that hair follicles play an important role in topical administration, but this hypothesis would not explain the enhancement seen with SC disruption. The likelihood that follicles are not significant antigen transit pathways is supported by the observation that out-bred CD1 mice with normal hair follicle development, and hairless SKH mice (same genetic background) with sparse, vestigial follicles, respond equally well to topical immunization and disruption of the SC (Glenn et al. 2003).

Robust immune responses to TCI are generally dependent on the presence of an adjuvant in the formulation (Baca-Estrada et al. 2000; Chen et al. 2001; Glenn et al 1999a; Güereña-Burgueño et al. 2002; Kenney et al 2004c; Scharton-Kersten et al. 2000), although some antigens may be immunogenic in sufficient doses by themselves. In general, adjuvants greatly augment the immune responses to co-administered antigens and there are a wide variety of adjuvants that may be used (Kenney and Edelman 2004). The bacterial ADP-ribosylating exotoxins (bAREs) are potent adjuvants in the context of the skin and include CT, LT, and their mutants and subunits. The bAREs have had extensive use as adjuvants via intranasal and oral routes, and are causative agents in the natural setting resulting in self-limiting diarrheal diseases, the latter finding suggesting that their topical use would not be accompanied by long-term side effects (Dickinson and Clements 1995; Freytag and Clements 1999; Glück et al. 2000; Kenney and Edelman 2003; Michetti et al. 1999; O'Hagan 2000; Scharton-Kersten et al. 2000; Snider 1995; Weltzin et al. 2000).

The adjuvanticity of the bAREs on the skin appears to correlate with the level of ribosyl-transferase activity as it does in oral and most nasal immunization studies (Lycke et al. 1992; Scharton-Kersten et al. 2000).Purified cholera toxin B-subunit (pCTB) and mutant toxins that retain ribosyl-transferase activity act as adjuvants on the skin, in contrast to recombinant CTB that is devoid of ribosyl-transferase activity and is subsequently far less potent as an adjuvant (Hammond et al. 2001a; Matousek et al. 1998; Scharton-Kersten et al. 2000; Simmons et al. 2001). Other adjuvants, including bacterial DNA, cytokines, lipopolysaccharide (LPS), and LPS analogs, have been shown to have activity in the context of the skin, but their comparative potency on the skin needs to be further evaluated (Scharton-Kersten et al. 2000).

TCI is similar to intranasal or oral immunization, as the simple admixture of LT with a co-administered antigen such as tetanus toxoid (TTx) or influenza hemagglutinin results in markedly higher antibody levels compared to the administration of antigens alone (Glenn et al. 1998; Güereña-Burgueño et al. 2002; Scharton-Kersten et al. 2000). Similarly, use of bAREs by TCI induces cell-mediated immunity to the co-administered antigens such as $CD4^+$ or $CD8^+$ T cells with a balanced T helper profile (Hammond et al. 2001b; Neidleman et al. 2000; Porgador et al. 1997; Seo et al. 2000).

4
The Safety and Immunogenicity of an Adjuvant on the Skin

4.1
Preclinical Safety

For specific product development, we have focused on the adjuvant LT, a member of the family of bARE adjuvants that includes CT, *Pseudomonas* exotoxin A, and diphtheria toxin. Each member has distinctive features, such as cell surface binding targets, size, and qualitative immune effects. LT is the causative agent in enterotoxigenic *E. coli* (ETEC) traveler's diarrhea. As an adjuvant, LT has a unique safety database since millions of persons are exposed yearly to this self-limiting disease with no short-term or long-term adverse events. In developing countries with endemic ETEC, a high proportion of the population develops anti-LT antibodies through repeated exposure to the pathogen, and adults in developed countries frequently have high levels of serum anti-LT IgG, suggesting local or travel-related exposure to ETEC. The immune responses to LT after challenge studies are similar in magnitude to responses elicited by transcutaneous immunization (D.N. Taylor, unpublished observations), suggesting that this level of exposure and response to LT occurs without significant effects beyond the self-limited diarrheal disease. Additionally, there exists a unique and extensive publication record on the safety/toxicology of LT, providing helpful guidance for reviewers and regulatory authorities.

LT and its mutants have been subjected to extensive formal toxicology studies (Peppoloni et al. 2003; Zurbriggen et al. 2003). This includes ferrets, rats, miniature pigs, NZW rabbits, and baboons using nasal, oral, and intravenous (IV) routes. The most invasive route, IV injection, required 630 human doses to reach an LD_{50}, whereas the oral route using equivalent doses did not induce mortality or clinical changes (Zurbriggen et al. 2003). Ocular exposure in New Zealand White mice and nasal use of LT in baboons resulted in no local or distal changes in a detailed CNS histopathologic study (Zurbriggen et al. 2003). Toxicology studies in guinea pigs using LT with a recombinant antigen, CS6, previously demonstrated the preclinical safety of LT as adjuvant on the skin (Yu et al. 1994). Six carefully controlled GLP toxicology studies in guinea pigs and rabbits have confirmed these findings (S.A. Frech, unpublished observations). Claims that CT may induce chronic diseases based on contrived mouse models (using spinal cord proteins as immunogens given in conjunction with IV infusion of pertussis toxin; Riminton et al. 2004) have been made. Previous similar claims have been made for oil-in-water adjuvants (autoimmune disease, cancer), and Hib vaccination (diabetes). These specific claims have been discounted with extensive, carefully conducted human studies showing that these models have no predictive value for safety in human vaccination studies (Graves et al. 1999; Offit and Hackett 2003; Page et al. 1993).

Although the native LT and CT toxins are highly sensitive to the low pH found in the stomach, the use of various mutant toxins as adjuvants are molecular approaches to address the potential concerns associated with oral vaccination, which can cause diarrhea upon ingestion in fasting subjects in whom the gastric acid has been neutralized (Levine et al. 1983; Michetti et al. 1999). The relevance of these concerns for topical use of adjuvants such as LT is doubtful. Given the common use of potentially toxic drugs in transdermal patches, such as nicotine, and the potential for misuse of other pharmaceuticals such as acetaminophen, when used as directed, patches are likely to have no significant side effects. The ability to safely use potent adjuvants on the skin that might not be used otherwise is precisely the strength of skin-targeting technologies.

4.2
Clinical Safety

In Phase I human trials, the use of LT on the skin appears to be safe and well tolerated (Glenn et al. 2000, 2003; Güereña-Burgueño et al. 2002). Local, mild rashes on the skin have been described in up to 74% of the subjects in conjunction with topical use of LT (Güereña-Burgueño et al. 2002). In contrast, the use of gene guns to deliver DNA to the skin resulted in mild, self-limiting local rashes in 100% of the subjects, but these do not appear to be a serious concern (Roy et al. 2000). Studies with smallpox and BCG result in local scarring, with the eschar of smallpox vaccination suggesting a clinical 'take' of the vaccine, but this clearly is not acceptable as a routine reaction for skin delivery of new vaccines. The oral use of LT or detoxified mutants appears to have enough side effects (including diarrhea) to discourage its use as an oral adjuvant (Kotloff et al. 2001), and the possible relationship between the increased incidence of Bell's Palsy in subjects and the administration of an intranasal flu vaccine with LT, and controversy suggesting LT may migrate along the olfactory bulb (Mutsch et al. 2004; Zurbriggen et al. 2003) suggests that the skin may be the most acceptable route by which LT may be used as an adjuvant. Others have pursued the use of mutant LT adjuvants for intranasal products and are in Phase I trials (Peppoloni et al. 2003). Our group has completed double-blind placebo controlled trials and repeat dosing trials that have confirmed the finding of the preclinical toxicology studies showing that LT may be safely used on the skin. These findings are in concert with the scientific data on the mechanism of adjuvanticity, the epidemiology of enteric diseases as toxin-based, self-limiting events with no long-term sequelae, and suggest that LT is an ideal adjuvant for use on the skin.

4.3
Immune Response to Transcutaneous Immunization

The ability of LT to act as antigen as well as adjuvant led us to conduct an initial clinical trial using LT alone in a simple patch on untreated skin in a dose escalation fashion to assess the safety and immune responses (Glenn and Alving 1999). Volunteers received an LT solution in a gauze pad under an adhesive patch, and were immunized at 0, 1, and 9 months. No serious vaccine-related adverse reactions were observed, and histological sections of biopsies taken at the dosing sites were normal, consistent with the absence of delayed type hypersensitivity (DTH) clinically. All subjects in the high dose group produced a greater than fourfold increase in serum antibodies against LT, along with IgG or IgA antibodies against LT in either the urine or stool. Antibodies against LT were durable and persisted long after the second immunization, with a clear booster response after the second and third dose. This was the first demonstration that a vaccine antigen passively delivered to the skin could elicit a systemic immune response in humans.

The importance of the role of an adjuvant in the induction of immune responses to a co-administered antigen was initially tested in the context of ETEC-related traveler's diarrhea using the colonization factor CS6, a multi-subunit intestinal epithelial cell-binding protein (Wolf et al. 1997). Volunteers were given CS6 with or without LT in a dose escalating fashion at 0, 1, and 3 months (Güereña-Burgueño et al. 2002). Mild DTH skin reactions occurred in 74% of volunteers in the combined groups with the second or third dose, possibly to the colonization factor CS6 or LPS in the CS6 buffer. No other adverse events correlated with vaccine administration. Only volunteers receiving LT as adjuvant produced serum anti-CS6 IgG and IgA. The anti-CS6 response compared favorably to responses seen after challenge infection using the live B7A ETEC strain, which results in full protection on rechallenge (Levine et al. 1983; Wolf et al. 1997). Antibody secreting cells (ASCs) to CS6 were also detected in the peripheral blood. The lack of response to CS6 without LT and clear responses in the presence of LT confirmed the universal finding in animal studies that the adjuvant plays a critical role in TCI. This study also confirmed that large antigens such as CS6 ($>1,500,000$ Da) can be readily delivered to the human skin immune system (Yu et al. 2002).

Preclinical studies suggested the dose of antigen could be reduced with retention of immunogenicity by disruption of the SC. The effect of mild disruption of the SC on the delivery of LT was explored with commercially available medical products, including abrasive pads used to enhance EKG signal conductivity, or adhesive tape used to evaluate skin hydration. These strategies are in clinical practice to enhance the flux of drugs for topical application or electrical conductivity to improve the quality of electrocardiograms. To evaluate the penetration enhancement of various skin pretreatment methods in humans, we conducted a Phase I study in healthy adults (Fig. 2). The skin was pretreated prior to vaccination with either a glycerol/isopropyl alcohol (IPA) solution (groups 1 and 5), tape-stripping followed by glycerol/IPA hydrating solution (group 2), a pumice-impregnated IPA pad (group 3), or with emery paper (group 4). Following pretreatment, all groups were then vaccinated twice, 21 days apart, with a patch composed of gauze containing 50 µg LT (groups 1–4) or 400 µg LT (group 5), covered by Tegaderm. No significant adverse events were observed after either LT vaccination, apart from a mild, self-limited maculopapular rash that occasionally developed with or without associated pruritus at the site of vaccination.

Results from this study demonstrate that pretreatment with either emery paper or tape-stripping delivered LT more efficiently than with glycerol/IPA hydration alone (Fig. 2). Following each vaccination, LT IgG showed greater

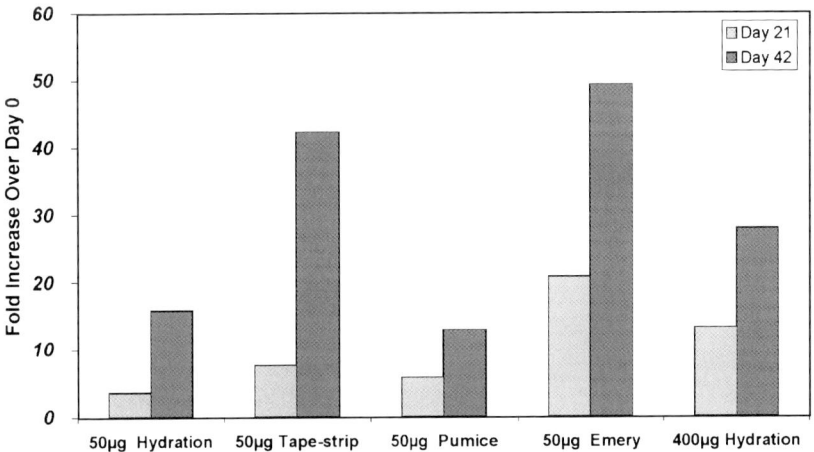

Fig. 2 Response to various skin pretreatments. Disruption of human stratum corneum can augment delivery of proteins to the Langerhans cells to provide substantial improvements in antibody titers. Eight subjects per group were dosed at days 0 and 21 with 50 µg or 400 µg LT on gauze patches following pretreatment with hydration alone, tape-stripping, pumice pads, or emery paper. Serum LT-specific IgG measured by ELISA is shown after the second dose at day 42 and the geometric mean was calculated. (Adapted from Glenn et al. 2003, with permission)

response following pretreatment with glycerol/alcohol hydration and emery paper (group 4) and tape-stripping (group 2) when compared to glycerol/IPA hydration alone (group 1). The improvements in LT IgG seen in the treatment groups (emery and tape-stripping), with respect to hydration alone, suggest improved LT delivery with SC disruption using emery pretreatment. Subjects pretreated with tape-stripping (group 2) or emery (group 4) and vaccinated with 50 µg showed no significant difference for LT IgG when compared to those receiving hydration alone and 400 µg LT (group 5). These data indicate that an eightfold reduction in LT from 400 µg to 50 µg is possible when emery pretreatment, or its equivalent, is used. This study established the general tolerability of various penetration enhancement techniques, as well as the potential dose-sparing such pretreatment can yield.

4.4
Transcutaneous Immunization Induces Functional Antibodies

Serum antibodies that block pathogenic factors are typically used as predictors of vaccine efficacy, even in the absence of validated correlates of protection. The most familiar example may be the influenza vaccine HAI assay, where a titer of 1:40 is commonly regarded as providing a degree of protection. Vaccination by TCI can induce potent mucosal neutralizing antibodies to LT in mice that block the induction of diarrhea by an oral challenge of LT. This effect can even be passively transferred by injection of immune serum into naïve mice, emphasizing the importance of circulating antibodies (Yu et al. 2002). Toxin neutralizing antibodies (TNA) were induced by TCI with the recombinant protective antigen (rPA) of anthrax in mice and rabbits, and were associated with protection from an anthrax spore challenge in the mice (Kenney et al 2004c).

We evaluated the ability of TCI to generate protective antibodies in humans in the anthrax system. Eight subjects per group were randomized to receive rPA without or co-administered with LT in a dry adhesive patch (groups 1–4) or as liquid antigens on gauze (group 5) following skin pretreatment with a nonwoven abrasive pad. Subjects were dosed at 0, 4, and 8 weeks and followed for safety and immunogenicity. Serum IgG antibodies to rPA were readily induced, particularly in the groups that also received LT (unpublished data). A moderate dose response was observed, although the response to the liquid antigens was stronger, suggesting the dry adhesive formulation will need further optimization. Functional antibodies were induced in groups that received the adjuvant (Fig. 3). The level of TNA that is required for protection in humans is unknown; however, the presence of significant toxin neutralization capacity in most subjects suggests this mode of vaccination

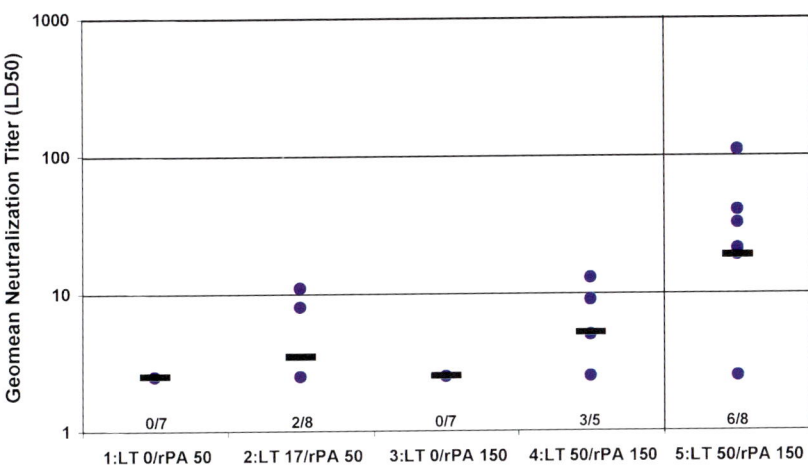

Fig. 3 Human toxin neutralization antibody responses to anthrax vaccination. Serum antibodies against rPA can neutralize the effect of anthrax lethal toxin on J774A.1 mouse macrophage cells. Eight subjects per group were pretreated with a non-woven abrasive pad and then immunized on days 0, 28, and 56 with 0 μg, 17 μg or 50 μg LT and 50 μg or 150 μg rPA as indicated. The titers of toxin neutralizing antibodies measured on day 84 are shown for the individuals in each group and a geometric mean is calculated. The number of subjects with detectable responses in each group is shown at the bottom. Groups 1–4 were vaccinated with dry adhesive patches and liquid antigen on gauze was used for group 5

could be developed as a means of rapid vaccination on a massive scale. The rPA also appears to be well stabilized in patch formulations. In pre-clinical studies, it is clear that a formulated dry patch provides improved delivery compared to the simple wet patch used in this study. These observations have led to a development program for a cold-chain-free, easily self-administered patch vaccine for anthrax that can improve delivery and reach immune responses that are superior or equal to those seen by the IM route.

4.5
Dose-Sparing and Immune Enhancement via a Universal Adjuvant Patch

The use of a 'universal' adjuvant patch as a nonspecific local immunostimulant (IS) is a dose-sparing and immune enhancement strategy to consider for vaccine supply crises or limitations in manufacturing. An LT patch added directly over the site of an injected vaccine greatly enhances the immune response to the injected vaccine (Frech et al. 2005; Guebre-Xabier et al. 2003, 2004). The simple placement of an adjuvant-laden patch on the skin results in trafficking of activated Langerhans cells to the draining lymph nodes where immune responses are generated as a part of normal host defense (Glenn et al. 2003; Hammond et al. 2001a). The presence of adjuvant-activated LCs in the draining lymph node appears to have positive bystander effects on both IM and ID injected vaccines (Glenn et al 2003; Guebre-Xabier et al. 2003). The IS patch was recently shown to enhance the immune responses to annual influenza vaccination in the elderly (Frech et al. 2005). Preclinical data suggests that intradermal, as opposed to intramuscular, immunization combined with the adjuvant patch may be the most efficient at improving the immune response to the injected vaccine up to tenfold. In a preclinical study using recombinant pandemic H5 antigen, mice were immunized by the ID route and given an IS patch. As shown in Fig. 4, significant dose-sparing was achieved by adding an LT patch at the time of immunization.

The adjuvant patch could fit simply into the vaccine administration protocol in that it can replace the 'bandaid' used at the injection site. Given the

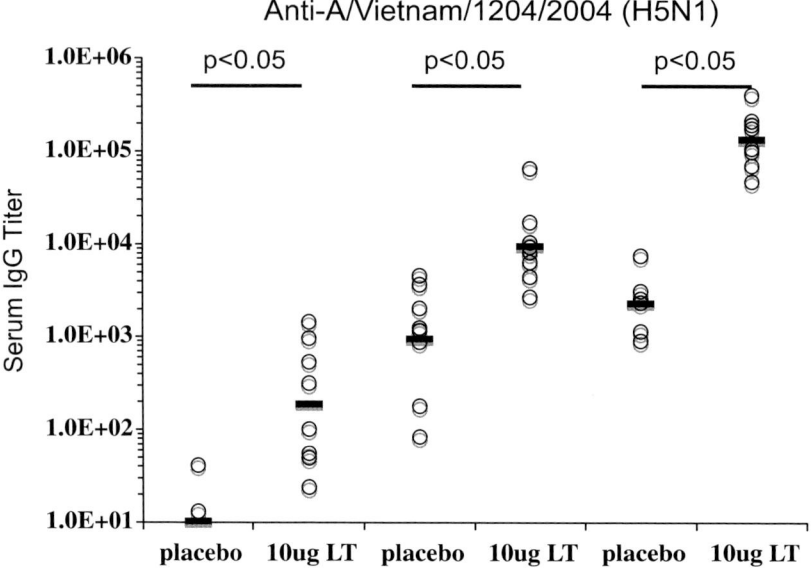

Fig. 4 Intradermal immunization with pandemic flu antigens can be augmented by an immunostimulant patch. C57Bl/6 mice were shaved near the base of the tail and the area was hydrated with saline and pretreated with emery paper. Mice were immunized by ID injection with the indicated doses of recombinant H5N1 influenza vaccine (A/Vietnam/1203/2004) and a 1-cm^2 gauze patch (with placebo or 10 μg LT) was applied over the injection site. Patches were removed the next day and the skin rinsed with water. The geometric mean titer is indicated for groups of 10

human data showing fivefold dose-sparing through use of ID injection (Kenney et al. 2004a), an additional five- to tenfold dose-sparing effect conferred by an IS patch (Guebre-Xabier et al. 2004) could potentially allow one million pandemic influenza vaccine doses to be used in 25–50 million subjects. Because a dry, formulated patch is an ideal format for LT stability, the adjuvant patch can be stockpiled in advance, unlike pandemic influenza vaccines. This strategy could greatly extend the supply and provide sufficient vaccine for the whole population in a pandemic event.

5
Mass Vaccination: Logistics of an Anthrax Patch

A major obstacle to the routine use of a vaccine for mass distribution is the overhead associated with its delivery, storage, and administration, as well as the safe disposal of the needles, all of which can account for 80% or more of the cost of a vaccine program. We have been developing an anthrax patch vaccine as a biodefense product (Kenney et al. 2004b; Matyas et al. 2004). In this situation, where the currently preferred approach is to stockpile the vaccine for local emergency use, it is critical to conserve packaging space and simplify conditions where the product is stored. The safe storage of a million glass syringes of a liquid vaccine requires substantial protection and careful handling to avoid breakage, as well as refrigerated warehouse space. Distribution invokes maintenance of the cold chain, delivery to personnel trained in injections, and organization of clinics for immunization. On the other hand, in the event of an anthrax exposure a dry, temperature-stabilized, self-administered patch that was being stored in much more efficient packaging in a standard warehouse could be rapidly shipped to the site and distributed broadly with relative ease. Needle disposal, which seems trivial in industrialized countries that routinely dispose of garbage in landfills, also becomes a major public health problem in areas without the necessary infrastructure.

The patch approach answers each of the major distribution and delivery needs associated with planning for a biodefense emergency, such as with anthrax. The benefits are actually amplified in truly massive vaccination campaigns, where immunization coverage becomes more important. Funds that are currently going toward expensive storage and distribution channels could be freed up to allow better organization and tracking of delivery. If injections are not required, public health authorities can depend on less well-trained personnel to be the actual providers, which simplifies planning for the campaign and enhances the ability to vaccinate everyone in each geographic area. Development of a patch that could be reliably self administered, like the various over-the-counter patches in use today, would simplify the approach even more.

6
Conclusions

Skin delivery techniques are promising technologies that can utilize the immune environment of the skin to confer clinically important immune responses. Given the success of smallpox eradication, it is unfortunate that the skin has generally been bypassed as the preferred approach for vaccination. Patch vaccination has the advantage of being simple to apply with minimal administrative overhead in its distribution, storage, and ultimate disposal, potentially making a vaccine campaign less expensive and assisting the general usage of the vaccine. The dose-sparing potential embodied in the immunostimulant patch approach may become a key element in increasing the vaccine supply for pandemic influenza responses where production capacity is severely limited. The simplified logistics associated with the TCI approach become readily apparent in the biodefense arena, such as with the anthrax vaccine that we are developing, where plans for stockpiling and ease of rapid distribution and self-administration become paramount. Developments in skin delivery techniques can meet the needs of mass vaccination campaigns in times of crisis in addition to addressing the challenges of disease control and eradication.

Acknowledgements We thank David Flyer, Mimi Guebre-Xabier, and Guoling Xi for research support and Wanda Hardy for administrative assistance. The authors point out that Mimi Guebre-Xabier has played a key role in demonstrating the use of the IS patch and generated the first pandemic dose-sparing data.

References

Baca-Estrada ME, Foldvari M, Ewen C, Badea I, and Babiuk LA (2000) Effects of IL-12 on immune responses induced by transcutaneous immunization with antigens formulated in a novel lipid-based biphasic delivery system. Vaccine 18:1847–1854

Briggs DJ, Banzhoff A, Nicolay U, Sirikwin S, Dumavibhat B, Tongswas S, Wasi C (2000) Antibody response of patients after postexposure rabies vaccination with small intradermal doses of purified chick embryo cell vaccine or purified Vero cell rabies vaccine. Bull World Health Organ 78:693–698

Bryan JP, Sjogren MH, Perine PL, Legters LJ (1992) Low-dose intradermal and intramuscular vaccination against hepatitis B. Clin Infect Dis 14:697–707

Chen D, Erickson CA, Endres RL, Periwal SB, Chu Q, Shu C, Maa YF, Payne LG (2001) Adjuvantation of epidermal powder immunization. Vaccine 19:2908–2917

Christoph T, Muller-Rover S, Audring H, Tobin DJ, Hermes B, Cotsarelis G, Ruckert R, Paus R (2000) The human hair follicle immune system: cellular composition and immune privilege. Br J Dermatol 142:862–873

Dickinson BL, Clements JD (1995) Dissociation of Escherichia coli heat-labile enterotoxin adjuvanticity from ADP-ribosyltransferase activity. Infect Immun 63:1617–1623

Frech SA, Kenney RT, Spyr CA, Lazar H, Viret JF, Herzog C, Gluck R, Glenn GM (2005) Improved immune responses to influenza vaccination in the elderly using an immunostimulant patch. Vaccine 23:946–950

Freytag LC, Clements JD (1999) Bacterial toxins as mucosal adjuvants. Curr Top Microbiol Immunol 236:215–236

Glenn GM, Rao M, Matyas GR, Alving CR (1998) Skin immunization made possible by cholera toxin. Nature 391:851

Glenn GM, Alving CR (1999a) Use of penetration enhancers and barrier disruption agents to enhance the transcutaneous immune response induced by ADP-ribosylating exotoxin. *European Patent No. 1061951*

Glenn GM, Alving CR (1999b) Adjuvant for transcutaneous immunization. *US Patent No. 5,980,898.* The United States of America as represented by the U.S. Army Medical Research & Material Command (Washington, DC)

Glenn GM, Taylor DN, Li X, Frankel S, Montemarano A, Alving CR (2000) Transcutaneous immunization: a human vaccine delivery strategy using a patch. Nat Med 6:1403–1406

Glenn GM, Kenney RT, Ellingsworth LR, Frech SA, Hammond SA, Zoeteweij JP (2003) Transcutaneous immunization and immunostimulant strategies: capitalizing on the immunocompetence of the skin. Expert Rev Vaccines 2:253–267

Glück R, Mischler R, Durrer P, Furer E, Lang AB, Herzog C, Cryz SJ, Jr. (2000) Safety and immunogenicity of intranasally administered inactivated trivalent virosome-formulated influenza vaccine containing *Escherichia coli* heat-labile toxin as a mucosal adjuvant. J Infect Dis 181:1129–1132

Graves PM, Barriga KJ, Norris JM, Hoffman MR, Yu L, Eisenbarth GS, Rewers M (1999) Lack of association between early childhood immunizations and beta-cell autoimmunity. Diabetes Care 22:1694–1697

Guebre-Xabier M, Hammond SA, Epperson DE, Yu J, Ellingsworth L, Glenn GM (2003) Immunostimulant patch containing heat-labile enterotoxin from *Escherichia coli* enhances immune responses to injected influenza virus vaccine through activation of skin dendritic cells. J Virol 77:5218–5225

Guebre-Xabier M, Hammond SA, Ellingsworth LR, Glenn GM (2004) Immunostimulant patch enhances immune responses to influenza virus vaccine in aged mice. J Virol 78:7610–7618

Güereña-Burgueño F, Hall ER, Taylor DN, Cassels FJ, Scott DA, Wolf MK, Roberts ZJ, Nesterova GV, Alving CR, Glenn GM (2002) Safety and immunogenicity of a prototype enterotoxigenic *Escherichia coli* vaccine administered transcutaneously. Infect Immun 70:1874–1880

Hammond SA, Tsonis C, Sellins K, Rushlow K, Scharton-Kersten T, Colditz I, Glenn GM (2000) Transcutaneous immunization of domestic animals: opportunities and challenges. Adv Drug Deliv Rev 43:45–55

Hammond SA, Guebre-Xabier M, Yu J, Glenn GM (2001a) Transcutaneous immunization: an emerging route of immunization and potent immunostimulation strategy. Crit Rev Ther Drug Carrier Syst 18:503–526

Hammond SA, Walwender D, Alving CR, Glenn GM (2001b) Transcutaneous immunization: T cell responses and boosting of existing immunity. Vaccine 19:2701–2707

Henderson DA, Borio LL, Lane JM (2004) Smallpox and vaccinia. In Plotkin SA and Orenstein WA (ed) Vaccines. Saunders, Philadelphia, pp 123–153

Jakob T, Udey MC (1999) Epidermal Langerhans cells: from neurons to nature's adjuvants. Adv Dermatol 14:209–258

Kenney RT, Edelman R (2003) Survey of human-use adjuvants. Expert Rev Vaccines 2:167–188

Kenney RT, Edelman R (2004a) Adjuvants for the future. In Levine MM (ed) New Generation Vaccines, 3rd Edition. Marcel Dekker, Inc., New York, pp 213–223

Kenney RT, Frech SA, Muenz LR, Villar CP, Glenn GM (2004b) Dose sparing with intradermal injection of influenza vaccine. N Engl J Med 351:2295–2301

Kenney RT, Yu J, Guebre-Xabier M, Frech SA, Lambert A, Heller BA, Ellingsworth LR, Eyles JE, Williamson ED, Glenn GM (2004c) Induction of protective immunity against lethal anthrax challenge with a patch. J Infect Dis 190:774–782

Kotloff KL, Sztein MB, Wasserman SS, Losonsky GA, DiLorenzo SC, Walker RI (2001) Safety and immunogenicity of oral inactivated whole-cell Helicobacter pylori vaccine with adjuvant among volunteers with or without subclinical infection. Infect Immun 69:3581–3590

La Montagne JR, Fauci AS (2004) Intradermal influenza vaccination–can less be more? N Engl J Med 351:2330–2332

Levine MM, Ristaino P, Sack RB, Kaper JB, Orskov F, Orskov I (1983) Colonization factor antigens I and II and type 1 somatic pili in enterotoxigenic Escherichia coli: relation to enterotoxin type. Infect Immun 39:889–897.

Lycke N, Tsuji T, Holmgren J (1992) The adjuvant effect of *Vibrio cholerae* and *Escherichia coli* heat-labile enterotoxins is linked to their ADP-ribosyltransferase activity. Eur J Immunol 22:2277–2281

Matousek MP, Nedrud JG, Cieplak W, Jr., Harding CV (1998) Inhibition of class II major histocompatibility complex antigen processing by *Escherichia coli* heat-labile enterotoxin requires an enzymatically active A subunit. Infect Immun 66:3480–3484

Matyas GR, Friedlander AM, Glenn GM, Little S, Yu J, Alving CR (2004) Needle-free skin patch vaccination method for anthrax. Infect Immun 72:1181–1183

Michetti P, Kreiss C, Kotloff KL, Porta N, Blanco JL, Bachmann D, Herranz M, Saldinger PF, Corthesy-Theulaz I, Losonsky G, Nichols R, Simon J, Stolte M, Ackerman S, Monath TP, Blum AL (1999) Oral immunization with urease and *Escherichia coli* heat-labile enterotoxin is safe and immunogenic in *Helicobacter pylori*-infected adults. Gastroenterology 116:804–812

Mikszta JA, Alarcon JB, Brittingham JM, Sutter DE, Pettis RJ, Harvey NG (2002) Improved genetic immunization via micromechanical disruption of skin-barrier function and targeted epidermal delivery. Nat Med 8:415–419

Mutsch M, Zhou W, Rhodes P, Bopp M, Chen RT, Linder T, Spyr C, Steffen R (2004) Use of the inactivated intranasal influenza vaccine and the risk of Bell's palsy in Switzerland. N Engl J Med 350:896–903

Neidleman JA, Ott G, O'Hagan D (2000) Mutant heat-labile enterotoxins as adjuvants for CTL induction. In O'Hagan D (ed) Vaccine Adjuvants: Preparation Methods and Research Protocols. Humana Press, Totowa, NJ, pp 327–336

O'Hagan DT, ed. (2000) Methods in Molecular Medicine, Humana Press, Inc., Totowa, NJ

Offit PA, Hackett CJ (2003) Addressing parents' concerns: do vaccines cause allergic or autoimmune diseases? Pediatrics 111:653–659

Page WF, Norman JE, Benenson AS (1993) Long-term follow-up of army recruits immunized with Freund's incomplete adjuvanted vaccine. Vaccine Research 2:141–149

Panchagnula R, Stemmer K, Ritschel WA (1997) Animal models for transdermal drug delivery. Methods Find Exp Clin Pharmacol 19:335–341

Peppoloni S, Ruggiero P, Contorni M, Morandi M, Pizza M, Rappuoli R, Podda A, Del Giudice G (2003) Mutants of the *Escherichia coli* heat-labile enterotoxin as safe and strong adjuvants for intranasal delivery of vaccines. Expert Rev Vaccines 2:285–293

Porgador A, Staats HF, Faiola B, Gilboa E, Palker TJ (1997) Intranasal immunization with CTL epitope peptides from HIV-1 or ovalbumin and the mucosal adjuvant cholera toxin induces peptide-specific CTLs and protection against tumor development in vivo. J Immunol 158:834–841

Redfield RR, Innis BL, Scott RM, Cannon HG, Bancroft WH (1985) Clinical evaluation of low-dose intradermally administered hepatitis B virus vaccine. A cost reduction strategy. JAMA 254:3203–3206

Richter T, Peuckert C, Sattler M, Koenig K, Riemann I, Hintze U, Wittern KP, Wiesendanger R, Wepf R (2004) Dead but highly dynamic–the stratum corneum is divided into three hydration zones. Skin Pharmacol Physiol 17:246–257

Riminton DS, Kandasamy R, Dravec D, Basten A, Baxter AG (2004) Dermal enhancement: bacterial products on intact skin induce and augment organ-specific autoimmune disease. J Immunol 172:302–309

Roberts MS, Walker M (1993) Water, the most natural penetration enhancer, Marcel Dekker, New York

Roy MJ, Wu MS, Barr LJ, Fuller JT, Tussey LG, Speller S, Culp J, Burkholder JK, Swain WF, Dixon RM, Widera G, Vessey R, King A, Ogg G, Gallimore A, Haynes JR, Heydenburg Fuller D (2000) Induction of antigen-specific CD8+ T cells, T helper cells, and protective levels of antibody in humans by particle-mediated administration of a hepatitis B virus DNA vaccine. Vaccine 19:764–778

Sandby-Moller J, Poulsen T, Wulf HC (2003) Epidermal thickness at different body sites: relationship to age, gender, pigmentation, blood content, skin type and smoking habits. Acta Derm Venereol 83:410–413

Scharton-Kersten T, Yu J, Vassell R, O'Hagan D, Alving CR, Glenn GM (2000) Transcutaneous immunization with bacterial ADP-ribosylating exotoxins, subunits, and unrelated adjuvants. Infect Immun 68:5306–5313

Seo N, Tokura Y, Nishijima T, Hashizume H, Furukawa F, Takigawa M (2000) Percutaneous peptide immunization via corneum barrier-disrupted murine skin for experimental tumor immunoprophylaxis. Proc Natl Acad Sci USA 97:371–376

Simmons CP, Ghaem-Magami M, Petrovska L, Lopes L, Chain BM, Williams NA, Dougan G (2001) Immunomodulation using bacterial enterotoxins. Scand J Immunol 53:218–226

Snider DP (1995) The mucosal adjuvant activities of ADP-ribosylating bacterial enterotoxins. Crit Rev Immunol 15:317–348

Udey MC (1997) Cadherins and Langerhans cell immunobiology. Clin Exp Immunol 107 Suppl 1:6–8

Weltzin R, Guy B, Thomas WD, Jr., Giannasca PJ, Monath TP (2000) Parenteral adjuvant activities of *Escherichia coli* heat-labile toxin and its B subunit for immunization of mice against gastric *Helicobacter pylori* infection. Infect Immun 68:2775–2782

Wolf M, Hall E, Taylor D, Coster T, Trespalacios F, Cassels F, deLorimier A, McQueen C (1999) Use of the human challenge model to characterize the immune response to the colonization factors of enterotoxigenic *Escherichia coli* (ETEC). *The 35th U.S.-Japan Cholera and Other Bacterial Enteric Infections Joint Panel Meeting.* Baltimore, MD.

Wolf MK, de Haan LA, Cassels FJ, Willshaw GA, Warren R, Boedeker EC, and Gaastra W (1997) The CS6 colonization factor of human enterotoxigenic *Escherichia coli* contains two heterologous major subunits. FEMS Microbiol Lett 148:35–42

Yu J, Cassels F, Scharton-Kersten T, Hammond SA, Hartman A, Angov E, Corthesy B, Alving C, Glenn G (2002) Transcutaneous immunization using colonization factor and heat-labile enterotoxin induces correlates of protective immunity for enterotoxigenic *Escherichia coli*. Infect Immun 70:1056–1068

Yu RC, Abrams DC, Alaibac M, Chu AC (1994) Morphological and quantitative analyses of normal epidermal Langerhans cells using confocal scanning laser microscopy. Br J Dermatol 131:843–848

Zurbriggen R, Metcalfe IC, Gluck R, Viret JF, Moser C (2003) Nonclinical safety evaluation of *Escherichia coli* heat-labile toxin mucosal adjuvant as a component of a nasal influenza vaccine. Expert Rev Vaccines 2:295–304

Subject Index

adjuvants
- bacterial   255, 256
- bacterial DNA   255
- cholera toxin B-subunit   255
- enterotoxigenic *E. coli* (ETEC)   256
- LT   255–257

ADP-ribosylating exotoxins (bAREs)   255, 256

adverse events   128

Advisory Committee on Immunization Practices (ACIP)   133

American Revolutionary War   37

anaphylaxis   46

animal models for transcutaneous immunization
- guinea pig   254
- mouse   254, 255

antigen
- anthrax   260
- CS6   258, 259
- enterotoxigenic *E. coli* (ETEC)   258
- LT   258, 260
- recombinant protective antigen (rPA)   260
- tetanus toxoid   253

Armed Forces Epidemiological Board (AFEB)   36

Behavioral Risk Factor Surveillance   135
blood exposures   127
Boer War   37

carriage rate of HBV   117
childhood infectious disease   71
children   125
cold chain   39
communication   146
confidence crisis   128
congenital rubella   222, 225
contact tracing   22
contacts   20
contagious outbreaks   34
continuous quality improvement   47
contraindications to immunization   45
cost effectiveness   137
coverage   125
customized immunization   45

demyelinating disorders   123
diphtheria disease   71
diphtheria epidemic   71, 82, 83, 87, 89–91
diphtheria epidemiology   75
diphtheria immunization schedules   75
diphtheria toxoid vaccine   74, 85, 89
displaced persons   9

epidemiology   20, 258
exercises   146
Expanded Programme on Immunization (EPI)   75

Franco-Prussian War   37

Guillain–Barré syndrome (GBS)   141, 147

health care workers   136, 137, 141, 142, 144
healthcare workers   120
hemagglutinin   132
hepatitis   100
hepatitis A   95–97, 99, 101–105, 107, 108
 - Europe   102
 - USA   106
hepatitis B immunization programme   120
herd immunity   18

immunization coverage rate   124
immunization histories   39
immunization registries   147
immunization services   40
immunization tracking   47
inactivated poliovirus vaccine (IPV)   196
incident command   143
indirect protection ("herd immunity")   134, 141, 142, 148
influenza   7, 8, 132–149
 - annual   132–138
 - antigenic drift   132
 - antigenic shift   132
 - avian   133, 142
 - pandemic   132, 138–149
 - swine influenza   138, 141, 147
 - universal vaccination   134, 148
 - vaccination clinic   134–137, 145, 149
 - vaccine   133
 - workplace vaccanation   135–138
influenza vaccine
 - adjuvant   149
 - antigen-sparing   149
 - intradermally   149
 - live-attenuated   148
 - monovalent   140, 141
 - trivalent   133, 134
IPV   201, 202, 214
isolation   22

jet guns   19
jet injectors   42

logistical requirements   40
long-term care facilities   136

mass immunization   32, 72
mass psychogenic illness   47
mass vaccination   18, 26
mathematical model   25
measles   18–20, 153–158, 160–163
 - aerosol
    aerosolization   168
    animal studies   172
    benefits   168
    booster   185
    cellular immunity   186
    challenges   188
    Classic Mexican Device   168
    clinical studies   176
    dose   169
    droplet size   171
    early studies   174
    in vitro studies   172
    initial studies   173
    local immune responses   186
    mass campaign   173
    Measles Aerosol Project   189
    measles–rubella   185
    Mexican studies   185
    potency   169
    primary immunization   186
    respirable fraction   170
    South African studies   185
    triple viral vaccine   188
    vaccine strain   171
 - surveillance   158, 160, 162
 - unsafe injections   167
 - vaccine coverage   155
 - vaccine strain
    Edmonston-Zagreb   171
    Schwarz   171
 - vaccine supply   167
meningococcal outbreaks   37, 43
military   137
military trainees   34
mother-to-infant   126

National Immunization Days   32
newborns   118

Subject Index

observation interval 46
oral poliovirus vaccine (OPV) 196–200

PAHO 161, 162
Pan American Health Organization (PAHO) 153
passive reporting 22
pharmacists 138
polemic 123
polio 196, 197
polio eradication 197, 198, 203, 214
polio vaccine associated paralysis 198
poliomyelitis 195
pregnant women 118

quality-improvement programs 48

rate-limiting steps 40
refugees 34
religious pilgrims 34
ring vaccination 20
routine immunization 35
rubella 221–226, 228
rubella campaigns 227
rubella vaccine safety 228

secular trend 23
simultaneous immunization 36
skin
- antigen-presenting cells 248, 250
- dendritic cells 248, 250
- dermis 250
- disruption 253, 254
- epidermis 250
- Langerhans cells 250
- penetration 252–254
- pretreatment 259, 260
- skin immune system 248, 250, 253
- stratum corneum 249
- stratum corneum thickness 249
- structure 249, 250
smallpox 1–4, 9, 18–21, 25, 26

Soviet Union infectious disease outbreaks 71
Spanish–American War 37
students 34
surveillance 18, 19, 23, 24
syncope 46

tetanus 4, 13
the marked seasonality 21
toxicology studies 256, 257
transcutaneous immunization
- clinical safety 248, 257, 258
- immune response 258, 260, 262
transmission 19, 20
Ty21a 233–235, 239–241
typhoid fever 231–239

US Public Health Service 140

vaccination coverage 122
vaccine administration 39
vaccine delivery
- dose-sparing 251, 252, 261
- gas-powered gun 252, 254
- immunostimulant patch 252, 253, 261, 263
- intradermal 251, 252
- intramuscular 252
- self-administration 261, 263, 264
- transcutaneous 251, 253, 254, 260
vaccine storage and handling 39
vaccine supply
- anthrax 264
- pandemic influenza 264
vaccine-associated adverse events 39
viral shedding 20, 21
virus 253

whole cell parenteral vaccine 233, 238
World Health Assembly 121
World War I 37
World War II 37

yellow fever 8, 9, 11

Current Topics in Microbiology and Immunology

Volumes published since 1989 (and still available)

Vol. 260: **Burton, Didier R. (Ed.):** Antibodies in Viral Infection. 2001. 51 figs. IX, 309 pp. ISBN 3-540-41611-0

Vol. 261: **Trono, Didier (Ed.):** Lentiviral Vectors. 2002. 32 figs. X, 258 pp. ISBN 3-540-42190-4

Vol. 262: **Oldstone, Michael B.A. (Ed.):** Arenaviruses I. 2002. 30 figs. XVIII, 197 pp. ISBN 3-540-42244-7

Vol. 263: **Oldstone, Michael B. A. (Ed.):** Arenaviruses II. 2002. 49 figs. XVIII, 268 pp. ISBN 3-540-42705-8

Vol. 264/I: **Hacker, Jörg; Kaper, James B. (Eds.):** Pathogenicity Islands and the Evolution of Microbes. 2002. 34 figs. XVIII, 232 pp. ISBN 3-540-42681-7

Vol. 264/II: **Hacker, Jörg; Kaper, James B. (Eds.):** Pathogenicity Islands and the Evolution of Microbes. 2002. 24 figs. XVIII, 228 pp. ISBN 3-540-42682-5

Vol. 265: **Dietzschold, Bernhard; Richt, Jürgen A. (Eds.):** Protective and Pathological Immune Responses in the CNS. 2002. 21 figs. X, 278 pp. ISBN 3-540-42668X

Vol. 266: **Cooper, Koproski (Eds.):** The Interface Between Innate and Acquired Immunity, 2002. 15 figs. XIV, 116 pp. ISBN 3-540-42894-X

Vol. 267: **Mackenzie, John S.; Barrett, Alan D. T.; Deubel, Vincent (Eds.):** Japanese Encephalitis and West Nile Viruses. 2002. 66 figs. X, 418 pp. ISBN 3-540-42783X

Vol. 268: **Zwickl, Peter; Baumeister, Wolfgang (Eds.):** The Proteasome-Ubiquitin Protein Degradation Pathway. 2002. 17 figs. X, 213 pp. ISBN 3-540-43096-2

Vol. 269: **Koszinowski, Ulrich H.; Hengel, Hartmut (Eds.):** Viral Proteins Counteracting Host Defenses. 2002. 47 figs. XII, 325 pp. ISBN 3-540-43261-2

Vol. 270: **Beutler, Bruce; Wagner, Hermann (Eds.):** Toll-Like Receptor Family Members and Their Ligands. 2002. 31 figs. X, 192 pp. ISBN 3-540-43560-3

Vol. 271: **Koehler, Theresa M. (Ed.):** Anthrax. 2002. 14 figs. X, 169 pp. ISBN 3-540-43497-6

Vol. 272: **Doerfler, Walter; Böhm, Petra (Eds.):** Adenoviruses: Model and Vectors in Virus-Host Interactions. Virion and Structure, Viral Replication, Host Cell Interactions. 2003. 63 figs., approx. 280 pp. ISBN 3-540-00154-9

Vol. 273: **Doerfler, Walter; Böhm, Petra (Eds.):** Adenoviruses: Model and Vectors in VirusHost Interactions. Immune System, Oncogenesis, Gene Therapy. 2004. 35 figs., approx. 280 pp. ISBN 3-540-06851-1

Vol. 274: **Workman, Jerry L. (Ed.):** Protein Complexes that Modify Chromatin. 2003. 38 figs., XII, 296 pp. ISBN 3-540-44208-1

Vol. 275: **Fan, Hung (Ed.):** Jaagsiekte Sheep Retrovirus and Lung Cancer. 2003. 63 figs., XII, 252 pp. ISBN 3-540-44096-3

Vol. 276: **Steinkasserer, Alexander (Ed.):** Dendritic Cells and Virus Infection. 2003. 24 figs., X, 296 pp. ISBN 3-540-44290-1

Vol. 277: **Rethwilm, Axel (Ed.):** Foamy Viruses. 2003. 40 figs., X, 214 pp. ISBN 3-540-44388-6

Vol. 278: **Salomon, Daniel R.; Wilson, Carolyn (Eds.):** Xenotransplantation. 2003. 22 figs., IX, 254 pp. ISBN 3-540-00210-3

Vol. 279: **Thomas, George; Sabatini, David; Hall, Michael N. (Eds.):** TOR. 2004. 49 figs., X, 364 pp. ISBN 3-540-00534X

Vol. 280: **Heber-Katz, Ellen (Ed.)**: Regeneration: Stem Cells and Beyond. 2004. 42 figs., XII, 194 pp. ISBN 3-540-02238-4

Vol. 281: **Young, John A. T. (Ed.)**: Cellular Factors Involved in Early Steps of Retroviral Replication. 2003. 21 figs., IX, 240 pp. ISBN 3-540-00844-6

Vol. 282: **Stenmark, Harald (Ed.)**: Phosphoinositides in Subcellular Targeting and Enzyme Activation. 2003. 20 figs., X, 210 pp. ISBN 3-540-00950-7

Vol. 283: **Kawaoka, Yoshihiro (Ed.)**: Biology of Negative Strand RNA Viruses: The Power of Reverse Genetics. 2004. 24 figs., IX, 350 pp. ISBN 3-540-40661-1

Vol. 284: **Harris, David (Ed.)**: Mad Cow Disease and Related Spongiform Encephalopathies. 2004. 34 figs., IX, 219 pp. ISBN 3-540-20107-6

Vol. 285: **Marsh, Mark (Ed.)**: Membrane Trafficking in Viral Replication. 2004. 19 figs., IX, 259 pp. ISBN 3-540-21430-5

Vol. 286: **Madshus, Inger H. (Ed.)**: Signalling from Internalized Growth Factor Receptors. 2004. 19 figs., IX, 187 pp. ISBN 3-540-21038-5

Vol. 287: **Enjuanes, Luis (Ed.)**: Coronavirus Replication and Reverse Genetics. 2005. 49 figs., XI, 257 pp. ISBN 3-540-21494-1

Vol. 288: **Mahy, Brain W. J. (Ed.)**: Foot-and-Mouth-Disease Virus. 2005. 16 figs., IX, 178 pp. ISBN 3-540-22419X

Vol. 289: **Griffin, Diane E. (Ed.)**: Role of Apoptosis in Infection. 2005. 40 figs., IX, 294 pp. ISBN 3-540-23006-8

Vol. 290: **Singh, Harinder; Grosschedl, Rudolf (Eds.)**: Molecular Analysis of B Lymphocyte Development and Activation. 2005. 28 figs., XI, 255 pp. ISBN 3-540-23090-4

Vol. 291: **Boquet, Patrice; Lemichez Emmanuel (Eds.)** Bacterial Virulence Factors and Rho GTPases. 2005. 28 figs., IX, 196 pp. ISBN 3-540-23865-4

Vol. 292: **Fu, Zhen F (Ed.)**: The World of Rhabdoviruses. 2005. 27 figs., X, 210 pp. ISBN 3-540-24011-X

Vol. 293: **Kyewski, Bruno; Suri-Payer, Elisabeth (Eds.)**: CD4+CD25+ Regulatory T Cells: Origin, Function and Therapeutic Potential. 2005. 22 figs., XII, 332 pp. ISBN 3-540-24444-1

Vol. 294: **Caligaris-Cappio, Federico, Dalla Favera, Ricardo (Eds.)**: Chronic Lymphocytic Leukemia. 2005. 25 figs., VIII, 187 pp. ISBN 3-540-25279-7

Vol. 295: **Sullivan, David J.; Krishna Sanjeew (Eds.)**: Malaria: Drugs, Disease and Post-genomic Biology. 2005. 40 figs., XI, 446 pp. ISBN 3-540-25363-7

Vol. 296: **Oldstone, Michael B. A. (Ed.)**: Molecular Mimicry: Infection Induced Autoimmune Disease. 2005. 28 figs., VIII, 167 pp. ISBN 3-540-25597-4

Vol. 297: **Langhorne, Jean (Ed.)**: Immunology and Immunopathogenesis of Malaria. 2005. 8 figs., XII, 236 pp. ISBN 3-540-25718-7

Vol. 298: **Vivier, Eric; Colonna, Marco (Eds.)**: Immunobiology of Natural Killer Cell Receptors. 2005. 27 figs., VIII, 286 pp. ISBN 3-540-26083-8

Vol. 299: **Domingo, Esteban (Ed.)**: Quasispecies: Concept and Implications. 2006. 44 figs., XII, 401 pp. ISBN 3-540-26395-0

Vol. 300: **Wiertz, Emmanuel J.H.J.; Kikkert, Marjolein (Eds.)**: Dislocation and Degradation of Proteins from the Endoplasmic Reticulum. 2006. 19 figs., VIII, 168 pp. ISBN 3-540-28006-5

Vol. 301: **Doerfler, Walter; Böhm, Petra (Eds.)**: DNA Methylation: Basic Mechanisms. 2006. 24 figs., VIII, 324 pp. ISBN 3-540-29114-8

Vol. 302: **Robert N. Eisenman (Ed.)**: The Myc/Max/Mad Transcription Factor Network. 2006. 28 figs. XII, 278 pp. ISBN 3-540-23968-5

Vol. 303: **Thomas E. Lane (Ed.)**: Chemokines and Viral Infection. 2006. 14 figs. XII, 154 pp. ISBN 3-540-29207-1

Printing: Krips bv, Meppel
Binding: Stürtz, Würzburg